Community-Acquired Pneumonia: Controversies and Questions

Editor

THOMAS M. FILE Jr

INFECTIOUS DISEASE CLINICS OF NORTH AMERICA

www.id.theclinics.com

Consulting Editor
HELEN W. BOUCHER

March 2013 • Volume 27 • Number 1

ELSEVIER

1600 John F. Kennedy Boulevard • Suite 1800 • Philadelphia, Pennsylvania, 19103-2899.

http://www.theclinics.com

INFECTIOUS DISEASE CLINICS OF NORTH AMERICA Volume 27, Number 1
March 2013 ISSN 0891–5520, ISBN-13: 978-1-4557-7106-6

Editor: Stephanie Donley
Developmental Editor: Teia Stone

Infectious Disease Clinics of North America (ISSN 0891–5520) is published in March, June, September, and December by Elsevier Inc., 360 Park Avenue South, New York, NY 10010-1710. Periodicals postage paid at New York, NY and additional mailing offices. Subscription prices are $282.00 per year for US individuals, $482.00 per year for US institutions, $139.00 per year for US students, $334.00 per year for Canadian individuals, $596.00 per year for Canadian institutions, $398.00 per year for international individuals, $596.00 per year for international institutions, and $192.00 per year for Canadian and international students. To receive student rate, orders must be accompanied by name of affiliated institution, date of term, and the *signature* of program/ residency coordinator on institution letterhead. Orders will be billed at individual rate until proof of status is received. Foreign air speed delivery is included in all *Clinics* subscription prices. All prices are subject to change without notice. **POSTMASTER:** Send address changes to *Infectious Disease Clinics of North America*, Elsevier Health Sciences Division, Subcription Customer Service, 3251 Riverport Lane, Maryland Heights, MO 63043. **Customer Service: 1-800-654-2452 (US). From outside of the US and Canada, call 1-314-447-8871. Fax: 1-314-447-8029. E-mail: JournalsCustomerService-usa@elsevier.com (print support) or JournalsOnlineSupport-usa@elsevier.com (online support).**

Infectious Disease Clinics of North America is also published in Spanish by Editorial Inter-MÅdica, Junin 917, 1ᵉʳ A 1113, Buenos Aires, Argentina.

Reprints. For copies of 100 or more, of articles in this publication, please contact the Commercial Reprints Department, Elsevier Inc., 360 Park Avenue South, New York, New York 10010-1710. Tel. (212) 633-3812, Fax: (212) 462-1935, E-mail: reprints@elsevier.com.

Infectious Disease Clinics of North America is covered in *MEDLINE/PubMed (Index Medicus), Current Contents/ Clinical Medicine, Science Citation Alert, SCISEARCH,* and *Research Alert.*

Printed and bound by CPI Group (UK) Ltd, Croydon, CR0 4YY
Transferred to Digital Printing, 2013

Contributors

CONSULTING EDITOR

HELEN W. BOUCHER, MD, FIDSA, FACP
Director, Infectious Diseases Fellowship Program; Associate Professor of Medicine, Division of Geographic Medicine and Infectious Diseases, Tufts Medical Center, Boston, Massachusetts

EDITOR

THOMAS M. FILE Jr, MD, MSc
Chair, Infectious Disease Division, Summa Health System, Akron, Ohio; Professor, Internal Medicine; Master Teacher, Chair, Infectious Disease Section, Northeast Ohio Medical University, Rootstown, Ohio

AUTHORS

ANTONIO ANZUETO, MD
University of Texas Health Science Center at San Antonio; South Texas Veterans Health Care System, San Antonio, Texas

EDINA AVDIC, PharmD, MBA
Infectious Disease Clinical Pharmacist, Department of Pharmacy, The Johns Hopkins Hospital, Baltimore, Maryland

JOHN G. BARTLETT, MD
Professor of Medicine, Johns Hopkins University School of Medicine, Baltimore, Maryland

SARA COSGROVE, MD, MS
Associate Professor, Division of Infectious Diseases, Department of Medicine, The Johns Hopkins University School of Medicine, Baltimore, Maryland

DEBAPRIYA DATTA, MD
Assistant Professor of Medicine, Division of Pulmonary and Critical Care Medicine, University of Connecticut Health Center, Farmington, Connecticut

THOMAS M. FILE Jr, MD, MSc
Chair, Infectious Disease Division, Summa Health System, Akron; Professor, Internal Medicine; Master Teacher, Chair, Infectious Disease Section, Northeast Ohio Medical University, Rootstown, Ohio

CHARLOTTE A. GAYDOS, MS, MPH, DrPH
Professor, Division of Infectious Diseases, Department of Medicine, Johns Hopkins University, Baltimore, Maryland

JENNIE JOHNSTONE, MD, FRCPC
Assistant Professor, Department of Medicine; Institute for Infectious Disease Research, McMaster University, Hamilton, Ontario, Canada

ROBERT KELLEY, PhD
Assistant Professor, Division of Infectious Diseases, University of Louisville, Louisville, Kentucky

ADAMANTIA LIAPIKOU, MD, PhD
3rd Pneumology Department, Sotiria Hospital, Athens, Greece

DONALD E. LOW, MD, FRCP(C)
Professor of Medicine and Microbiology, Department of Microbiology, Mount Sinai Hospital/University Health Network and University of Toronto, Toronto, Ontario, Canada

LIONEL MANDELL, MD, FRCPC
Professor, Department of Medicine, McMaster University, Hamilton, Ontario, Canada

THOMAS J. MARRIE, MD
Dean, Faculty of Medicine, Dalhousie University, Halifax, Nova Scotia, Canada

MARK L. METERSKY, MD
Professor of Medicine, Division of Pulmonary and Critical Care Medicine, University of Connecticut Health Center, Farmington, Connecticut

DONNA MILDVAN, MD
Chief, Division of Infectious Diseases, Beth Israel Medical Center, Professor of Medicine, Albert Einstein College of Medicine, New York, New York

DANIEL M. MUSHER, MD
Professor of Medicine and Distinguished Service Professor, Baylor College of Medicine; Member, Infectious Disease Section, Michael E. DeBakey VA Medical Center, Houston, Texas

MICHAEL S. NIEDERMAN, MD
Professor of Medicine, The State University of New York, Stony Brook, New York; Chairman, Departments of Medicine, Pulmonary and Critical Care Medicine, Winthrop-University Hospital, Mineola, New York

VERONIQUE NUSSENBLATT, MD, MHS
Fellow, Division of Infectious Diseases, Department of Medicine, The Johns Hopkins University School of Medicine, Baltimore, Maryland

ANDREW T. PAVIA, MD
George and Esther Gross Presidential Professor and Chief, Division of Pediatric Infectious Diseases, Department of Pediatrics, University of Utah, Salt Lake City, Utah

PAULA PEYRANI, MD
Instructor of Medicine, Division of Infectious Diseases, University of Louisville, Louisville, Kentucky

JULIO RAMIREZ, MD
Professor of Medicine, Division of Infectious Diseases, University of Louisville, Louisville, Kentucky

MARCOS I. RESTREPO, MD, MSc
University of Texas Health Science Center at San Antonio, San Antonio; South Texas Veterans Health Care System, San Antonio, Texas; Veterans Evidence Based Research Dissemination and Implementation Center (VERDICT)

JÖRG RUHE, MD, MPH
Division of Infectious Diseases, Beth Israel Medical Center, Assistant Professor of Medicine, Albert Einstein College of Medicine, New York, New York

SALVADOR SIALER, MD
Pneumology Department, Clinic Institute of Thorax (ICT), Hospital Clinic of Barcelona, Barcelona, Spain

ORIOL SIBILA, MD
University of Texas Health Science Center at San Antonio, San Antonio, Texas; Servei de Pneumologia, Hospital de la Santa Creu i Sant Pau, Barcelona, Spain

ANTONI TORRES, MD, PhD
Pneumology Department, Clinic Institute of Thorax (ICT), Hospital Clinic of Barcelona; Insitut d'investigacions biomèdiques August Pi i Sunyer (IDIBAPS), University of Barcelona (UB), CIBERES, Barcelona, Spain

SHWETA UPADHYAY, MD
Fellow, Pulmonary and Critical Care Medicine, Winthrop-University Hospital, Mineola, New York

TIMOTHY WIEMKEN, PhD, MPH, CIC
Assistant Professor, Division of Infectious Diseases, University of Louisville, Louisville, Kentucky

RICHARD G. WUNDERINK, MD
Professor of Medicine, Pulmonary and Critical Care Division, Northwestern University Feinberg School of Medicine, Chicago, Illinois

VANESSA YAP, MD
Resident in Internal Medicine, University of Connecticut Health Center, Farmington, Connecticut

Contents

Health care-associated pneumonia (HCAP) is associated with an increased risk of infection with multidrug-resistant pathogens compared
with community-acquired pneumonia. Recent studies suggest that the
designation of HCAP is a poor predictor of resistant pathogens and that
antibiotic coverage for multidrug-resistant pathogens is not necessary in
all patients with HCAP. This article reviews existing literature on HCAP,
discusses the utility of the current definition of HCAP in identifying patients
at risk for potentially drug-resistant pathogens, and compares how well the
current HCAP designation predicts the risk of drug-resistant pathogens
with other proposed algorithms for doing so.

Biomarkers have been proposed as tools that can guide the management
of patients with community-acquired pneumonia, providing information
that supplements the usually available clinical data. Among the available
biomarkers, procalcitonin has been studied extensively and seems promising for several purposes. The use of biomarkers needs further study, to
validate their utility in daily practice, especially given the limitations of
the current tools for identifying the need for antibiotic therapy in patients
with influenza and secondary bacterial pneumonia, in patients with aspiration syndromes, and in those infected with atypical pathogens.

During the initial management of patients with community-acquired pneumonia (CAP), physicians need to assess severity of the disease and predict
likely clinical outcomes of the patient. This information is used to make
important clinical decisions, such as site of care, extent of laboratory
work-up, and therapeutic interventions. CAP prediction scores were
developed to help physicians define severity of disease and likely clinical
outcomes of their patients. This article reviews the most relevant clinical
outcomes in hospitalized patients with CAP and outlines the role of these
scores as tools to help physicians predict these outcomes.

Community-acquired pneumonia (CAP) accounts for major morbidity and mortality in the United States. With improved broad-spectrum antibiotics, the implementation of diagnostic studies has declined and most patients do not have an etiologic pathogen of CAP identified. To enhance the appropriate use of antiviral agents and prevent overuse of antibiotics, the successful management of CAP requires rapid and accurate diagnosis of the etiologic agent of CAP. This article provides an overview of the new rapid molecular tests for the diagnosis of influenza, other respiratory viruses, and bacteria compared with nonmolecular tests and how their use for directed therapy can enhance and improve the management of CAP.

Community-acquired pneumonia (CAP) has a significant impact in terms of morbidity, mortality, and cost of care. Guidelines play an important role in the management of this disease, and evidence supporting the positive effects of guidelines on outcomes in patients with CAP is substantial. However, evidence supporting many of the CAP quality indicators is low, and pay-for-performance measures do not seem to influence clinically important outcomes. Future CAP quality indicators should incorporate evidence-based interventions.

Multidrug-resistant pneumococci continue to increase worldwide. Although there are still questions regarding the relevance of β-lactam resistance, the recommendation for the use of the macrolides as monotherapy for mild community-acquired pneumonia should be revisited in view of high rates of resistance, the association of clinical failures with low-level and high-level resistance, and the lack of clinical data to support their need for empirical therapy for the atypicals.

The present controversy regarding the need to cover atypical pathogens in the empiric therapy of community-acquired pneumonia is related to several issues, including the relevance of terminology, imprecise diagnostic methods, and perceived contradictory results of published evidence. Studies evaluating the time to clinical recovery and the use of earlier endpoints for evaluation suggest that appropriate therapy provides a benefit if an atypical pathogen is a pathogen. Because recent surveillance studies suggest these pathogens are common and until there is the availability of accurate, cost-effective, and easily interpreted laboratory tests to provide the etiologic diagnosis at the time of point of care, empiric therapy of atypical pathogens is supported.

Community-acquired pneumonia (CAP) is a frequent cause of morbidity and mortality in the United States and worldwide, in particular among older patients and those with significant comorbid conditions. Current guidelines recommend therapy with a fluoroquinolone or a β-lactam plus a macrolide for the treatment of hospitalized adults with CAP who do not require admission to an intensive care unit. This article provides a brief summary and overview of the existing literature on this topic categorized by the main results; the potential implications for future clinical practice and research are discussed.

Community-acquired pneumonia (CAP) is the leading cause of death from infectious diseases in the United States. The mortality rate due to severe CAP has shown little improvement over the past few years, with a rate as high as 50% mainly in patients admitted to intensive care units. Death and adverse outcomes from CAP result from a complex interplay between the pathogen and the host. Several therapies have been tested in patients with severe CAP in recent years. This article reviews recent data regarding different treatments including antimicrobials and adjunctive therapies in patients with severe CAP.

Anaerobic bacteria are infrequent pulmonary pathogens, and, even then they are, they are almost never recovered due to the need for specimens uncontaminated by the upper airway flora and failure to do adequate anaerobic bacteriology. These bacteria are relatively common in selected types of lung infections including aspiration pneumonia, lung abscess, necrotizing pneumonia and emphyema. Preferred antibiotics for these infections based on clinical experience are clindamycin and any betalactam-betalactamase inhibitor.

Respiratory viruses have long been appreciated as a cause of community acquired pneumonia (CAP), particularly among children, people with serious medical comorbidities, and military recruits. They are increasingly recognized as a cause of CAP among adults. Polymerase chain reaction–based testing has allowed detection of newer agents and improved the ability to detect such viral infections as influenza virus and rhinovirus. Coinfection with viruses and bacteria is common and it remains challenging to determine which patients have only viral infection as the cause of CAP. Better ways to diagnose viral CAP and to integrate detection into management, and better treatment options for noninfluenza respiratory viral infections are needed.

The emergence of methicillin-resistant strains of *Staphylococcus aureus* has raised issues regarding the importance of methicillin-resistant *S aureus* (MRSA) in community-acquired pneumonia (CAP) and its optimal treatment. Community-acquired MRSA (CA-MRSA) is an important cause of CAP because of the high mortality if not suspected early, and its occurrence in young patients with long life expectancy. Certain clinical features can increase the probability of CA-MRSA as a cause of CAP. The consistent trend toward better outcomes for documented MRSA pneumonia suggests that linezolid be considered the drug of choice for documented MRSA CAP, especially for CA-MRSA.

Treatment failure in community-acquired pneumonia (CAP) is the failure to normalize the clinical features (eg, fever, cough, sputum production), or nonresolving image in chest radiograph, despite antimicrobial therapy. The incidence of treatment failure in CAP has not been clearly established; according to several studies it ranges between 6% and 15%. The rate of mortality increases significantly, especially in those patients with severe CAP. It is important to be able to identify what patients are at risk for progressive or treatment failure pneumonia that may make them candidates for a more careful monitoring.

Cardiovascular disease is the leading cause of morbidity and mortality in the United States. Several investigators recently reported an increased risk of cardiovascular events (CVEs) in hospitalized patients with community-acquired pneumonia (CAP). CVEs may be the primary determinant of clinical failure in hospitalized patients with CAP. Future research may be necessary to identify patients at risk of CVEs during or after an episode of CAP. In these patients, therapeutics beyond antibiotics (eg, heparin or aspirin) may be indicated during and after hospitalization.

INFECTIOUS DISEASE CLINICS
OF NORTH AMERICA

Preface

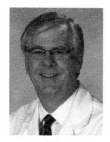

Thomas M. File Jr, MD, MSc
Editor

Despite significant advances in management and prevention, community-acquired pneumonia (CAP) remains a common and serious infection. The burden of CAP is significant and the mortality among patients requiring hospitalization remains relatively high with little change in the past 4 decades.[1,2] The economic burden associated with CAP is substantial at greater than $17 billion annually in the United States.[1] Although there is extensive clinical experience in the care of CAP as well as numerous published clinical practice guidelines, there remain several controversial areas and unanswered questions.

The objective of this issue is to provide an overview of many of the controversial questions that are clinically relevant to the management or prevention of CAP. I am grateful to the distinguished group of colleagues who have contributed their expertise to this issue. Controversial issues that are addressed in this issue include those regarding the following general topics:

- Pneumonia classification: the relevance of the definition of health care–associated pneumonia
- New diagnostic tests and prognostic markers/scoring systems including the utility of biomarkers (especially procalcitonin and cardiac markers)
- Etiologic agents: specifically the relevance of viruses, anaerobes ("aspiration pneumonia"), and methicillin-resistant *Staphylococcus aureus*
- Therapy: the benefit of guideline recommendations and quality measures, relevance of pneumococcal resistance (including utility of the macrolides in light of macrolide resistance, need to cover "atypical pathogens" empirically, the relative benefit of fluoroquinolone versus β-lactam/macrolide therapy, best therapy for severe CAP, and the role of antimicrobial stewardship)
- Outcomes: approach to management of the nonresponding patient, and the association of cardiovascular events and CAP
- Prevention: the benefit of pneumococcal vaccines and the role of conjugate vaccine for adults

While there may not be definitive answers to each of the questions or controversial issues, the authors provide expert commentary relevant to the available information and provide recommendations based on the present evidence.

Infect Dis Clin N Am 27 (2013) xiii–xiv
http://dx.doi.org/10.1016/j.idc.2012.11.017
0891-5520/13/$ – see front matter © 2013 Published by Elsevier Inc.

id.theclinics.com

I thank Helen Boucher for inviting me to guest edit this issue and Stephanie Donley for her expert assistance.

Thomas M. File Jr, MD, MSc
Infectious Disease Division
Summa Health System
Akron, OH
Internal Medicine; Infectious Disease Section
Northeast Ohio Medical University
Rootstown, OH

E-mail address:
filet@summahealth.org

REFERENCES

1. File TM Jr, Marrie TJ. Burden of community-acquired pneumonia in North American adults. Postgrad Med 2010;122(2):130–41.
2. Waterer GW, Rello J, Wundrink RG. Management of community-acquired pneumonia in adults. Am J Respir Crit Care Med 2011;183:157–64.

Erratum

Errors were made in the December 2012 issue of *Infectious Disease Clinics (IDC 26.4)*.

1. In the abstract it states 'systemic vascular resistance' when it should be 'sustained virologic response.'
2. In the keywords the same problem, should state 'sustained virologic respinse' not 'systemic vascular resistance.'

Infect Dis Clin N Am 27 (2013) xv
http://dx.doi.org/10.1016/j.idc.2013.01.001
0891-5520/13/$ – see front matter © 2013 Elsevier Inc. All rights reserved.

Is the Present Definition of Health Care–Associated Pneumonia the Best Way to Define Risk of Infection with Antibiotic-Resistant Pathogens?

Vanessa Yap, MD, Debapriya Datta, MD, Mark L. Metersky, MD*

KEYWORDS

- Health care–associated pneumonia • Community-acquired pneumonia
- Antibiotic resistance • Risk score

KEY POINTS

- Guidelines on health care–associated pneumonia (HCAP), which is defined as pneumonia in outpatients in contact with the health care system, are a valid attempt at targeting a population at risk of infection with multidrug-resistant pathogens; however, there is significant heterogeneity in terms of the magnitude of risk as well as the type of risk.
- HCAP is a poor predictor of multidrug-resistant pathogens. The definition of HCAP needs further modification so that adequate coverage can consistently be provided while avoiding excessive antibiotic use.
- Recent studies indicate that HCAP guideline compliance did not result in better outcomes than noncompliance.
- Individualization of therapy is necessary in patients with HCAP. Patients need to be risk stratified for drug-resistant pathogens based on comorbidities, functional status, and severity of disease to better categorize which patients would benefit from broad-spectrum antibiotic therapy. Various clinical algorithms are available for this purpose but need to be validated in prospective studies.
- Recent hospitalization within 90 days, recent antibiotic therapy within the last 30 days, severe pneumonia, immunosuppression, and poor functional status are associated with increased risk of drug-resistant pathogens. Broad-spectrum antibiotic therapy should be used in such patients.
- Appropriate monotherapy or guideline-concordant community-acquired pneumonia therapy is probably as efficacious as combination therapy for HCAP which is not associated with risk factors for multidrug-resistant pathogens.

Disclosures: V.Y., D.D.: None. Dr Metersky has previously served as a consultant and speaker for Wyeth and Pfizer. He has received funding from Bayer for clinical trials unrelated to pneumonia.
Division of Pulmonary & Critical Care Medicine, University of Connecticut Health Center, 263 Farmington Avenue, Farmington, CT 06030-1321, USA
* Corresponding author.
E-mail addresses: metersky@uchc.edu; metersky@nso.uchc.edu

Infect Dis Clin N Am 27 (2013) 1–18
http://dx.doi.org/10.1016/j.idc.2012.11.002
0891-5520/13/$ – see front matter © 2013 Elsevier Inc. All rights reserved.

id.theclinics.com

INTRODUCTION

Health care–associated pneumonia (HCAP) was introduced as a new category of pneumonia in the 2005 update of American Thoracic Society (ATS)/Infectious Disease Society of America's (IDSA) guidelines on nosocomial pneumonia.[1] This category of pneumonia was characterized as pneumonia occurring in outpatients in contact with the health care system who were at risk of infections with resistant pathogens. Specifically, HCAP was defined by the ATS guidelines as pneumonia occurring in the setting of any of the following risk factors: (1) hospitalization for more than 2 days in an acute care hospital in the last 90 days; (2) residence in a skilled nursing facility; (3) recent intravenous antibiotic therapy, chemotherapy, or wound care in the last 30 days; (4) attending a hospital or hemodialysis clinic; and (5) immunosuppression.

This entity was defined based on evidence that these health care–associated infections may have a different epidemiology and that the causative pathogens are different from those causing community-acquired pneumonia (CAP) and are more often caused by potentially drug-resistant pathogens such as those commonly seen in hospital-acquired infections. This group of patients was, hence, thought to require antibiotic coverage broader than that for CAP to reduce the risk of initially inadequate antibiotic therapy and subsequent worsened outcomes.

Although the concept of HCAP may enable the initiation of appropriate antibiotic therapy by identifying patients at risk for infection with resistant organisms, prospective studies have not validated the need for this practice in all of the subcategories of HCAP. Thus, there has been concern that the use of broad-spectrum antibiotic therapy for all patients with HCAP might be unnecessary and could increase costs and promote selection for more resistant pathogens. More recently, guideline-concordant (GC) therapy was associated with increased mortality in patients with possible multidrug-resistant (MDR) pneumonia, including HCAP,[2,3] although unmeasured confounders likely played a role in this finding. Comparison of GC-HCAP versus GC-CAP therapy for patients meeting the criteria for nonsevere HCAP was also not associated with improved survival.[4] For all of these reasons, attempts are now being made to refine the definition of HCAP.[5,6]

The objective of this article is to review existing literature on the subject of HCAP and discuss the accuracy of the current definition of HCAP in identifying patients at risk for potentially drug-resistant pathogens. The authors compare how well the current HCAP designation predicts the risk of drug-resistant pathogens with other proposed algorithms for doing so. Although some experts have proposed entirely eliminating the designation of HCAP, the authors avoid that debate. Although the population that the authors are concerned about in this article could accurately be designated as either patients with HCAP or patients with CAP at risk of infection with drug-resistant pathogens, the authors think that the more important issue is how best to determine which patients are at risk of developing pneumonia caused by antibiotic-resistant pathogens.

THE CONCEPT OF HCAP

The concept of HCAP was introduced by the authors of the 2005 ATS and IDSA's guidelines for the management of adults with hospital-acquired pneumonia (HAP), ventilator-associated pneumonia (VAP), and health care–associated pneumonia to address the concern of the shifting microbiology[5] of patients presenting to the hospital with pneumonia. Recent or chronic contact with the health care system seemed to be a risk factor of infection with MDR pathogens.[6] Data supporting the concept were first published in a large retrospective study.[7] This study examined more than 4000 patients with culture-positive (CP) pneumonia acquired outside of the hospital admitted to 59 hospitals in the United States. The defining criteria for HCAP in this study differed from the ATS guidelines in including only the following: (1) admission to the hospital in the prior 3 months, (2) transfer from a skilled nursing facility (SNF), and (3) long-term hemodialysis. The results demonstrated a high frequency of HCAP; 21.9%, of all patients with pneumonia, and a high mortality rate of 19.8%, comparable to that associated with ventilator-associated pneumonia, and much higher than that of patients with CAP (10%). The microbiologic spectrum was also different from CAP, with the following organisms frequently isolated on culture: Enterobacteriaceae (25.8%), *Pseudomonas aeruginosa* (25.3%), methicillin-resistant *Staphylococcus aureus* (MRSA) (26.5%), and *Acinetobacter* (2.6%). A subsequent retrospective study of patients admitted to the hospital with pneumonia[6] examined other patients with potential risks for antibiotic-resistant pathogens, such as admission to the hospital in the past 12 months; immunocompromised, including human immunodeficiency virus (HIV) infection, organ transplant, and radiation or chemotherapy in the preceding 6 months; as well as the ATS HCAP criteria. This study found a higher incidence of HCAP (67%), but the microbiologic spectrum and mortality were similar to the study by Kollef.[8] However, other investigators have questioned the generalizability of these results. The definition of health care facility was unclear in these studies. The microbial pattern of patients with CAP consisted of an incidence of MDR pathogens that was higher than previously reported. Only patients with CP results were included in the study. Although this was entirely appropriate given the goals of the studies, this may have resulted in bias because physicians may be more likely to pursue diagnostic studies in patients at a greater risk of resistant pathogens and/or poor outcomes.[9]

The results of the studies from the United States have not been validated by subsequent studies. A retrospective study[10] used the ATS definition of HCAP and reported the occurrence of HCAP to be 38% of 371 patients hospitalized with pneumonia in a Japanese community hospital. Mortality from HCAP was higher in this study (11.1%) than CAP (1.9%). Drug-resistant pathogens were isolated in only 12% of patients with HCAP and 2.9% of patients with CAP. Forty-five percent of patients had no pathogen identified. Among patients with drug-resistant pathogens, the mortality rate was reported to be similar in CAP and HCAP. A study from Spain[11] reported a prospective analysis of 727 patients and determined the presence of HCAP (based on the criteria of recent hospitalization, nursing home residence, long-term hemodialysis, and immunosuppression) in 17.3%. The frequency of specific pathogens isolated in these 2 studies was different from the earlier studies performed in the United States. There was a lower incidence of MDR pathogens, with *Streptococcus pneumoniae* and methicillin-sensitive *S aureus* (MSSA) being the most common organism isolated in the Japanese study, and the Spanish study showing a higher incidence of *Haemophilus influenza*. Another European study[12] using the diagnostic criteria for HCAP of hemodialysis in the past 30 days, nursing home residence, and admission to the hospital in the past 30 to 180 days reported an HCAP incidence of 24.9% and had a higher mortality rate of 17.8% but did not assess the impact of MDR pathogens on mortality. A study by Rello and colleagues[13] revealed a higher mortality rate in HCAP (29.5%) despite appropriate antibiotic therapy, resulting in the conclusion that increased mortality in HCAP was independent of bacterial susceptibility and was caused by advanced age, comorbidities, and limitations on aggressive interventions.

PATTERN OF MICROBIOLOGICAL INVOLVEMENT IN HCAP

A wide variation in the frequency of potentially resistant microorganisms causing HCAP has been reported (**Table 1**). In the study by Kollef and colleagues,[7] the most

4 Yap et al

Table 1
Reported bacterial cause of HCAP

Author, Year	Kollef et al,[7] 2005[a]	Carratala et al,[11] 2007	Micek et al,[52] 2007[a]	Shindo et al,[10] 2009[a]	Schreiber et al,[5] 2010[a]	Park et al,[15] 2010[a]	Chalmers et al,[17] 2011[a]	Grenier et al,[53] 2011[a]	Park et al,[18] 2012[a]
Country	United States	Spain	United States	Japan	United States	Korea	United Kingdom	Canada	Korea
n	988	126	431	141	94	182	277	563	167
Pathogen									
MSSA	21	2	14	6	11	4	4	2	7
MRSA	27	1	31	5	22	3	1	1	11
P aeruginosa	25	2	26	6	23	5	1	3	21
S pneumonia	6	28	10	14	6	14	20	13	13
Haemophilus sp	6	12	4	3	b	2	6	6	1
Others	36	30	30	30	46	12	9	16	50
No pathogen	0	33	0	45	0	64	68	67	0

All data are presented in percent per total population.
Abbreviation: MSSA, methicillin-susceptible *Staphylococcus aureus*.
[a] Indicates the studies detecting mixed infections in study population in which numbers may add to more than 100%.
[b] Indicates that number was not specified in the study.

common pathogens isolated were S aureus and P aeruginosa, very similar to that in the HAP and VAP populations, with a high rate of methicillin resistance (56.8%) in HCAP with S aureus. The single-center review by Micek and colleagues[6] had similar findings wherein S aureus was again the most frequently isolated pathogen (44.5%, with 68.8% being MRSA), followed by P aeruginosa.

In contrast, in the study by Carratala and colleagues,[11] the cause was similar for both CAP and HCAP cohorts. S pneumonia was the most frequent organism identified in the patients with HCAP, and strains resistant to penicillin and erythromycin were more commonly isolated from patients with HCAP. Among only 3 isolates of S aureus, only one causing HCAP was methicillin resistant. This study documented that prior antibiotic use was more frequent among patients with HCAP, which may explain the high rates of drug resistance among the S pneumonia isolates. Aspiration pneumonia was also found to be a common cause of HCAP because the population was older and more often had cerebrovascular disease and impaired consciousness.[14]

In the study by Shindo[10] of patients with HCAP and CAP, S pneumonia was also the most common pathogen identified in patients with HCAP. Gram-negative pathogens, Streptococci other than S pneumonia, P aeruginosa, and MRSA, were isolated more frequently in patients with HCAP than patients with CAP. There was a higher proportion of patients with severe pneumonia who had HCAP, but it was in the moderate severity class that in-hospital mortality was found to be significantly higher than among patients with CAP. It was also in moderate-severity patients that MDR pathogens were isolated more frequently than from the CAP group. On the other hand, there were no significant differences between HCAP and CAP in the severe class in occurrence of MDR pathogens and in-hospital mortality. This study further showed that the occurrence of MDR organisms was associated with a higher proportion of inappropriate initial antibiotic treatment and treatment failure.[10]

A retrospective analysis of patients presenting to the hospital with pneumonia complicated by respiratory failure requiring mechanical ventilation concurred with prior studies from the United States showing high rates of MDR pathogens, traditionally implicated in nosocomial infections.[5] P aeruginosa (23.4%) was the most commonly isolated pathogen followed by MRSA (22.3%).

A retrospective observational study by Park and colleagues[15] revealed that S pneumonia was the most frequently isolated pathogen in both HCAP and CAP populations, with no significant difference in terms of occurrence of S aureus, either methicillin-susceptible S aureus (MSSA) or MRSA. Gram-negative pathogens were more commonly isolated in HCAP than those in CAP and occurrence of potentially drug-resistant pathogens (29.3% vs 13.0%) was significantly higher in patients with HCAP.[15] Inappropriate initial antimicrobial treatment (24.6% vs 8.7%) was also significantly higher in patients with HCAP. However, the main predictive factor for in-hospital mortality among patients admitted with pneumonia through the emergency department was severity of illness rather than cause of pneumonia.[15]

The incidence of resistant organisms seen in a recent British study[16] was low in both HCAP and CAP groups, similar to other studies from Europe, validating the doubts over the concept of HCAP expressed in the 2009 British Thoracic Society guidelines for the management of CAP in adults in which HCAP was not recognized as a distinct entity.[17] S pneumoniae was the most frequent pathogen; gram-negative Enterobacteriaceae (2.9%), P aeruginosa (0.7%), and MRSA (1.0%) were all infrequent in both groups. These organisms were more frequent in the HCAP group, although these differences were not statistically significant.[16]

The more recent retrospective analysis of CP pneumonia from Korea showed that P aeruginosa (21%), Klebsiella pneumonia (26.9%), and S aureus were common among patients with HCAP[18] and MDR organisms were more common in patients with HCAP than patients with CAP. Logistic regression of the risk factors associated with HCAP revealed that prior hospitalization within 90 days of pneumonia, recent treatment with antimicrobials, and nasogastric tube feeding were independently associated with MDR pathogens.[18]

In summary, there has been a wide variation in the frequency of antibiotic-resistant pathogens or potentially resistant pathogens detected in studies of HCAP (see **Table 1**). Examining the prevalence of the most common pathogens in HCAP demonstrates that just as the severity of illness varies between studies, so does the prevalence of these pathogens. Factors explaining this variation are the significant heterogeneity among the patients classified as having HCAP caused by differences in the definition of HCAP used; local microbiology; individual risk factors, such as functional status or prior antibiotic exposure[19]; as well as inclusion of only severe pneumonia in the Schreiber study.[6]

It is well known that in most cases of CAP and HCAP, a pathogen is never identified. Thus, patients in whom a pathogen is identified likely differ from most patients. The identification of a pathogen might be a correlate of a sicker patient in whom more aggressive attempts to obtain a respiratory sample are made, or perhaps such patients are more likely to grow resistant organisms merely because their organism survived to grow in a clinical sample despite an initial dose of antibiotics received in the emergency department. Indeed, a retrospective cohort study of adult patients with HCAP found differences in demographics and risk factors for HCAP between CP and culture-negative (CN) patients.[20] Those with CP HCAP had greater severity of illness, hospital mortality, and a longer hospital stay compared with patients with CN HCAP. These results suggest that patients with CN HCAP may differ substantially from patients with HCAP with positive microbiologic cultures and that the findings from studies of CP patients cannot necessarily be applied to most patients in whom a pathogen is not detected.

EVIDENCE FOR AND AGAINST INCREASED RISK OF DRUG-RESISTANT PATHOGENS IN SUBCATEGORIES OF HCAP

The concept of HCAP was created to identify the group of patients that are more likely to be infected with resistant pathogens and commonly includes the following risk factors:

1. Hospitalization for 2 days or more in the preceding 90 days
2. Residence in a nursing home or extended care facility
3. Home infusion therapy (including antibiotics)
4. Chronic dialysis within 30 days
5. Home wound care
6. Family member with MDR pathogen[1]

These risk factors were derived by extrapolation from the study by Friedman and colleagues[21,22] on health care–associated bloodstream infections in adults whereby bloodstream infection was defined by a positive blood culture obtained from a patient at the time of hospital admission or within 48 hours of admission if the patient fulfilled any of the following criteria:

1. Received intravenous therapy at home; received wound care or specialized nursing care through a health care agency, family, or friends; or had self-administered intravenous medical therapy in the 30 days before the bloodstream infection (Patients whose only home therapy was oxygen use were excluded.)

2. Attended a hospital or hemodialysis clinic or received intravenous chemotherapy in the 30 days before the bloodstream infection
3. Was hospitalized in an acute care hospital for 2 or more days in the 90 days before the bloodstream infection
4. Resided in a nursing home or long-term care facility

Immunosuppression has been included as a risk factor in many studies,[6] but this subset was excluded from the ATS/IDSA's guidelines.[23-25]

Recent Hospitalization

The definition of recent hospitalization varies by investigator but is most commonly defined as hospital admission during the previous 90 days.[24,26] This reason is the most common cause for classification as HCAP,[11,24] applying to up to 63% of patients with HCAP.[26] Hospitalization within 90 days of the pneumonia was identified as an independent variable associated with the identification of patients with MDR pathogens (odds ratio [OR] = 2.51; 95% confidence interval [CI] [1.36–4.63]; P = .003).[18] There are no specific studies identifying reasons for hospitalization, length of hospital stay, and antibiotic exposure during the prior hospitalization.

Admission from a Nursing Home

Patients with pneumonia admitted from a nursing home or long-term care facility constitutes a large subgroup, constituting 10% to 61% of patients with HCAP.[24,27,28] The incidence of nursing home–associated pneumonia (NHAP) has been progressively increasing and is expected to increase worldwide.[27]

An article reviewing the primary studies of NHAP published between 1978 and 1994 showed that the most common pathogens were gram-negative bacilli (18%), S pneumonia (16%), H influenza (11%), and S aureus (6%).[8] A more recent study on very elderly patients requiring mechanical ventilation showed higher rates of S aureus than their CAP counterparts (30% vs 7%) and fewer S pneumonia isolates (9% vs 14%). All Staphylococcus isolates from patients with CAP were methicillin susceptible, whereas 79% from patients with NHAP were methicillin resistant.[29] In a subsequent study by the same investigators in 2004, S aureus accounted for the most isolates (31%), followed by enteric gram-negative bacilli (28%) and S pneumoniae (25%).[30]

In a study of nonintubated patients comparing NHAP and HAP, S pneumonia was predominant (37.3%) and more common in NHAP, followed by S aureus (33.3%), which was mostly methicillin sensitive. There was also a high rate of Chlamydophila infection noted.[31] In another study differentiating bacteriologic findings among subgroups of Japanese patients with HCAP, MRSA and K pneumonia were most frequently identified in patients with NHAP.[32] Four recent studies from Europe[23,27,33] found S pneumonia to be the most frequently isolated pathogen, with low prevalence of MDR organisms.[23,27,33,34] The microbiologic pattern of involvement in NHAP in various studies is summarized in **Table 2**.

Mortality

Mortality rates in NHAP have been reported to be less than in patients with HAP[31] but higher than in CAP or even other subgroups included in HCAP.[32] Thirty-day[23,27,32] as well as long-term mortality rates (6 months) in NHAP also tend to be higher than in patients with CAP.[23]

The effect of cause of NHAP on mortality is probably slight because in one study, the microbial pattern did not differ between survivors and deceased patients.[27] This finding was similar to that from the German study[23] in which S pneumonia was the predominant organism isolated; although the short-term mortality was fourfold and

Table 2
Bacterial cause of patients with NHAP

Authors	El Solh et al,[29] 2001[b]	Maruyama et al,[31] 2008[b]	Polverino et al,[27] 2010	Umeki et al,[32] 2011	Garcia- Vidal et al,[34] 2011[b]	Klapdor et al,[33] 2012	
Country	United States	Japan	Spain	Japan	Spain	Germany	
Age						≥65	≤65
n	47	75	57	46	131	518	100
Pathogen							
S pneumonia	9	37	22	13	37	7	11
MSSA	23	3	0	3	1	2	2
MRSA	6	1	2	17	[a]	0	0
P aeruginosa	4	1	1	4	1	1	4
H influenza	2	0	1	2	2	0	2
Others	20	72	12	35	48	10	13
No pathogen	47	28	62	30	27	77	68

All data are presented in percent per total population.
  [a] Indicates that number was not specified in the study.
  [b] Indicates the studies detecting mixed infections in study population and numbers may add to more than 100%.

long-term mortality threefold higher than for patients with CAP aged 65 years or older across all common pathogens, this was seemingly unrelated to MDR pathogens.[23]

Factors affecting outcomes in NHAP
A study from Germany on NHAP in younger nursing home residents included 100 patients aged younger than 65 years out of 618 patients with NHAP.[33] The rate of potential MDR pathogens was low both in patients aged younger than 65 years and in those aged older than 65 years, and the NHAP presentation was less severe in the younger patients based on the confusion, respiratory rate, blood urea nitrogen-65 score (CRB-65) score. Short- and long-term mortality was twice as low in the younger patients. All these findings suggest that age and associated comorbidities are the main determinants of clinical presentation and outcomes.

Patients with NHAP are the only HCAP subgroup whereby functional status has been consistently evaluated.[24] Many investigators have shown that patients' premorbid functional status is one of the important prognostic factors for mortality.[24,27] The Spanish study showed that advanced age, comorbidities (particularly neurologic disorders), and functional status (up to 70% were totally or partially dependent) were similar in both patients with NHAP and patients with HAP, although mortality and microbiological data in NHAP are more similar to those with CAP.[27] The German study reported mortality rates in patients with NHAP much higher than their CAP counterparts across all common pathogens, suggesting that comorbidity, severe disability, and treatment restrictions (eg, do not resuscitate [DNR] and other hidden restrictions, including *do not transfer to intensive care unit* [ICU] or *do not reevaluate extensively in case of treatment failure*) are the reasons behind increased mortality.[28] In fact, a study from Belgium showed that residence in a nursing home or chronic health care facility was an independent predictor for increased mortality, again citing observed differences in the management between patients with CAP and HCAP. It is important to note that patients with HCAP in this study were older, had more comorbidity, and more severe pneumonia in comparison with patients with CAP. More patients with HCAP were not admitted to the ICU because of DNR codes related to the higher prevalence of malignant disease, dementia, or advanced age in these patients.[35]

In the Spanish study, empiric treatment of NHAP was mainly concordant with CAP guidelines[36] and, depending on the antibiotic resistance, was inappropriate only in a few cases, with no increased mortality.[27] A cluster randomized controlled trial of 680 nursing home residents aged 65 years or older in Canada demonstrated that using a clinical pathway for on-site monotherapy with levofloxacin for pneumonia and other lower respiratory tract infections in nursing homes resulted in no significant differences in health-related quality of life or functional status compared with the usual care group.[37] The presence of other risk factors for MDR infections (eg, previous antibiotic treatment and recent hospitalization), risk of aspiration and severity of disease, presence of wounds and decubitus ulcers,[19] comorbid illness[19] should always be assessed on an individual basis to guide the selection of broad-spectrum antibiotic treatment.[24,27]

Much of the heterogeneity within the literature is caused by vast differences between nursing homes and the services they provide. There is no unique definition of nursing homes available worldwide and it may not be possible given the organizational differences in local health care systems in different countries. Some may cater to bedridden patients and include tube feeding, full nursing, or merely support if necessary.

Hemodialysis

Infection is a major complication affecting both prognosis and survival of patients with end-stage renal disease and is ranked as the second leading cause of death in Japanese patients undergoing hemodialysis, following cardiovascular disease.[38–40] Hemodialysis-associated pneumonia (HDAP) is among the most common infection, and mortality rates from HDAP are 14 to 16 times higher than those from pneumonia in the general population.[38,41] One in 5 patients were diagnosed with pneumonia in the 1-year period following inception of dialysis therapy, and higher rates were found among patients undergoing hemodialysis (29%) than in patients undergoing peritoneal dialysis (18.2%).[41] Increased susceptibility to infection has been attributed partly to old age, high prevalence of diabetes mellitus, defective phagocytic function of granulocytes, and frequent exposure to potential infectious risk factors during the normal course of dialysis therapy.[40]

Two large retrospective studies of Medicare data provide the limited data on the cause of pneumonia in patients undergoing dialysis.[4,39] The microbiologic pattern of involvement in HDAP in various studies is summarized in **Table 3**. In 2006, a historical cohort study conducted by the United Stated Renal Data System revealed that among patients undergoing long-term hemodialysis, S pneumonia and P aeruginosa were the most common pathogens isolated from hospitalized patients undergoing dialysis.[39] Despite high rates of colonization with MRSA in the dialysis population, Staphylococcus species were found in only 2.2% of the CP study population, less than 1% of which were caused by S aureus.[7,24,39] However, this study had a large number of cases without identification of a bacterial cause (81.8%), indicating that the risk of MDR pathogens causing pneumonia has not yet been adequately studied among patients undergoing dialysis. In a subsequent study in 2008,[41] S pneumonia remained the most common organism isolated, followed by Staphylococcus species and P aeruginosa.[41]

A prospective cohort study from Spain showed that among the patients undergoing dialysis, the most common causative pathogen was S pneumonia, followed by H influenza and Legionella, with no S aureus isolated from the 44 patients with HDAP. There

Table 3
Bacterial cause of hemodialysis-associated pneumonia

Pathogen	Slinin et al,[39] 2006	Guo et al,[41] 2008	Kawasaki et al,[43] 2011[a]	Viasus et al,[42] 2011
Country	United States	United States	Japan	Spain
n	3101	60 610	69	44
S pneumoniae	3	3	10	34
MSSA	0	2	12	0
MRSA	b	b	28	0
P aeruginosa	3	1	3	0
H influenzae	2	0	7	7
Others	10	10	35	9
No organism identified	82	84	26	50

All data are presented in percent per total population.
 [a] Indicates the studies detecting mixed infections in study population and numbers may add to more than 100%.
 [b] Indicates that number was not specified in the study.

were no significant differences in the frequency of pathogens compared with patients without dialysis. The frequency of gram-negative bacilli and S aureus were quite low in this subgroup of patients. Findings from this study suggest that empiric antibiotic treatment of pneumonia in patients undergoing hemodialysis likely can be safely based on the CAP guidelines.[36,42]

More recent data on HDAP from Japan[43] retrospectively analyzed 69 patients, 42 with moderate and 27 with severe pneumonia based on A-DROP (age, dehydration, respiratory failure, orientation disturbance, and low blood pressure). The most common pathogens were S aureus (38%), 28% of which were MRSA, followed by S pneumoniae (10.1%), K pneumonia (8.7%), H influenzae (7.2%), and Moraxella catarrhalis (5.8%). There were no differences in microbiological findings, including the incidence of MDR pathogens, between the moderate and severe groups. Most cases in the study (82.6%) received only monotherapy, and outcomes and in-hospital mortality and 30-day mortality rates were similar to previous HCAP studies.[43] The question remains of how to predict the possibility of MDR pathogens and how to choose the antibiotics for each group. Unlike the Spanish study, this study suggests that HDAP should be included in the HCAP category, realizing that analysis of the severity of illness is crucial in the treatment strategy of HDAP.[43]

Home Health Care

Patients using home health care is the smallest cohort of patients with HCAP. There are no epidemiologic studies specific for patients receiving home health care. A case control study in 2006 comparing MSSA and MRSA infections isolated within the first 48 hours of hospitalization determined home nursing care to be an independent risk factor for isolation of MRSA.[24] There were no specific studies identified that investigated home infusion care or patients receiving wound care as a risk factor for HCAP.

Immunosuppression

Immunosuppression is not listed in the ATS-IDSA guidelines as a HCAP risk factor; however, many studies have included it as an HCAP criterion.[24] It is comprised of a diverse group of patients, including but not limited to patients with neutropenia during the index hospitalization, HIV-infection, history of any solid organ or hematopoietic stem cell transplantation or prednisone use (>20 mg) for more than 3 weeks in the year before hospitalization,[44] treatment of malignancy, and the use of immunosuppressive medications.[24]

The 2 largest groups under this category, patients with cancer and patients with HIV, both have specialty-specific guidelines.[24] The data are limited on the cause of pneumonia in such patients. The current combination antiretroviral therapy era for patients with HIV has decreased the incidence of pneumonia and other opportunistic infections.[45] A study on nosocomial pneumonia in patients with HIV in 2006 may overlap with the current HCAP definition because nosocomial pneumonia was defined as pneumonia that developed after 48 hours of hospitalization or within 14 days of previous hospitalization. The more common pathogens were P aeruginosa (33%), S aureus (25%) with high prevalence of methicillin resistance (65%), and S pneumonia (21%). This study identified only having MRSA as the etiologic agent to be associated with lower survival.[46]

Patients with cancer are unique in that they frequently have implantable devices and are relatively immunocompromised, even without overt neutropenia. In a study of non-neutropenic patients with cancer with S aureus infections, pneumonia was the second most common type of infection, with a prevalence of MRSA of 67.3% in S aureus pneumonia. The findings of this observational study also demonstrated that even in these non-neutropenic patients, S aureus had a high mortality rate.[47]

Pneumonia in patients with a relative harboring MDR pathogens

The anterior nares are known reservoirs for S aureus, with up to 80% of the general population constantly or intermittently harboring the bacteria. It can be carried for more than 1 year with a half-life colonization of MRSA around 40 months. MRSA colonization was associated with a 4- to 10-fold increased risk of infection, including pneumonia.[48] However, no specific studies were identified assessing pneumonia in patients who have a relative with known MDR pathogens.

ALTERNATIVES TO THE HCAP DEFINITION FOR IDENTIFYING PATIENTS WITH PNEUMONIA AT RISK FOR ANTIBIOTIC-RESISTANT PATHOGENS

Several studies have demonstrated that potentially resistant organisms are now commonly encountered in patients with HCAP with severe pneumonia, highlighting a group of patients at risk of infection with organisms traditionally confined to the hospital. A study by Shorr[49] on 639 patients admitted with pneumonia identified resistant pathogens in 45.2% of the population. The following independent variables were found to be associated with HCAP caused by resistant pathogens: recent hospitalization, SNF resident, long-term hemodialysis, and ICU admission. The likelihood of developing a resistant infection was 4 times (adjusted OR 4.21, 95% CI) higher in patients with recent hospitalization and 2 times higher in patients on hemodialysis or who were SNF residents. The need for ICU admission also increased the risk of resistant infection (adjusted OR 1.62, CI 95%). Based on the logistic regression, the investigators created a scoring system and assigned points to each of these variables: recent hospitalization, 4 points; residence in SNF, 3 points; long-term hemodialysis, 2 points; and ICU admission, 1 point. Moderate predictive risk for this model was demonstrated by the receiver operating characteristic curve. For scores less than 3 points, the prevalence of resistant organisms was less than 20%; for scores between 3 and 5 points, the prevalence was 55%; and for scores more than 6, it was75%. Although this risk stratification scoring system provided a simple tool to predict the need for broader spectrum antibiotic treatment, it is noteworthy that in this cohort, even the low-risk patients had a risk of resistant organisms of less than 20%. Hence, when caring for a population with as high a risk of resistant organisms as this cohort, the usefulness of this tool is not clear.

A subsequent study in 2010 by Schreiber[5] demonstrated that there was no difference in either demographics or severity of illness between individuals with infection caused by an MDR organism and those with a traditionally susceptible isolate. There was also no difference in the prevalence of comorbid illness across the 2 cohorts, and HCAP alone performed poorly as a screening test. A clinical scoring tool was developed based on logistic regression analysis wherein points were assigned as follows: immunosuppression, 3; admission from long-term care, 2; and prior antibiotics, 1; with a maximum score of 6. A higher score was associated with an increase in infection with MDR pathogens. Patients with 2 or more points had a more than 40% chance of harboring a resistant pathogen. It was noted that about 17% patients with none of these risk factors had infection with resistant organisms.

Based on risk factors for resistant organisms in HCAP identified by various studies, another algorithm was devised by Brito and Niederman[25] (**Fig. 1**) for initial antibiotic therapy for patients with HCAP. According to this algorithm, all patients with HCAP should be identified and then divided by severity of illness to guide initial therapy. Patients should then be divided into groups based on an assessment of severity of illness (need for ventilatory support or ICU admission) and presence of risk factors for MDR organisms. Risk factors for drug-resistant pathogens include recent antibiotic therapy in the past 6 months, recent hospitalization in the past 3 months, the presence

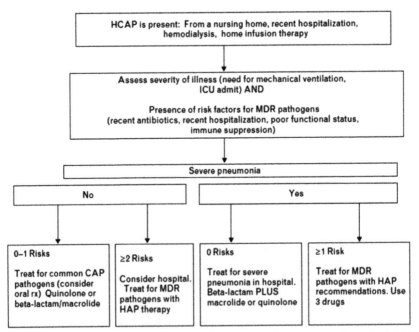

Fig. 1. Clinical algorithm for treatment of HCAP. ICU, intensive care unit. (*Data from* Brito V, Niederman MS. Healthcare-associated pneumonia is a heterogeneous disease, and all patients do not need the same broad-spectrum antibiotic therapy as complex nosocomial pneumonia. Curr Opin Infect Dis 2009;22(3):316–25.)

of immunosuppression, or poor functional status as defined by activities of daily living. Patients with severe pneumonia and the presence of zero risk factors should be treated with antibiotics for CAP, such as a beta-lactam plus macrolide or quinolone. Patients with severe pneumonia with one or more risk factors should be treated for resistant pathogens with a broader spectrum of coverage. Patients with nonsevere pneumonia with 0 to 1 risk factors should be treated for common CAP pathogens; those with 2 or more risk factors should be treated for resistant pathogens. The investigators reiterate that in addition to these risk factors, it is important to consider local patterns of microbiology because each hospital setting and nursing home has unique bacteriology, and therapy choices must be modified with such local data in mind. This scheme represents an attempt to balance the risk of MDR pathogens with the potential negative consequences of antibiotic overuse. A multicenter prospective study to evaluate the frequency of initial inappropriate antibiotic use with the use of this scheme would yield important knowledge. Specific issues that require testing are the safety of not including hemodialysis or nursing home residence as a risk factor in patients with severe pneumonia and the variation of results among various centers in the setting of a well-designed prospective study in which systematic bias can be minimized. Furthermore, although the importance of considering local patterns of infection and resistance cannot be underestimated, it is unclear how often clinicians actually do this. With the increasing use of electronic health records and computerized physician order entry systems that encompass decision support, it seems likely that local patterns of resistance could increasingly be made available to clinicians at the bedside.

El Sohl and colleagues[30] constructed a classification tree for predicting the risk of drug-resistant pathogen-related pneumonia among nursing home patients. The variables used in this tree were previous use of antibiotics and an activities of daily living (ADL) score. The ADL score took into account 6 major areas of activity, including transfer, feeding, bathing, toileting, and continence. Patients were assigned a score of 1 if they were fully independent, 2 if they were partially dependent, and 3 if they were completely dependent in each area of activity. A score of 6 indicated that a patient was fully functional and independent, and a score of 16 indicated total dependence. Previous use of antibiotics was defined as the receipt of antimicrobial therapy for 3 or more consecutive days in the preceding 6 months of hospital admission.

The decision tree predicted that patients with an ADL score less than 12.5 and no prior antibiotic exposure had no drug-resistant pathogens in cultures of protected bronchoalveolar lavage (BAL) fluid. Patients with an ADL score greater than 12.5 and a prior history of antibiotic exposure showed a 90% probability of having drug-resistant pathogens on culture of BAL. The validity of this predictive tree was tested prospectively in a separate cohort of patients. The model was reported to perform with 100% sensitivity (95% CI, 71.3%–100%) and 69.4% specificity for resistant pathogens. One limitation is the fact that patients do not always present to the hospital with all of the necessary data to allow scoring of a 6-component ADL scale.

Another scoring system was proposed recently by Park and colleagues[18] to identify patients with MDR pathogens using identified risk factors. Points were assigned based on the logistic regression: 5 points for nasogastric tube feeding; 3 points for recent hospitalization within 90 days of diagnosed pneumonia; 2 points for intravenous antibiotics within 30 days of diagnosed pneumonia; and 1 point each for residence in a nursing home or extended care facility, chemotherapy, wound care within 30 days of diagnosed pneumonia, or undergoing chronic dialysis. When the total score of 3 points was established as the cutoff point, the sensitivity was 68% (95% CI, 60.7–74.7%) and specificity 67.3% (95% CI 63.2%–71.0%).[18]

In another recent study, Shorr and colleagues[49] derived a tool for predicting the risk of MRSA in patients with pneumonia presenting to the hospital. The risk score consisted of 7 variables, each of which were assigned points as follows: recent hospitalization in last 90 days, 3 points; ICU admission, 2 points; and age younger than 30 years or older than 79 years, hospital-based wound care in last 30 days, dementia, cirrhosis, female with diabetes, 1 point each. The potential total score ranged from 0 to 10. The prevalence of MRSA increased as the score increased, ranging from 8% in those with a score of 0% to 33% in patients with a score of 7 or more. For simplification, the score was divided into 3 groups: score of 0 (low), 1 to 4 (moderate), 5 or more (high risk). MRSA rates were 8%, 17%, and 27%, respectively, in this simplified scheme. The areas under the receiver operating curves (AUROC) for the validation cohort was 0.63, whereas a model using HCAP alone had a lower AUROC (0.57, $P<.001$).

The clinical scoring system devised by Shorr and colleagues[49] in 2008 was validated to determine the risk for any resistant pathogen and compare it with the HCAP definition.[50] The cohort included 977 patients, and MDR organisms were isolated in 46.7% of them, with the most common organisms being MRSA (22.7%), *P aeruginosa* (19.1%), and *S pneumonia* (19.1%). The risk score was higher in those with MDR pathogens (median score of 4 vs 1, $P<.001$). The risk score was higher in those with an MDR pathogen (median score, 4 vs 1, $P<.001$). As a screening test for MDR organisms, a risk score of 0 had a high negative predictive value (84.5%) and could result in less use of unnecessary broad-spectrum antibiotics.[50]

These models may help identify patients with pneumonia at risk for MDR pathogens who require broad-spectrum antibiotic coverage; however, they need to be validated in large prospective studies performed in hospitals with a broad range of patient populations.

INTERPRETATION OF EVIDENCE AND RECOMMENDATIONS

It has become increasingly clear that not all patients with HCAP are at a high risk for MDR pathogens. There is geographic variation in resistance patterns as well as variation related to patient populations studied and institutional resistance patterns. Overall, no consistent pattern of antibiotic resistance has been delineated in HCAP. Concerns about overuse of broad-spectrum antibiotic treatment of patients with HCAP and a consequent effect on antibiotic resistance are, hence, warranted. Recent studies that have indicated that GC therapy has not been associated with improved outcomes in patients with HCAP, although clearly subject to the confounding by indication associated with these types of retrospective studies, have increased concern regarding the appropriateness of the systematic use of broad-spectrum antibiotics in patients with HCAP.[2–4]

Recent studies indicate that in patients with HCAP, the factors most closely associated with an increased risk of infection with MDR pathogens include recent hospitalization within 90 days,[25,51] recent antibiotic therapy within the last 30 days,[18,49] severe pneumonia,[30,49] immunosuppression, and poor functional status.[25,30] However, the last characteristic has generally been studied in nursing home patients and it is unclear if it would apply in countries besides the United States where nursing home use is less prevalent. Individualization of therapy is necessary in patients with HCAP. Patients need to be risk stratified for drug-resistant pathogens based on these characteristics to better categorize which patients would benefit from broad-spectrum antibiotic therapy. Given the wide variation in the frequency of drug-resistant pathogens in the various studies, none of the schema for predicting the risk of drug-resistant pathogens can be recommended for routine use in all hospitals. Rather, HCAP remains a condition whereby careful consideration of the evidence presented in this review in combination with knowledge of local antibiotic resistance patterns should inform empiric antibiotic choices. However, certain general statements can be made. In severely ill patients with one or more other risk factors for resistant organisms, coverage for resistant gram-negative bacilli and MRSA should be strongly considered. For non–severely ill patients with one or more risk factors for resistant organisms, there are numerous antibiotics that have efficacy against typical CAP pathogens and many gram-negative bacilli (for example, respiratory quinolones and advanced generation cephalosporins); it seems appropriate to use one of these in such patients. Making a recommendation regarding whether to add an additional antibiotic for MRSA coverage is more difficult, given the wide range of the frequency of MRSA isolation in studies across the world. It should go without saying that a gram stain of noninvasively obtained samples of respiratory tract secretions and/or knowledge of patients' prior isolates can often help to guide initial antibiotic therapy.

NEED FOR FURTHER STUDIES

- Prospective epidemiologic studies directly comparing the accuracy of the HCAP designation and various other schemes in determining the risk of resistant organisms
- Identification of risk factors for MRSA versus resistant gram-negative bacilli in HCAP
- Identify the role of geographic variation in HCAP by means of multinational and multicenter studies
- Comparative effectiveness studies to determine how relevant all of these issues are to patient outcomes

SUMMARY

- The HCAP designation is a poor predictor of infection with MDR pathogens. The definition of HCAP needs further modification so that adequate coverage can consistently be provided while avoiding excessive antibiotic.
- Recent studies indicate that HCAP guideline compliance did not result in better outcomes than noncompliance.
- Individualization of therapy is necessary in patients with HCAP. Patients need to be risk stratified for drug-resistant pathogens based on severity of illness, comorbidities, and functional status to better categorize which patients would benefit from broad-spectrum antibiotic therapy. Various clinical algorithms are available for this purpose but need to be validated in prospective studies.
- Hospitalization within 90 days, recent antibiotic therapy within the last 30 days, severity of pneumonia, immunosuppression, and poor functional status are associated with an increased risk of drug-resistant pathogens and merits broad-spectrum antibiotic therapy.
- Appropriate monotherapy is probably as efficacious as combination therapy for patients with HCAP who are not severely ill and have no risk factors for MDR pathogens.

REFERENCES

1. American Thoracic Society, Infectious Diseases Society of America. Guidelines for the management of adults with hospital-acquired, ventilator-associated, and

healthcare-associated pneumonia. Am J Respir Crit Care Med 2005;171(4): 388–416.

2. Madaras-Kelly KJ, Remington RE, Sloan KL, et al. Guideline-based antibiotics and mortality in healthcare-associated pneumonia. J Gen Intern Med 2012; 27(7):845–52.

3. Kett DH, Cano E, Quartin AA, et al. Implementation of guidelines for management of possible multidrug-resistant pneumonia in intensive care: an observational, multicentre cohort study. Lancet Infect Dis 2011;11(3):181–9.

4. Attridge RT, Frei CR, Restrepo MI, et al. Guideline-concordant therapy and outcomes in healthcare-associated pneumonia. Eur Respir J 2011;38(4):878–87.

5. Schreiber MP, Chan CM, Shorr AF. Resistant pathogens in nonnosocomial pneumonia and respiratory failure: is it time to refine the definition of health-care-associated pneumonia? Chest 2010;137(6):1283–8.

6. Micek ST, Reichley RM, Kollef MH. Health care-associated pneumonia (HCAP): empiric antibiotics targeting methicillin-resistant Staphylococcus aureus (MRSA) and Pseudomonas aeruginosa predict optimal outcome. Medicine (Baltimore) 2011;90(6):390–5.

7. Kollef MH, Shorr A, Tabak YP, et al. Epidemiology and outcomes of health-care-associated pneumonia: results from a large US database of culture-positive pneumonia. Chest 2005;128(6):3854–62.

8. Kollef MH, Morrow LE, Baughman RP, et al. Health care-associated pneumonia (HCAP): a critical appraisal to improve identification, management, and outcomes–proceedings of the HCAP Summit. Clin Infect Dis 2008;46(Suppl 4):S296–334 [quiz: 335–8].

9. Ewig S, Welte T, Chastre J, et al. Rethinking the concepts of community-acquired and health-care-associated pneumonia. Lancet Infect Dis 2010;10(4):279–87.

10. Shindo Y, Sato S, Maruyama E, et al. Health-care-associated pneumonia among hospitalized patients in a Japanese community hospital. Chest 2009;135(3): 633–40.

11. Carratala J, Mykietiuk A, Fernandez-Sabe N, et al. Health care-associated pneumonia requiring hospital admission: epidemiology, antibiotic therapy, and clinical outcomes. Arch Intern Med 2007;167(13):1393–9.

12. Venditti M, Falcone M, Corrao S, et al. Outcomes of patients hospitalized with community-acquired, health care-associated, and hospital-acquired pneumonia. Ann Intern Med 2009;150(1):19–26.

13. Rello J, Lujan M, Gallego M, et al. Why mortality is increased in health-care-associated pneumonia: lessons from pneumococcal bacteremic pneumonia. Chest 2010;137(5):1138–44.

14. Carratala J, Garcia-Vidal C. What is healthcare-associated pneumonia and how is it managed? Curr Opin Infect Dis 2008;21(2):168–73.

15. Park HK, Song JU, Um SW, et al. Clinical characteristics of health care-associated pneumonia in a Korean teaching hospital. Respir Med 2010;104(11):1729–35.

16. Chalmers JD, Taylor JK, Singanayagam A, et al. Epidemiology, antibiotic therapy, and clinical outcomes in health care-associated pneumonia: a UK cohort study. Clin Infect Dis 2011;53(2):107–13.

17. Lim WS, Baudouin SV, George RC, et al. BTS guidelines for the management of community acquired pneumonia in adults: update 2009. Thorax 2009;64(Suppl 3): iii1–55.

18. Park SC, Kang YA, Park BH, et al. Poor prediction of potentially drug-resistant pathogens using current criteria of health care-associated pneumonia. Respir Med 2012;106(9):1311–9.

19. Poch DS, Ost DE. What are the important risk factors for healthcare-associated pneumonia? Semin Respir Crit Care Med 2009;30(1):26–35.
20. Labelle AJ, Arnold H, Reichley RM, et al. A comparison of culture-positive and culture-negative health-care-associated pneumonia. Chest 2010;137(5):1130–7.
21. Friedman ND, Kaye KS, Stout JE, et al. Health care–associated bloodstream infections in adults: a reason to change the accepted definition of community-acquired infections. Ann Intern Med 2002;137(10):791–7.
22. Gaynes R. Health care–associated bloodstream infections: a change in thinking. Ann Intern Med 2002;137(10):850–1.
23. Ewig S, Klapdor B, Pletz MW, et al. Nursing-home-acquired pneumonia in Germany: an 8-year prospective multicentre study. Thorax 2012;67(2):132–8.
24. Attridge RT, Frei CR. Health care-associated pneumonia: an evidence-based review. Am J Med 2011;124(8):689–97.
25. Brito V, Niederman MS. Healthcare-associated pneumonia is a heterogeneous disease, and all patients do not need the same broad-spectrum antibiotic therapy as complex nosocomial pneumonia. Curr Opin Infect Dis 2009;22(3): 316–25.
26. Sugisaki M, Enomoto T, Shibuya Y, et al. Clinical characteristics of healthcare-associated pneumonia in a public hospital in a metropolitan area of Japan. J Infect Chemother 2012;18(3):352–60.
27. Polverino E, Dambrava P, Cilloniz C, et al. Nursing home-acquired pneumonia: a 10 year single-centre experience. Thorax 2010;65(4):354–9.
28. Ewig S, Welte T, Torres A. Is healthcare-associated pneumonia a distinct entity needing specific therapy? Curr Opin Infect Dis 2012;25(2):166–75.
29. El-Solh AA, Sikka P, Ramadan F, et al. Etiology of severe pneumonia in the very elderly. Am J Respir Crit Care Med 2001;163(3 Pt 1):645–51.
30. El Solh AA, Pietrantoni C, Bhat A, et al. Indicators of potentially drug-resistant bacteria in severe nursing home-acquired pneumonia. Clin Infect Dis 2004; 39(4):474–80.
31. Maruyama T, Niederman MS, Kobayashi T, et al. A prospective comparison of nursing home-acquired pneumonia with hospital-acquired pneumonia in non-intubated elderly. Respir Med 2008;102(9):1287–95.
32. Umeki K, Tokimatsu I, Yasuda C, et al. Clinical features of healthcare-associated pneumonia (HCAP) in a Japanese community hospital: comparisons among nursing home-acquired pneumonia (NHAP), HCAP other than NHAP, and community-acquired pneumonia. Respirology 2011;16(5):856–61.
33. Klapdor B, Ewig S, Schaberg T, et al. Presentation, etiology and outcome of pneumonia in younger nursing home residents. J Infect 2012;65(1):32–8.
34. Garcia-Vidal C, Viasus D, Roset A, et al. Low incidence of multidrug-resistant organisms in patients with healthcare-associated pneumonia requiring hospitalization. Clin Microbiol Infect 2011;17(11):1659–65.
35. Depuydt P, Putman B, Benoit D, et al. Nursing home residence is the main risk factor for increased mortality in healthcare-associated pneumonia. J Hosp Infect 2011;77(2):138–42.
36. Mandell LA, Wunderink RG, Anzueto A, et al. Infectious Diseases Society of America/American Thoracic Society consensus guidelines on the management of community-acquired pneumonia in adults. Clin Infect Dis 2007;44(Suppl 2): S27–72.
37. Loeb M, Carusone SC, Goeree R, et al. Effect of a clinical pathway to reduce hospitalizations in nursing home residents with pneumonia: a randomized controlled trial. JAMA 2006;295(21):2503–10.

38. Wakasugi M, Kawamura K, Yamamoto S, et al. High mortality rate of infectious diseases in dialysis patients: a comparison with the general population in Japan. Ther Apher Dial 2012;16(3):226–31.

39. Slinin Y, Foley RN, Collins AJ. Clinical epidemiology of pneumonia in hemodialysis patients: the USRDS waves 1, 3, and 4 study. Kidney Int 2006;70(6):1135–41.

40. Wakino S, Imai E, Yoshioka K, et al. Clinical importance of Stenotrophomonas maltophilia nosocomial pneumonia due to its high mortality in hemodialysis patients. Ther Apher Dial 2009;13(3):193–8.

41. Guo H, Liu J, Collins AJ, et al. Pneumonia in incident dialysis patients–the United States Renal Data System. Nephrol Dial Transplant 2008;23(2):680–6.

42. Viasus D, Garcia-Vidal C, Cruzado JM, et al. Epidemiology, clinical features and outcomes of pneumonia in patients with chronic kidney disease. Nephrol Dial Transplant 2011;26(9):2899–906.

43. Kawasaki S, Aoki N, Kikuchi H, et al. Clinical and microbiological evaluation of hemodialysis-associated pneumonia (HDAP): should HDAP be included in healthcare-associated pneumonia? J Infect Chemother 2011;17(5):640–5.

44. Hsu JL, Siroka AM, Smith MW, et al. One-year outcomes of community-acquired and healthcare-associated pneumonia in the Veterans Affairs Healthcare System. Int J Infect Dis 2011;15(6):e382–7.

45. Crothers K, Huang L, Goulet JL, et al. HIV infection and risk for incident pulmonary diseases in the combination antiretroviral therapy era. Am J Respir Crit Care Med 2011;183(3):388–95.

46. Franzetti F, Grassini A, Piazza M, et al. Nosocomial bacterial pneumonia in HIV-infected patients: risk factors for adverse outcome and implications for rational empiric antibiotic therapy. Infection 2006;34(1):9–16.

47. Kang CI, Song JH, Ko KS, et al. Clinical features and outcomes of Staphylococcus aureus infections in non-neutropenic cancer patients. Support Care Cancer 2012;20(3):483–8.

48. Lam AP, Wunderink RG. The role of MRSA in healthcare-associated pneumonia. Semin Respir Crit Care Med 2009;30(1):52–60.

49. Shorr AF, Zilberberg MD, Micek ST, et al. Prediction of infection due to antibiotic-resistant bacteria by select risk factors for health care-associated pneumonia. Arch Intern Med 2008;168(20):2205–10.

50. Shorr AF, Zilberberg MD, Reichley R, et al. Validation of a clinical score for assessing the risk of resistant pathogens in patients with pneumonia presenting to the emergency department. Clin Infect Dis 2012;54(2):193–8.

51. Lescure FX, Locher G, Eveillard M, et al. Community-acquired infection with healthcare-associated methicillin-resistant Staphylococcus aureus: the role of home nursing care. Infect Control Hosp Epidemiol 2006;27(11):1213–8.

52. Micek ST, Kollef KE, Reichley RM, et al. Health care-associated pneumonia and community-acquired pneumonia: a single-center experience. Antimicrob Agents Chemother 2007;51(10):3568–73.

53. Grenier C, Pepin J, Nault V, et al. Impact of guideline-consistent therapy on outcome of patients with healthcare-associated and community-acquired pneumonia. J Antimicrob Chemother 2011;66(7):1617–24.

Biomarkers

What is Their Benefit in the Identification of Infection, Severity Assessment, and Management of Community-acquired Pneumonia?

Shweta Upadhyay, MD[a], Michael S. Niederman, MD[a,b,c],*

KEYWORDS

- Biomarkers • Procalcitonin • C-reactive protein • Duration of therapy
- Community-acquired pneumonia • Severity of illness

KEY POINTS

- Information from measurement of levels of inflammatory biomarkers such as procalcitonin (PCT) at the time of admission with radiographic community-acquired pneumonia (CAP) can help to define the need for antibiotic therapy because levels are high with bacterial infection but not with viral infection.
- Measurement of PCT levels on admission and serially can help to define the prognosis of CAP and the likelihood of developing pneumonia complications.
- Serial measurement of PCT levels can be used to define the optimal duration of antibiotic therapy in CAP, and a PCT-guided approach has led to good outcomes, with a shorter duration of therapy than a standard clinical approach.
- Measurement of PCT levels may not be valuable in the setting of partially treated CAP and cannot always recognize whether influenza is complicated by secondary bacterial pneumonia.
- In patients with CAP and a low PCT value on admission, treatment in the intensive care unit (ICU) may not be necessary, even if the patient falls into the high-risk group by traditional prognostic scoring tools.
- Cardiac biomarkers may be more valuable than inflammatory biomarkers for predicting the long-term mortality risk in patients with CAP.

CAP is one of the most common reasons for hospitalization and is associated with significant morbidity and mortality. It is one of the most common infections for which antibiotics are prescribed and is the leading cause of death from infection in the United States. The annual incidence of CAP is between 5 and 11 per 1000 population, with the

[a] Pulmonary and Critical Care Medicine, Winthrop-University Hospital, Mineola, NY 11501, USA; [b] The State University of New York, Stony Brook, NY, USA; [c] Department of Medicine, Winthrop-University Hospital, Mineola, NY 11501, USA
* Corresponding author. 222 Station Plaza North, Suite 509, Mineola, NY 11501.
E-mail address: mniederman@winthrop.org

Infect Dis Clin N Am 27 (2013) 19–31
http://dx.doi.org/10.1016/j.idc.2012.11.003
0891-5520/13/$ – see front matter © 2013 Elsevier Inc. All rights reserved.

id.theclinics.com

frequency rising in elderly patients. In 2006, 1.2 million people in the United States were hospitalized with pneumonia and 55,477 people died of the disease.[1] The mortality varies according to the severity of disease. Among outpatients, the mortality is less than 5%, whereas in the hospital, the mortality increases to more than 10%, but can exceed 30% when patients are admitted to the ICU.[2,3]

Early identification of patients with CAP with severe illness can lead to proper site-of-care decisions, and recent data have shown that delayed transfer to the ICU is a risk factor for poor outcome.[4] The Joint Commission on Accreditation of Healthcare Organizations and the Centers for Medicare and Medicaid services have in the past included rapid treatment of CAP as a performance measure, which has added pressure to start antibiotics rapidly, in the emergency department (ED), often before a firm diagnosis is established, and this practice has led to antibiotic complications such as *Clostridium difficile* colitis.[5] At present, we rely on several clinical scoring systems to define the severity of illness, and we use clinical and radiographic assessment to define the presence of pneumonia, the severity of illness, and the need for antibiotic therapy. Several new biomarkers have been developed that can supplement the current approach, by helping to define the presence of pneumonia, assisting in the assessment of disease severity, and guiding the duration of antibiotic therapy.[6,7] It remains controversial whether the use of biomarkers to manage patients with CAP is an improvement over the standard approach, using clinical assessment.

USING BIOMARKERS TO DIAGNOSE THE PRESENCE OF CAP AND THE NEED FOR ANTIBIOTIC THERAPY
Available Biomarkers and Their Advantages

Biomarkers include several proinflammatory cytokines such as tumor necrosis factor (TNF)-α, interleukin (IL)-1, and IL-6, which can not only reflect the degree of acute inflammation in the patient with CAP but also be direct stimulants of acute-phase reactants such as C-reactive protein (CRP) and PCT (**Box 1**). The levels of antiinflammatory cytokines can also be measured and include IL-1 receptor antagonist and IL-10. PCT is currently one of the most widely studied biomarkers and is produced in large quantities by parenchymal cells such as the liver in response to bacterial toxins or proinflammatory cytokines, but is downregulated in the presence of viral infection.[8] Serum levels of PCT rise within 2 hours of a bacterial infection stimulus, which is faster than the rise in CRP levels. The appeal of studying a biomarker in patients with CAP, when compared with a clinical assessment (fever, white blood cell [WBC] count, chest radiograph, and vital signs) is that it may give accurate information, rapidly, that is specific to bacterial infection and at an early time point in illness. Clinical features of CAP vary with the host inflammatory response, which can be a reflection of either the type of patient infected or the etiologic pathogen, and the data may not be specific for infection. In addition, clinical features can be attenuated by the presence of prior antibiotic therapy and may not be valuable early in the course of illness, as is the case in patients with initial chest radiographs with negative results in early CAP. In trying to use clinical features and laboratory testing to separate viral from bacterial CAP, Gram stain could be helpful, but its result needs to be correlated with cultures of sputum and other microbiological data such as blood cultures, which can take at least 24 to 48 hours to yield results. On the other hand, biomarkers measured in serum may give an indication about the presence of bacterial infection in a rapid and reliable manner, guiding the need for antibiotic therapy. In addition, as therapy leads to clinical improvement, levels of inflammatory biomarkers may decline, and serial monitoring can be used to guide when to stop antibiotic therapy.

Box 1
Advantages and disadvantages of using biomarkers to help in CAP management

Advantages

Provides information that is specific to infections needing antibiotic therapy

    Levels can be high with bacterial infection and not viral infection

    Levels rise rapidly with bacterial infection

    Response is usually not organism dependent

    May be more specific for bacterial infection than clinical assessment

Results available rapidly

Levels may be abnormal early in the course of illness, before abnormal clinical and radiographic findings

Can help define short-term and long-term prognoses

Can supplement the information provided by prognostic scoring tools

Can help define the response to therapy

Can help determine the need for continuing antibiotic therapy

    Can reduce antibiotic usage without adverse consequences

Disadvantages

Results may be misleading and conflict with careful clinical assessment

Prior (effective) antibiotic therapy can lower levels rapidly and lead to false-negative findings

May not always distinguish atypical pathogen pneumonia from viral pneumonia

Cannot always recognize if influenza is complicated by secondary bacterial infection

Cannot separate aspiration chemical pneumonitis from aspiration bacterial pneumonia

---

Using Biomarkers to Define the Need for Antibiotic Therapy in CAP

In one study, patients with confirmed CAP were compared with those with respiratory tract infection (RTI) without CAP and to a group of healthy controls. Serum levels of CRP were highest in the CAP group, but those with pneumococcal or *Legionella* infection had higher CRP levels than those with viral or atypical pathogen infection and than those with negative results of microbiologic tests.[9] In this early study of biomarkers, there was also a correlation of CRP levels with the severity of illness, with the levels being higher in those who were hospitalized than in those treated at home. Many investigators have used CRP to define the need for antibiotic therapy in patients with CAP, but most of the recent data have come from studies of PCT, which seems to be more sensitive and specific for this purpose than CRP.

A group of Swiss investigators have carefully studied several biomarkers in patients with RTI, but have relied heavily on PCT levels measured with the highly sensitive Kryptor assay.[10–12] This assay is based on using a sheep polyclonal antibody, which can detect levels as low as 0.06 µg/L, which is far more sensitive than the previously popular commercially available Immunoluminometric assay (LUMI assay), which detected levels only as low as 0.3 to 0.5 µg/L. The group has performed several randomized interventions, including the Pro RESP, Pro CAP, and Pro HOSP studies, which studied patients with RTIs coming to the ED, patients with CAP, and patients with RTIs seen in the ED, respectively.[10–12] In the Pro RESP study, there were 87 patients with CAP and fewer who were randomized to PCT guidance received antibiotic therapy than those randomized to standard care. Also, 1 patient with radiographic CAP received no antibiotics based on the PCT results, and recovered, in spite of being bacteriologically positive.[10] The safety of using serum PCT levels to guide antibiotic therapy led to the next study, the Pro CAP study, in which 302 patients with radiographic CAP were randomized either to receive standard care or to use admission and serial PCT levels guide the use of antibiotics. In the PCT group, therapy was strongly discouraged for levels less than 0.1 μg/L, discouraged if the value was 0.25 μg/L or less, encouraged if the level was greater than 0.25 μg/L, and strongly encouraged if the level was greater than 0.5 μg/L. However, clinical judgment was always allowed to override the guidance suggested by measurement of PCT levels. In the study, 15% with radiographic CAP had antibiotics withheld in the PCT group, compared with 1% in the standard care group, with no adverse outcomes in those not receiving therapy.[11] This observation led the investigators to suggest that PCT levels could be used to separate bacterial from nonbacterial causes of lung infiltrates; that patients with a favorable clinical picture, and a PCT level less than 0.25 μg/mL, could safely have antibiotics withheld; and that this decision was more reliably made when adding a biomarker to clinical assessment than by using clinical judgment alone. The Pro HOSP study extended the data from the earlier findings, which came from a single center, by including 6 different Swiss hospitals in a multicenter intervention study. This study also confirmed that by using PCT levels to guide the use of antibiotics less therapy was initiated, compared with standard care.[12]

In a subsequent analysis, the investigators combined patients from the Pro RESP and Pro CAP studies, which included 373 patients with radiographic CAP. Of these patients, 20 ultimately had noninfectious diagnoses and another 24 recovered without antibiotic therapy.[13] The investigators found that both PCT and highly sensitive CRP (hsCRP) were similarly accurate for predicting the presence of an abnormality in chest radiograph, with both being more useful than clinical signs such as fever, leukocyte count, abnormal lung examination, sputum production, cough, and dyspnea ($P<.001$). A clinical model alone had an area under the curve (of sensitivity vs 1 − specificity) of 0.79 to predict an abnormal result of radiography, compared with a value of 0.88 and 0.92, respectively, when PCT was added or when both PCT and hsCRP were added to the clinical assessment. PCT was more accurate than hsCRP or clinical features to predict the presence of bacteremia ($P<.01$) and to predict the severity of pneumonia, as defined by the Pneumonia Severity Index (PSI). Stolz and colleagues[14] have demonstrated that CRP levels can also predict radiographic pneumonia at a CRP cutoff value of 100 mg/mL with 91% specificity.[14] The advantages of using CRP include low cost, easy availability, historic use, and familiarity with the test, particularly in Europe, but currently, the data with PCT seem more robust for determining when to use antibiotic therapy in patients with suspected CAP.[13,15]

Limitations of Using Biomarkers to Define the Need for Antibiotic Therapy in CAP

Although the Swiss studies have shown that PCT may be able to separate patients with radiographic CAP who need antibiotics from those who do not, it is uncertain if PCT can reliably recognize the presence of atypical pathogen CAP versus bacterial CAP. A small study evaluated 30 patients with CAP, 20 with bacterial pneumonia, and 10 with infection involving *Chlamydophila pneumoniae*, *Mycoplasma pneumoniae*, or *Legionella pneumophila*.[16] Unlike the Swiss studies, this study used the less-sensitive LUMI assay for PCT, rather than the Kryptor assay. PCT levels were high for bacterial pneumonia versus atypical pathogen infection (7.64 vs 0.8 μg/L, $P = .03$). However, clinical parameters and CRP levels were not able to differentiate bacterial from atypical pathogen CAP, and from a practical perspective, one would want PCT data to recommend antibiotic therapy for patients with atypical pathogen CAP. The German Competence

Network, Community Acquired Pneumonia (CAPNETZ) study evaluated the cause of CAP in 1337 patients and did not find that PCT levels could reliably separate individual patients with bacterial CAP from those with atypical pathogen CAP, although groups of patients with bacterial CAP tended to have higher PCT levels than those with atypical pathogen infections.[17] In the recent H1N1 epidemic, PCT levels in patients with pure viral infection tended to be lower than in those with bacterial pneumonia, but still, some patients with severe viral pneumonia had relatively high levels, which overlapped with levels found in patients with bacterial infection.[18] Using a PCT level of 0.1 μg/mL as the threshold, pneumococcal pneumonia was 8.3-fold more likely than CAP due to atypical or viral cause if PCT was increased. Using a PCT level of 0.25 μg/mL as threshold was not as effective; however, the likelihood of *Streptococcus pneumoniae* CAP compared with the other causes was still more than threefold if PCT exceeded this level. There were no significant differences in PCT levels, CRP levels, and WBC count in patients with atypical or viral cause of CAP.

One of the reasons that PCT may not be useful in defining the cause of CAP in individual patients is that levels are influenced not only by the identity of the pathogen but also by the severity of illness, and thus patients with severe nonbacterial pneumonia may have relatively high levels. In The CAPNETZ study, in contrast to CRP levels and WBC count, there was a marked increase in PCT levels with increasing severity of CAP.[17] In addition, bacteremia may lead to an increased level of PCT, and in one CAP study, a cutoff value of 0.25 μg/L for the initial PCT measurement identified 96% of patients with positive results of blood cultures.[19] However, a low level, as discussed above, may still indicate the safety of withholding antibiotic therapy. A confounding factor to this general rule is the use of antibiotic pretreatment. Kruger and colleagues[20] have shown that PCT and copeptin levels (pro-arginine vasopressin, a cardiac biomarker) fall rapidly after antibiotic therapy, and thus the levels of these markers may be falsely low in the setting of treated bacterial pneumonia.

One potential application of PCT would be in patients with suspected aspiration pneumonia, to separate chemical pneumonitis from bacterial pneumonia, the former possibly not requiring antibiotic therapy. In one study of 65 patients with aspiration syndrome, 32 were bacteriologically positive using bronchoalveolar lavage, but their PCT levels did not differ from that of the bacteriologically negative patients.[21] It is possible that PCT was not useful in this clinical setting, because even chemical pneumonitis is associated with a high level of inflammation, and some patients with initial chemical aspiration may still get subsequent secondary bacterial infection.[22]

BIOMARKERS TO HELP DEFINE PROGNOSIS AND SITE-OF-CARE DECISIONS IN PATIENTS WITH CAP
Predicting Prognosis and Complications

The most widely used prognostic scoring systems are the PSI and modifications of the British Thoracic Society rule, the CURB-65 and CRB-65 scores. Other tools, such as the Infectious Disease Society of America/American Thoracic Society (IDSA/ATS) criteria for severe CAP and the SMART-COP system are designed to assess the severity of illness along with the need for ICU admission or intensive respiratory and vasopressor support.[23] These systems are useful for assessing the short-term mortality of CAP, but there may also be long-term mortality consequences of this illness, which are not the result of acute infection and inflammation.[24] Several studies have evaluated the role of biomarkers alone and also in conjunction with scoring systems in predicting prognosis.

Some early investigations established the idea that PCT levels were highest in patients with more severe illness and in those who developed complications.[25] In a group of inpatients and outpatients with CAP, PCT levels measured within 24 hours of admission were higher for those in the highest mortality risk groups (PSI classes III–V) than for those in the lowest mortality risk groups (classes I–II). In addition, PCT levels were higher in patients with pneumonia complications and mortality than in those without these consequences of infection. In general, PCT levels in this study were not influenced by the cause of CAP.[25] Similarly, serial measurements of PCT may have prognostic significance. In a study of 100 ICU-admitted patients with CAP, PCT levels were measured on days 1 and 3, and both levels were higher in non-survivors than in survivors.[26] In addition, levels increased over time in the nonsurvivors, whereas they decreased in survivors. In a multivariate model, an increase in PCT level from day 1 to day 3 was associated with a 4.5 odds ratio (OR) for death.

Another study examined 75 patients with radiographic CAP and found that initial PCT levels were highest in those with higher PSI class, pneumococcal infection, and bacteremia.[27] Those who developed complications (ICU admission or death) had higher PCT levels initially and serially than those who did not. In addition, midregional pro-Atrial Natriuretic Peptide (ANP), a cardiac biomarker, was better than PCT to predict mortality, and its levels also remained high on serial measurement in those with complications. The biomarkers in this study were comparable to clinical scoring systems (CURB-65 and PSI) for predicting mortality, and levels tended to be higher with higher clinical severity scores.

Levels of inflammatory biomarkers may also correlate with long-term outcomes in CAP. In a report of 1799 patients with CAP, Yende and colleagues[28] found that 17.1% died within 1 year of admission and that the risk of dying was associated with persistent inflammation at discharge, as reflected by high levels of IL-6 and IL-10. Menendez and colleagues[29] found a correlation between inflammation and treatment failure, with higher IL-6, PCT, and CRP levels on days 1 and 3 and higher IL-8 levels on day 3 as predictors of this specific complication. Similarly, Reade and colleagues[30] found that higher levels of IL-6 and IL-10 on admission correlated with a higher risk of mortality at 6 months, whereas higher TNF and d-dimer levels correlated with 1-year mortality. More recently, Kruger and colleagues[31] examined the 28-day and 180-day mortalities in 728 patients with CAP. Although PCT, CRB-65 scoring system, midregional pro-ANP, copeptin, and pro-endothelin were all predictors of mortality, the best predictor of both short-term and long-term mortalities was midregional pro-adrenomedullin (MR-proADM). MR-proADM was independent of the CRB-65 score for predicting short-term and long-term mortalities.[31] Adrenomedullin is a peptide biomarker with several biologic effects, including vasodilatation, immune modulation, and bactericidal activity and has been shown to be a prognostic marker in CAP. Levels of adrenomedullin are increased in sepsis, and levels of proADM are increased in heart failure. The finding that cardiac biomarkers, such as MR-proADM, were more predictive of mortality than inflammatory biomarkers is consistent with recent observations about the high frequency and importance of cardiac complications of CAP. Approximately 6% to 7% of patients with CAP have a concomitant myocardial infarction, and these patients have an increased mortality compared with patients without this type of event. The proinflammatory and procoagulant effects of infection may destabilize atheromatous plaque in the coronary arteries, and this may account for the high frequency of myocardial infarction and the usefulness of a cardiovascular marker such as MR-proADM for predicting long-term prognosis in patients with CAP.[32–34]

Other investigations have established a role for biomarkers in predicting the prognosis of patients with CAP. Menendez and colleagues[7] evaluated the impact of adding biomarkers to prognostic scoring, using the PSI and CURB-65, in 453 patients with CAP. They found that measurements of levels of CRP at admission added to the prediction of prognosis from scoring systems, whereas using PCT levels did not. However, they did find that PCT levels and CRP levels both increased significantly as the severity of illness increased, as measured by the PSI and CURB-65 scoring tools. Another study of 384 patients with CAP also found that CRP levels on admission had prognostic value and that levels were higher in patients with more severe illness, as measured by the PSI. An increment of 50 mg/L CRP on admission was associated with a 1.22-fold odds for a patient to be in PSI classes III–V as compared with classes I and II. In addition, levels were higher in patients with bacteremia than in those without and in those with complications (empyema, ICU admission, and death) than in those without.[35] In addition, if CRP levels were greater than 100 mg/L on day 4 after the admission, there was a significant increase in the rate of complications ($P<.01$).

Other studies of biomarkers to define the prognosis in CAP have evaluated the relative value of the prognostic information provided by PCT and CRP levels. One study found that among 1671 patients in the German CAPNETZ study, elevated PCT levels on admission helped to identify patients who had a high risk of dying up to 28 days and that the predictive value of PCT was comparable to that of CRB-65 and more accurate than measurements of levels of CRP.[36] In addition, PCT had a high negative predictive value, and when levels were less than 0.228 ng/mL, there was an almost 99% predictive value that the patient would not die. In addition, another study of 88 patients with CAP found that PCT levels on admission were more valuable than CRP levels to predict severity of illness.[37] In that study, although the sensitivity of CRP for predicting severe illness was higher than that of PCT, the specificity and positive and negative predictive values of PCT were substantially higher than the respective values for CRP. Similarly, a Korean study found that measurement of PCT in the ED was useful for predicting 28-day mortality and that it added to the predictive value of prognostic scoring tools to a much greater extent than measuring the levels of CRP was able to do.[38]

Thus, many studies have shown that measurement of levels of CRP on admission has limited prognostic information. However, as suggested above, serial measurements of CRP levels may be more valuable, especially in patients with severe CAP. Investigators from Portugal[39] have used serial measurements to define 3 patterns of CRP response to therapy: fast decline, slow decline, and nonresponse. They have found that survival was related to the rate of decline in CRP levels and that a level at day 5 that exceeds 50% of the level at day 1 was associated with increased mortality. In this study, of 191 patients in the ICU with CAP, 66 had a fast decline in CRP levels and a 4.8% mortality, 81 had a slow decline and a 17.3% mortality, and 44 had no response and a mortality rate of 36.4%.

Although PCT may be more valuable for predicting CAP prognosis than CRP, other biomarkers have also been studied and shown to be of value for this purpose. Studies have shown that increased levels of pro-adrenomedullin, copeptin, natriuretic peptides, and cortisol are significantly related to mortality in CAP, along with other prohormones such as pro-atrial natriuretic peptide and coagulation markers.[40] Bello and colleagues[41] performed a prospective study of 228 patients to assess the prognostic value of MR-proADM and found that levels of this biomarker increased with increasing disease severity and that the prognostic information provided was independent of the cause. PCT was the only biomarker that showed significant differences ($P<.0001$) between bacterial and viral/atypical CAP. In the study, MR-proADM predicted both short-term and long-term mortalities and was the only biomarker that discriminated between patients who died versus those who survived at 30, 90, and 180 days and 1 year. Thus, whereas PCT has value in deciding when to start antibiotics (with levels being higher in bacterial vs viral infection), MR-proADM cannot serve this purpose but provides much more discriminating information about the prognosis in CAP, both short and long term.

Defining Site of Care

The ability of biomarkers to refine the prognostic information provided by scoring systems may also be valuable in deciding whether an admitted patient needs to be treated in the ICU or on a medical floor. Ramirez and colleagues[42] evaluated 627 patients with CAP admitted to a medical ward and 58 additional patients admitted to the ICU. The investigators found that admission levels of PCT, CRP, IL-6, and TNF-α were higher in patients in the ICU than in those in the ward. However, for predicting the need for ICU admission, the IDSA/ATS criteria were the most accurate, with an OR of 12, but of all the biomarkers, PCT (value >0.35 ng/mL) was the most accurate with an OR of 6.9. Interestingly, of the 78 patients who met 3 of the IDSA/ATS minor criteria for severe CAP, no patient needed ICU admission if the PCT level was less than 0.35 ng/mL, but 23% with elevated PCT levels in this group did need ICU admission. There were also 10 patients admitted to the ICU without severe CAP criteria present, and 8 of them had elevated PCT levels. Of the group admitted to the ICU, 36 were admitted directly and had a 17% mortality, compared with the 27% mortality in the 22 with delayed admission. The patients with delayed ICU admission had higher PCT values than those who remained in the ward. Thus, admission PCT levels might be examined along with other clinical criteria for ICU admission and could be used to potentially avoid delayed ICU admission for patients with high levels and also to avoid using the ICU for low-risk patients who have low PCT levels, in spite of the presence of other clinical signs of severe CAP.

The finding that low levels of biomarkers could be used to avoid ICU admission for patients who have clinical signs of more severe illness was also corroborated in several other studies. Kruger and colleagues[36] found that when the PCT level was 0.228 ng/mL or less, mortality was low, regardless of the score on the CRB-65 scale, and that the negative predictive value for mortality of PCT at this level was 98.9%. Similarly, Huang and colleagues[43] found 546 patients with CAP in PSI class IV and V, but there were 126 who had PCT levels in the lowest quartile (<0.1 ng/mL) and only 2 of these patients (1.6%) died. When MR-proADM levels were measured in the same population, the finding of a level in the lowest quartile was less useful than the finding of a PCT level in the lowest quartile for defining patients at low risk of death.[44]

USING BIOMARKERS TO GUIDE THE DURATION OF CAP THERAPY

As discussed, measurement of levels of biomarkers, especially PCT, can help clinicians decide when to use antibiotics in a patient with CAP and levels measured at the time of admission, and serially, can help to define prognosis and the likelihood of disease-related complications (**Table 1**). Because a reduction in PCT indicates a good prognosis and a good response to therapy, several studies have examined whether serial measurements of PCT can be used to define the optimal duration of antibiotic therapy for CAP. In general, these studies have shown that PCT guidance can reduce the duration of antibiotic therapy, without adverse effects on the patient, compared with the use of clinical assessment to define the duration of CAP therapy.[44,45]

In the ProCAP study, 302 patients with radiographic pneumonia in a single center were randomized to either PCT-guided duration of antibiotic therapy or a control group with clinical guidance only.[11] In the 151 PCT patients, duration of therapy was based on serial PCT levels measured on admission, at 6 to 24 hours (if therapy was initially withheld) and days 4, 6, and 8. Using PCT values, therapy was strongly discouraged if the level was less than 0.1 μg/L, discouraged if the levels was 0.25 μg/L, encouraged if the

Table 1
Randomized controlled trials of PCT to guide duration of therapy in patients with CAP seen in the hospital

Author (Year) (Reference)	Number of Patients PCT (P) Control (C)	Setting	Duration of Therapy PCT	Duration of Therapy Control	Mortality
Christ-Crain et al,[10] 2004	42 (P) 45 (C)	Single center, ED	90.4% given antibiotics	97.8% given antibiotics	<5% in both groups
Christ-Crain et al,[11] 2006	151 (P) 151 (C)	Single center, ED	5 days (median)	12 days (median)	10% (P) 10% (C) Pneumonia related
Schuetz et al,[12] 2009	460 (P) 465 (C)	6 hospitals ED	7 days (median)	10 days (median)	5.2% (P) 5.6% (C)
Bouadma et al,[46] 2010	79 (P) 101 (C)	7 ICUs, Infection suspect	5.5 days (P) (mean)	10.5 days (mean)	16.9% (P) 19.0% (C) Not all were pneumonia in these data

levels 0.25 µg/L or more, and strongly encouraged if the level was 0.5 µg/L or more. In all instances, clinical assessment could be used to override the guidance suggested by the PCT measurement. Patients in the PCT group had a duration of therapy that was 55% shorter than that of the control population and the median duration was reduced to 5 days, compared with 12 days for the control population. After 4 days, approximately 50% of patients in the PCT group were receiving therapy, compared with over 90% in the control group; after 8 days, less than 20% in the PCT group were receiving therapy compared with greater than 80% in the control group. In patients with CAP of varying severity, PCT guidance led to a shorter duration of therapy than was seen in the control group, but for patients with mild CAP (PSI class I–III), duration of therapy was lower with PCT guidance than for patients with moderate to severe CAP (PSI classes IV and V) who had PCT guidance. At follow-up 4 to 6 weeks after admission, failure rates were the same for patients with PCT guidance as for the control group.

A similar randomized trial design was used in the multicenter (6 Swiss hospitals) proHOSP study, which included 925 patients with CAP.[12] When using PCT guidance, serial measures were used in the manner listed for the proCAP study and for patients with a high initial level, greater than 10 µg/L, therapy was urged to be stopped when the value decreased by more than 80% from the initial value. For patients with severe CAP, clinical assessment could lead to overriding the recommendation that followed from PCT measurement. In that study, 78% of the PCT-guided group and 90% of the control group, who were hospitalized, were initially treated with antibiotics. At day 5, 60% of the PCT-guided group and 90% of the control group were receiving antibiotics and the duration of therapy was reduced from 10.7 days for the control group to 7.2 days for the PCT group. Adverse outcomes occurred at the same rate in both groups, and mortality was low, approximately 5% to 6% in both groups. A similar approach has been used in a prospective randomized study of critically ill patients that included nearly 200 patients with CAP.[46] In that study, PCT guidance led to a reduction in antibiotic duration to 5.5 days, compared with 10.5 days for the control group.

In all these studies, there were no adverse events that could be related to the reduced duration of therapy that followed PCT guidance. Similarly, in a recent meta-analysis, Schuetz and colleagues[47,48] used individual patient data to perform a meta-analysis and concluded that in more than 2000 patients with CAP (inpatients and outpatients) studied with a randomized trial design, PCT guidance led to significantly fewer patients being started on antibiotics (90% vs 99%) as well as a substantial reduction in antibiotic use (7 days vs 10 days median duration), but that it had no impact on mortality and was associated with a significant reduction in the rate of treatment failure (19% vs 23.4%).

CONCLUSIONS: HOW AND WHEN TO USE BIOMARKERS IN CAP

Biomarkers are a promising tool for the management of CAP and can supplement the information provided by routine clinical assessment and commonly used prognostic scoring tools. Among the available biomarkers, PCT has been studied extensively in recent years, and several clinical trials have established its utility in CAP management, particularly if the highly sensitive Kryptor assay is used. PCT levels can be measured at the time of initial evaluation, and values can help to predict the presence of radiographic CAP and the need for antibiotic therapy. The latter is driven by the general finding that levels of PCT, an acute-phase reactant produced by many cell types, particularly the liver, rise with bacterial infection and fall with viral illness. However, PCT levels do rise with severe illness and may not be able to distinguish whether influenza is, or is not, complicated by secondary bacterial infection, and similarly, may not be able to distinguish chemical from bacterial aspiration syndromes. In the management of pneumonia, serial measurements of PCT levels can be used to guide duration of therapy, and the use of PCT guidance has led to a reduction in antibiotic use and duration, without adverse consequences to the patient.

Several biomarkers have been measured on admission and serially, to define the prognosis of patients with CAP, and the findings can supplement the information provided by traditional prognostic scoring tools. Levels of biomarkers tend to be higher in patients with more severe illness, and the pattern of serial change may have prognostic value, a finding that has been demonstrated for CRP. When PCT levels are low, prognosis in CAP is generally good, regardless of the severity of illness as defined by prognostic scoring tools such as the PSI. In predicting the long-term prognosis of patients with CAP, cardiac biomarkers, such as MR-proADM, are more valuable than inflammatory biomarkers, pointing to the important interaction between pneumonia and secondary heart disease.

In the future, biomarkers may help to streamline the care of patients with CAP, but as with any laboratory tool, the findings need to be moderated by clinical assessment and the results of biomarker testing need to be ignored if in conflict with a careful clinical evaluation.

REFERENCES

1. Kochanek KD, Xu J, Murphy SL, et al. Deaths: preliminary data for 2009. National Vital Statistics Reports; 59. No.4. CDC2011. Available at: http://www.cdc.gov/nchs/data/nvsr/nvsr59/nvsr59_04.pdf. Accessed June 30, 2011.
2. Heron MP, Hoyert DL, Murphy SL, et al. Deaths: final data for 2006. National Vital Statistics Reports; 57. 2009. Available at: http://www.cdc.gov/nchs/fastats/pneumonia.htm. Accessed July 10, 2011.
3. Welte T, Kohnlein T. Global and local epidemiology of community-acquired pneumonia: the experience of the CAPNETZ network. Semin Respir Crit Care Med 2009;30:127–35.
4. Restrepo MI, Mortensen EM, Rello J, et al. Late admission to the ICU in patients with community-acquired pneumonia is associated with higher mortality. Chest 2010;137:552–7.
5. Polgreen PM, Chen YY, Cavanaugh JE, et al. An outbreak of severe *Clostridium difficile*–associated disease possibly related to inappropriate antimicrobial therapy for community-acquired pneumonia. Infect Control Hosp Epidemiol 2007;28:212–4.
6. Niederman MS. Biological markers to determine eligibility in trials for community acquired pneumonia: a focus on procalcitonin. Clin Infect Dis 2008;47:S127–32.
7. Menendez R, Martinez R, Reyes S, et al. Biomarkers improve mortality prediction by prognostic scales in community-acquired pneumonia. Thorax 2009;64:587–91.
8. Christ Crain M, Muller B. Biomarkers in respiratory tract infections: diagnostic guides to antibiotic prescription, prognostic markers and mediators. Euo Respir J 2007;30:556–73.
9. Almirall J, Bolibar I, Toran P, et al. Contribution of C-reactive protein to the diagnosis and assessment of severity of community-acquired pneumonia. Chest 2004;125:1335–42.
10. Christ-Crain M, Jaccard-Stolz D, Bingisser R, et al. Effect of procalcitonin-guided treatment on antibiotic use and outcome in lower respiratory tract infections: cluster-randomized, single-blinded intervention trial. Lancet 2004;363:600–7.

11. Christ-Crain M, Stolz D, Bingisser R, et al. Procalcitonin guidance of antibiotic therapy in community-acquired pneumonia: a randomized trial. Am J Respir Crit Care Med 2006;174:84–93.
12. Schuetz P, Christ Crain M, Thomann R, et al. Effect of procalcitonin-based guidelines vs standard guidelines on antibiotic use in lower respiratory tract infections: the ProHOSP randomized controlled trial. JAMA 2009;302:1059–66.
13. Muller B, Harbarth S, Stolz D, et al. Diagnostic and prognostic accuracy of clinical and laboratory parameters in community-acquired pneumonia. BMC Infect Dis 2007;7:10.
14. Stolz D, Christ-Crain M, Gencay MM, et al. Diagnostic value of signs, symptoms and laboratory values in lower respiratory tract infection. Swiss Med Wkly 2006; 136:434–40.
15. Holm A, Nexoe J, Bistrup LA, et al. Aetiology and prediction of pneumonia in lower respiratory tract infection in primary care. Br J Gen Pract 2007;57:547–54.
16. Jereb M, Kotar T. Usefulness of procalcitonin to differentiate typical from atypical community-acquired pneumonia. Wien Klin Wochenschr 2006;118:170–4.
17. Krüger S, Ewig S, Papassotiriou J, et al. Inflammatory parameters predict etiologic patterns but do not allow for individual prediction of etiology in patients with CAP - results from the German competence network CAPNETZ. Respir Res 2009;10:65. http://dx.doi.org/10.1186/1465-9921-10-65.
18. Ingram PR, Inglis T, Moxon D, et al. Procalcitonin and C-reactive protein in severe 2009 H1N1 influenza infection. Intensive Care Med 2010;36:528–32.
19. Müller F, Christ-Crain M, Bregenzer T, et al. Procalcitonin levels predict bacteremia in patients with community-acquired pneumonia: a prospective cohort trial. Chest 2010;138:121–9.
20. Krüger S, Ewig S, Kunde J, et al. Pro-vasopressin (copeptin) in patients with community-acquired pneumonia - influence of antibiotic pre-treatment: results from the German competence network CAPNETZ. J Antimicrob Chemother 2009;64:159–62.
21. El-Solh AA, Vora H, Knight PR 3rd, et al. Diagnostic use of serum procalcitonin levels in pulmonary aspiration syndromes. Crit Care Med 2011;39:1251–6.
22. Niederman MS. Distinguishing chemical pneumonitis from bacterial aspiration: still a clinical determination. Crit Care Med 2011;39:1543–4.
23. Niederman MS. Making sense of scoring systems in community acquired pneumonia. Respirology 2009;14:327–35.
24. Kaplan V, Clermont G, Griffin MF, et al. Pneumonia: still the old man's friend? Arch Intern Med 2003;163:317–23.
25. Masia M, Gutierrez F, Shum C, et al. Usefulness of procalcitonin levels in community-acquired pneumonia according to the patients outcome research team pneumonia severity index. Chest 2005;128:2223–9.
26. Boussekey N, Leroy O, Alfandari S, et al. Procalcitonin kinetics in the prognosis of severe community-acquired pneumonia. Intensive Care Med 2006;32:469–72.
27. Lacoma A, Rodriguez N, Prat C, et al. Usefulness of consecutive biomarkers measurement in the management of community-acquired pneumonia. Eur J Clin Microbiol Infect Dis 2012;31:825–33.
28. Yende S, D'Angelo G, Kellum JA, et al. Inflammatory markers at hospital discharge predicts subsequent mortality after pneumonia and sepsis. Am J Respir Crit Care Med 2008;177:1242–7.
29. Menendez R, Cavalcanti M, Reyes S, et al. Markers of treatment failure in hospitalised community acquired pneumonia. Thorax 2008;63:447–52.
30. Reade MC, Yende S, D'Angelo G, et al. Differences in immune response may explain lower survival among older men with pneumonia. Crit Care Med 2009;37:1655–62.

31. Kruger S, Ewig S, Giersdorf S, et al. Cardiovascular and inflammatory biomarkers to predict short- and long-term survival in community-acquired pneumonia: results from the German Competence Network, CAPNETZ. Am J Respir Crit Care Med 2010;182:1426–34.

32. Ramirez J, Aliberti S, Mirsaeidi M, et al. Acute myocardial infarction in hospitalized patients with community-acquired pneumonia. Clin Infect Dis 2008;47: 182–7.

33. Musher DM, Rueda AM, Kaka AS, et al. The association between pneumococcal pneumonia and acute cardiac events. Clin Infect Dis 2007;45:158–65.

34. Koivula I, Sten M, Makela PH. Prognosis after community-acquired pneumonia in the elderly: a population-based 12-year follow-up study. Arch Intern Med 1999; 159:1550–5.

35. Hohenthal U, Hurme S, Helenius H, et al. Utility of C-reactive protein in assessing the disease severity and complications of community-acquired pneumonia. Clin Microbiol Infect 2009;15:1026–32.

36. Krüger S, Ewig S, Marre R, et al. Procalcitonin predicts patients at low risk of death from community-acquired pneumonia. Eur Respir J 2008;31:349–55.

37. Hirakata Y, Yanagihara K, Kurihara S, et al. Comparison of usefulness of plasma procalcitonin and C-reactive protein measurements for estimation of severity in adults with community-acquired pneumonia. Diagn Microbiol Infect Dis 2008; 61:170–4.

38. Park JH, Wee JH, Choi SP, et al. The value of procalcitonin level in community-acquired pneumonia in the ED. Am J Emerg Med 2012;36:1248–54.

39. Coelho LM, Salluh JI, Soares M, et al. Patterns of c-reactive protein RATIO response in severe community-acquired pneumonia: a cohort study. Crit Care 2012;16:R53.

40. Christ-Crain M, Opal SM. Clinical review: the role of biomarkers in the diagnosis and management of community-acquired pneumonia. Crit Care 2010;14:203.

41. Bello S, Lasierra A, Minchole E, et al. Prognostic power of proadrenomedullin in community-acquired pneumonia is independent of aetiology. Eur Respir J 2012; 39:1144–55.

42. Ramirez P, Ferrer M, Marti V, et al. Inflammatory biomarkers and prediction for intensive care unit admission in severe community-acquired pneumonia. Crit Care Med 2011;39:2211–7.

43. Huang DT, Weissfeld LA, Kellum JA, et al. Risk prediction with procalcitonin and clinical rules in community-acquired pneumonia. Ann Emerg Med 2008;52: 48–58.

44. Huang DT, Angus DC, Kellum JA, et al. Midregional proadrenomedullin as a prognostic tool in community-acquired pneumonia. Chest 2009;136:823–31.

45. Torres A, Ramirez P, Montull B, et al. Biomarkers and community-acquired pneumonia: tailoring management with biological data. Semin Respir Crit Care Med 2012;33:266–71.

46. Bouadma L, Luyt CE, Tubach F, et al. Use of procalcitonin to reduce patients' exposure to antibiotics in intensive care units (PRORATA trial): a multicentre randomised controlled trial. Lancet 2010;375:463–74.

47. Schuetz P, Chiappa V, Briel M, et al. Procalcitonin algorithms for antibiotic therapy decisions, a systematic review of randomized controlled trials and recommendations for clinical algorithms. Arch Intern Med 2011;171:1322–31.

48. Schuetz P, Briel M, Christ-Crain M, et al. Procalcitonin to guide initiation and duration of antibiotic treatment in acute respiratory infections: an individual patient data meta-analysis. Clin Infect Dis 2012;55:651–62.

Clinical Scoring Tools
Which Is Best to Predict Clinical Response and Long-Term Outcomes?

Timothy Wiemken, PhD, MPH, CIC*, Robert Kelley, PhD,
Julio Ramirez, MD

KEYWORDS

- Severity scores • Prediction scores • Outcomes • Mortality • Pneumonia
- Site of care

KEY POINTS

- One important aspect of the initial evaluation of a patient with CAP is to assess severity of the disease and to attempt to predict the likely clinical outcomes of the patient.
- This information is used to make important clinical decisions, such as site of care, extent of laboratory work-up, and therapeutic interventions.
- Clinical judgment has been the primary tool to define severity of disease and likely clinical outcomes in hospitalized patients with CAP, but has poor predictive value.
- CAP prediction scores were developed to help physicians define severity of disease and likely clinical outcomes of their patients.

THE NEED FOR PREDICTION SCORES

During the initial management of patients with community-acquired pneumonia (CAP), physicians need to assess severity of the disease and predict the likely clinical outcomes of the patient. This information is used to make important clinical decisions, such as site of care, extent of laboratory work-up, and therapeutic interventions. Clinical judgment is the primary tool to define severity of disease and likely clinical outcomes in hospitalized patients with CAP. However, it has been documented that using clinical judgment as the primary tool has poor predictive value.[1] Because of this, CAP prediction scores were developed to help physicians define severity of disease and likely clinical outcomes of their patients. CAP prediction scores are also important in clinical research. They are used to stratify patients on disease severity or the likelihood of a particular outcome in the design of the study, and to adjust for confounding bias during the analysis phase of the study.

Division of Infectious Diseases, University of Louisville, 501 East Broadway, Suite 120, Louisville, KY 40202, USA
* Corresponding author.
E-mail address: tlwiem01@louisville.edu

Infect Dis Clin N Am 27 (2013) 33–48
http://dx.doi.org/10.1016/j.idc.2012.11.015
0891-5520/13/$ – see front matter © 2013 Elsevier Inc. All rights reserved.

id.theclinics.com

The first prediction score for patients with CAP was the Pneumonia Severity Index (PSI). This prediction score was developed to predict 30-day mortality.[2] Because of the complexity in its calculation, investigators began to develop more simple scores to predict this outcome. Today, there are a multitude of prediction scores for CAP, and most of these scores were developed to predict 30-day mortality. **Table 1** outlines a few selected CAP prediction scores described in this article. Data on the use of these scores to predict clinical outcomes other than 30-day mortality are limited. This article reviews the most relevant clinical outcomes in hospitalized patients with CAP and outlines the role of these scores as tools to help physicians predict outcomes.

CAP CLINICAL OUTCOMES

The clinical outcomes of hospitalized patients with CAP can be classified as (1) outcomes during hospitalization (usually within the first 7 days after hospital admission); (2) outcomes during 30-day follow-up; and (3) outcomes occurring years after hospital discharge (long-term outcomes). **Fig. 1** depicts each outcome in chronologic order.

Outcomes During Hospitalization

Clinical failure

Clinical failure is associated with increased complications, length of hospital stay, and mortality (see **Fig. 1**, point 1).[6,7] These complications also increase the total direct cost of care for hospitalized patients with CAP, adding to strain on the health care system.

Definitions of clinical failure vary significantly from study to study. The simplest definition of failure is the lack of response to therapy associated with clinical deterioration.[6] This early outcome can occur in up to one-quarter of patients with CAP and nearly one-third of patients with severe CAP.[7–12] Although investigators increasingly examine clinical failure as an outcome for hospitalized patients with CAP, few studies have maintained a constant, comprehensive definition. Aliberti and Blasi provide an excellent overview of various failure definitions used in many of these studies.[13] Our group recently reported a comprehensive definition of clinical failure consisting of the following criteria: (1) acute pulmonary deterioration with the need for invasive or noninvasive mechanical ventilation; (2) acute hemodynamic deterioration with the need for aggressive fluid resuscitation (eg, >40 mL/kg colloids or crystalloids), vasopressors, or invasive procedures (eg, pericardial drainage or electrical cardioversion); and (3) in-hospital mortality up to 28 days after hospital admission.[6] It is hoped that this will be used as a basis for a consistently reported definition of clinical failure.

The ability to predict clinical failure in hospitalized patients with CAP is hampered by the lack of consistent definitions. Therefore, little work has been done to predict failure in hospitalized patients with CAP. One study suggested that the PSI and CURB-65 were inferior to SCAP in the prediction of treatment failure, although the areas under the receiver operating characteristic (ROC) curves (AUC) for all of these scores were very low (0.52–0.61).[14] Using data from a subset of 500 patients enrolled in the Community-Acquired Pneumonia Organization (CAPO) international cohort study,[15,16] we used ROC curves to examine the ability of PSI and CRB-65 to accurately predict clinical failure using the definition described previously. **Fig. 2** depicts the results of this analysis. We calculated AUC to be 0.62 and 0.63 ($P = .786$), respectively. These data do not support the use of these scores to accurately predict clinical failure.

Intensive care unit admission

Early identification of hospitalized patients with CAP in need of intensive care is important to improve outcomes and reduce health care costs (see **Fig. 1**, point 2). Improving

Table 1 Selected CAP prediction scores	
Name	**Variables/Points**
Pneumonia Severity Index[2]	If male/age (y)
	If female/age (y) – 10
	Nursing home resident/10
	Neoplastic disease/30
	Liver disease/20
	Congestive heart failure/10
	Cerebrovascular disease/10
	Renal disease/10
	Altered mental status/20
	Heart rate $\geq$125 beats per min/20
	Respiratory rate >30 breaths per min/20
	Systolic blood pressure <90 mm Hg/15
	Temperature <35°C or $\geq$40°C/10
	Arterial pH <7.35/30
	Blood urea nitrogen $\geq$30 mg/dL/20
	Sodium <130 mmol/L/20
	Glucose $\geq$250 mg/dL/10
	Hematocrit <30%/10
	Pao_2 <60 mm Hg/10
	Pleural effusion/10
CURB-65[3]	Confusion/1
	Urea >7 mmol/L/1
	Respiratory rate $\geq$30 breaths per min/1
	Systolic blood pressure <90 mm Hg or diastolic blood pressure $\leq$60 mm Hg/1
	Age $\geq$65/1
CRB-65[3]	Confusion/1
	Respiratory rate/1
	Systolic blood pressure/1
	Age $\geq$65/1
SMART-COP[4]	Systolic blood pressure <90 mm Hg/2
	Multilobar infiltrates/1
	Albumin <2.5 g/dL/1
	Respiratory rate $\geq$25 breaths per min if $\leq$50 y; $\geq$30 breaths per min if >50 y/1
	Heart rate (tachycardia) $\geq$125 beats/min/1
	Confusion/1
	Pao_2 <70 mm Hg, O_2 saturation <93% or Pao_2/Fio_2 <333 if $\leq$50 y; <60 mm Hg, $\leq$90%, <250 if >50 y/2
	Arterial pH <7.35/2
SCAP (severe CAP)[5]	Arterial pH <7.30/2.38
	Systolic blood pressure <90 mm Hg/2.19
	Respiratory rate >30 breaths per min/1.83
	Altered mental status/0.87
	Blood urea nitrogen >30 mg/dL/0.92
	Pao_2 <54 mm Hg or Pao_2/Fio_2 <250 mm Hg/1.12
	Age $\geq$80 y/0.86
	Multilobar infiltrates/0.68

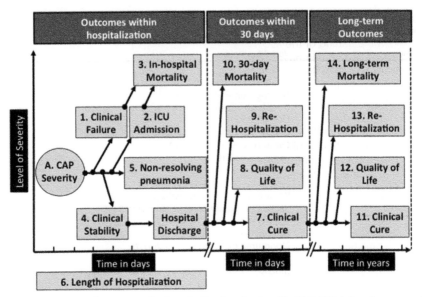

Fig. 1. Chronology of outcomes for hospitalized patients with CAP. ICU, intensive care unit.

outcomes is a necessary goal for all practitioners; however, the reduction in health care costs is only of recent interest.

The "need for intensive care" can be defined directly, in terms of the need for admission or transfer to the intensive care unit (ICU) per physician's orders, or indirectly

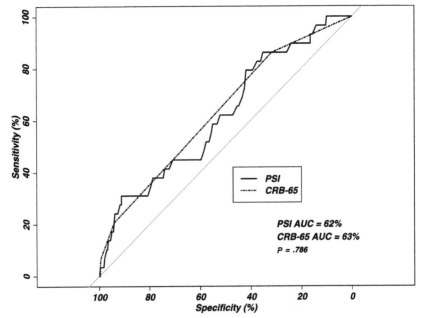

Fig. 2. Diagnostic accuracy of the PSI and the CRB-65 for the prediction of clinical failure in hospitalized patients with CAP. AUC, area under the receiver operating characteristic curve.

through assessing the patient's need for intensive respiratory or vasopressor support.[4] These indirect variables are proxy measures because they are often only provided in the setting of the ICU.

CAP prediction scores have been evaluated or developed to predict the need for intensive care on admission to the hospital. The SMART-COP score developed by Charles and colleagues[4] is the best studied of these scores. In the original study, the investigators found that SMART-COP was very good at predicting the need for ICU admission (AUC, 0.87). This prediction was much better than the next best score evaluated, the PSI, with an AUC of 0.69. Other studies have also shown that SMART-COP is a useful predictor of the need for ICU admission.[17,18] Investigators evaluating scores to predict ICU admission, such as REA-ICU, CURXO-80, PSI, CURB-65, and the 2007 International Diseases Society of America (IDSA)/American Thoracic Society (ATS) minor criteria for predicting ICU admission, have reported widely varied results.[5,17,18] Although many of these scores have relatively high AUCs for the prediction of the need for ICU admission, they often result in very low positive predictive values because of the low prevalence of severe CAP.[19] Although patients in the ICU may obtain the highest level of care, using a score with a low positive predictive value to define if a patient should be admitted to the ICU leads to unnecessary ICU admissions and increased costs of care.

In-hospital mortality

Mortality is arguably the worst possible outcome for patients with CAP (see **Fig. 1**, point 3). The burden on society is also significant with respect to lost productivity and cost. Mortality can be evaluated at any time point, although in-hospital mortality is the first time point of interest for hospitalized patients with CAP. However, in-hospital mortality has not been evaluated as a clinical outcome to a great extent.

In-hospital mortality is simply defined as death during hospitalization. Few investigators separate specific causes of death (eg, related to CAP vs not related to CAP) because of the difficulty in defining the actual cause. Some investigators have examined the predictive accuracy of various scores to predict this outcome. Ewig and colleagues[20] reported an AUC of 0.68 for the CRB-65 prediction of in-hospital mortality. Furthermore, they suggested that varying the age groups of the CRB score could enhance its ability to predict in-hospital mortality.[20] Similarly, Richards and colleagues[21] reported an AUC of 0.65 for CURB-65 and PSI for the prediction of in-hospital mortality. Karmakar and Wilsher[22] reported a dose-response relationship of CURB-65 scores on increasing in-hospital mortality rates (1% for CURB-65 of 0 or 1, 2% for CURB-65 of 2, and 13% for CURB-65 of >2).

The prediction of various outcomes, including in-hospital mortality, may also vary based on the cause of pneumonia. We reported for hospitalized patients with CAP caused by 2009 H1N1 influenza A virus, the PSI, CRB-65, and the CURB-65 were not adequate for predicting in-hospital mortality.[23] Although those scores, which weight advanced age heavily, should intuitively predict mortality at a later date, the prediction of in-hospital death may be more closely linked to acute decompensation rather than advanced age. During the time of the initial wave of the pandemic, we created a score using data from the CAPO international cohort study to assist with the prediction of in-hospital death for our patients with 2009 H1N1 influenza A virus pneumonia: the CROMI score (comorbidity, respiratory rate, oxygen saturation, mental status changes, and infiltrates at chest radiograph) (**Figs. 3** and **4**). This score had an AUC for the prediction of in-hospital mortality of 0.83, whereas the PSI, CURB-65, and CRB-65 had AUCs in the low 0.70s (data not shown).

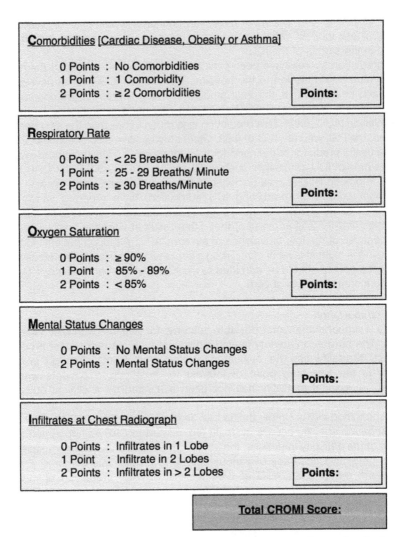

Fig. 3. Outline of the CROMI score for the prediction of in-hospital mortality for hospitalized patients with CAP caused by 2009 H1N1 influenza A virus.

Using data from our multicenter study for lower respiratory tract infections titled Rapid Empiric Treatment with Oseltamivir Study, we recently evaluated the diagnostic accuracy of the PSI and CRB-65 scores for predicting in-hospital mortality for all hospitalized patients with CAP in seven hospitals in the Louisville metropolitan area. As **Fig. 5** depicts, these two scores do not accurately predict in-hospital mortality (AUC, 0.68 vs 0.59, respectively; $P = .197$).

Clinical stability
Clinical stability is one of the most essential outcomes for hospitalized patients with CAP because it can assist in the direction of the management of these patients (see **Fig. 1**, point 4).[13] Use of clinical stability criteria can also assist the physician in the

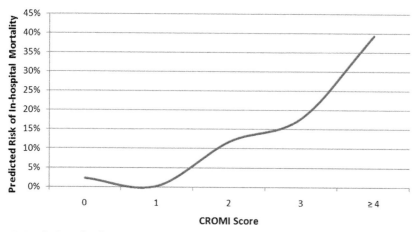

Fig. 4. Prediction of in-hospital mortality due to 2009 H1N1 influenza A virus by the CROMI score.

timely discharge of hospitalized patients with CAP, leading to lower health care resource use and lower costs of care.

Clinical stability is defined as the time at which the patient has improved enough to be switched from intravenous antibiotics to oral antibiotics. This is also known as the number of days to switch therapy, or the time to clinical stability (TCS).[24,25] Understanding what factors may predict TCS can be a critical factor in site-of-care decisions, improving clinical outcomes, and decreasing the overall cost of care.

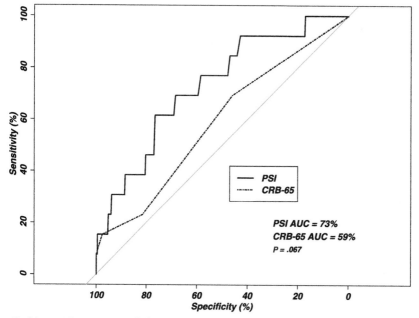

Fig. 5. Diagnostic accuracy of the PSI and the CRB-65 for the prediction of in-hospital mortality in hospitalized patients with CAP.

Two major definitions exist for evaluating when patients have improved enough to be considered clinically stable. These two criteria have been offered as recommendations by the ATS and IDSA in their guidelines for the management of patients with CAP. In 2001, the Ramirez criteria[25] were suggested,[26] and in 2007 the Halm criteria[27] were suggested.[28] These criteria can be found in **Table 2**.

Scores for predicting TCS have not been well defined. Our group previously evaluated the use of the PSI and CRB-65[3] for predicting TCS within the first week of hospitalization using the Ramirez criteria.[29] We found statistically equivalent prediction for the two scores (95% confidence interval for the difference in AUC, -0.03 to 0.01). More importantly, we identified the poor predictive accuracy of both scores with AUC values of 0.64 and 0.65, respectively.[30] Menendez and colleagues[31] reported that severe CAP, as defined by a PSI risk class of 3, 4, or 5, was associated with a longer TCS; however, the predictive accuracy of the score was not calculated. These investigators used the Halm (ATS/IDSA 2007) definition of clinical stability. These are the only studies evaluating a CAP score for the prediction of clinical stability. To add to this body of evidence, we used data from the more than 7000 patients enrolled in the CAPO international cohort study to construct ROC curves. These curves evaluated the accuracy of PSI and CRB-65 for predicting TCS in the first week of hospitalization using the Ramirez criteria and the Halm criteria (**Figs. 6** and **7**, respectively). These data suggest that these two scores are very poor methods for predicting both definitions of clinical stability.

Nonresolving pneumonia

Nonresolving pneumonia is a relevant outcome for the practicing physician (see **Fig. 1**, point 5). Approximately 15% of hospitalized patients with CAP may have nonresolving pneumonia.[32] Nonresolving or nonresponding pneumonia can be defined as patients who do not improve within 1 week to 10 days after initiation of antimicrobial therapy[13,33]; however "resolution" of pneumonia may not be easily defined. This creates difficulties for studying this outcome. Furthermore, a noninfectious cause of nonresolving CAP has been documented to play a role in up to 20% of hospitalized patients with CAP.[12] To date, no investigations have evaluated the accuracy of any score for the prediction of nonresolving pneumonia.

Length of hospitalization

Decreasing the length of hospitalization of patients with CAP is essential for decreasing the overall costs of care (see **Fig. 1**, point 6). Prompt discharge of patients who are able to improve at home may also decrease the risk of other poor outcomes, such as falls or health care–associated infections.

Table 2	
Clinical stability criteria	
Criteria	**Variables**
Ramirez et al,[25] 1995	1. Subjective cough and shortness of air improving 2. Afebrile for at least 8 h 3. White blood cell count returning to normal
Halm et al,[27] 1998	1. Temperature $\leq 38.3°C$ 2. O_2 saturation >90% 3. Respiratory rate ≤ 24 breaths per min 4. Systolic blood pressure ≥ 90 mm Hg 5. Normal mental status

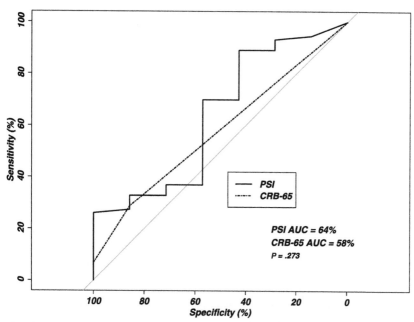

Fig. 6. Diagnostic accuracy of the PSI and the CRB-65 for the prediction of 2001 clinical stability criteria in hospitalized patients with CAP.

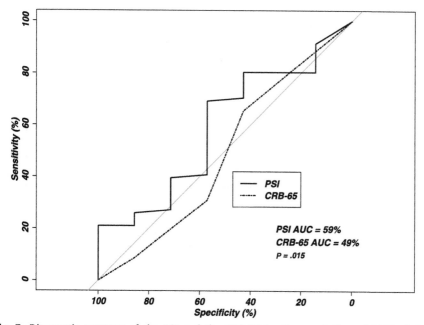

Fig. 7. Diagnostic accuracy of the PSI and the CRB-65 for the prediction of 2007 clinical stability criteria in hospitalized patients with CAP.

Length of hospitalization for patients with CAP is defined as the number of days between hospital admission and discharge. This outcome can be used as a proxy measure for the cost of care, because a reasonable fixed price can be assigned to a patient per day of hospitalization. However, this measure can be biased significantly because of several factors. For example, if a score is to predict how many days a patient will be hospitalized, a significant confounding effect is the number of days the patient is ill before hospitalization. Regardless, limited data have been reported examining the prediction of length of stay using pneumonia severity scores. In 2010, our group presented data suggesting the poor predictive accuracy of PSI (AUC, 0.65) and CRB-65 (AUC, 0.60) for this outcome.[30]

Outcomes During 30-Day Follow-Up

Clinical cure at 30 days

Clinical cure can be defined as complete resolution of signs and symptoms of respiratory infection (see **Fig. 1**, point 7). Resolution of signs and symptoms include the lack of fever; shortness of air; leukocytosis; pulmonary infiltrate; and cough (or return to the level of cough present before the episode of pneumonia in patients with chronic obstructive pulmonary disease). This results in the patient's respiratory function returning to the level present before the development of pneumonia.

In some patients, the primary signs and symptoms of pneumonia may resolve, but organ functions do not return to baseline levels. These patients are clinically cured, but their general well-being is not back to baseline. In this regard, evaluation of "quality of life" after an episode of pneumonia may be a more relevant outcome that "clinical cure" after pneumonia.

The ultimate goal of pneumonia therapy is not only to cure the pneumonia but also to restore quality of life to the level present before the pulmonary infection. Regardless, no data are available for the accuracy of CAP scores to predict clinical cure at 30 days postdischarge.

Quality of life at 30 days

Quality of life, as previously described, is arguably the most important outcome for hospitalized patients with CAP because the goal of quality medical care should be to cure the patient and improve the patient's overall quality of life (see **Fig. 1**, point 8). Quality of life for patients with CAP is defined using standardized instruments, such as the Short Form-36.[34] These measures can include absence of pain, ability to perform daily tasks, and various measures of physical abilities. However, little work has focused on the ability to predict the patient's quality of life at 30 days based on their disease severity on admission. One study reported that patients with pneumonia had significantly worse quality of life (as measured by the Short Form-36) compared with an age- and gender-matched nonpneumonia cohort shortly after hospitalization; however, differences based on initial disease severity were not thoroughly analyzed.[35] Our group is currently collecting data on 30-day quality of life measures for hospitalized patients with CAP as part of a multicenter, randomized, clinical trial entitled Rapid Empiric Treatment with Oseltamivir Study. These data will be used to examine the accuracy of various severity scores to predict quality of life as they become available.

Rehospitalization at 30 days

Rehospitalization has recently become a significant clinical outcome, particularly because of the risk of limited reimbursement from insurance agencies (see **Fig. 1**, point 9). In 2005, it was shown that the cost of preventable rehospitalizations was approximately $12 billion for Medicare beneficiaries.[36] Because of the extreme costs of preventable rehospitalizations, this outcome will be a focus of health care for years to come.

Approximately 20% of patients with CAP are rehospitalized within 30 days, with 30% of these patients reporting pneumonia to be the reason for readmission.[37] These data emphasize the need to be able to predict which patients may be at risk for preventable rehospitalization so they can be evaluated before discharge. However, no studies have evaluated the accuracy of CAP scoring tools to predict readmission at 30-days. To help fill this gap, we analyzed data from the CAPO international cohort study. As depicted in **Fig. 8**, it is clear that neither the PSI (AUC, 0.56) nor the CRB-65 (AUC, 0.49) is able to help assess the need for rehospitalization.

Thirty-day mortality

As outlined for in-hospital mortality, 30-day mortality is a critical outcome for hospital-ized patients with CAP (see **Fig. 1**, point 10). This outcome is also used as a quality measure for the Centers for Medicare and Medicaid Services in the United States.

In terms of outcome prediction, 30-day mortality is the outcome for which most of the CAP scores (severity scores) were developed. However, it is clear that up to 50% of CAP deaths are unrelated to the initial severity of disease.[38,39] These data question the use of predicting 30-day mortality in hospitalized patients with CAP. Regardless, numerous authors have published data on the use of nearly every pneumonia severity score to predict this outcome. Recently, Chalmers and colleagues[40] reported data on a meta-analysis of CAP scores to predict 30-day mortality. **Table 3** depicts the wide range of AUCs calculated for many different prediction scores. These data vary signif-icantly and suggest that a maximum AUC of 0.89 for all severity scores falls below the established cutoff of 90% for an excellent discriminatory test. Some authors have rec-ommended recalibrating these scores to account for differences in various

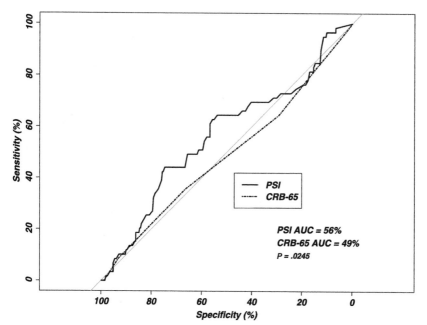

Fig. 8. Diagnostic accuracy of the PSI and the CRB-65 for the prediction of 30-day rehospi-talization in hospitalized patients with CAP.

Table 3
Predictive accuracy of five pneumonia severity scores for 30-day mortality

Severity Score	AUC Range
PSI	0.70–0.89
CURB-65	0.73–0.87
CRB-65	0.69–0.74
ATS 2001, sensitivity/specificity	41%–94%/71%–93%
IDSA/ATS 2007, sensitivity/specificity	45%–81%/75%–83%

Data from Chalmers JD, Mandal P, Singanayagam A, et al. Severity assessment tools to guide ICU admission in community-acquired pneumonia: systematic review and meta-analysis. Intensive Care Med 2011;37(9):1409–20.

populations under study.[41] Recalibration may change the AUCs for many of the published studies, although the methods and use of recalibration of severity scores in the clinical setting (eg, outside of research) are not well defined.

Clinical cure at 1 year or 5 years

No data are available defining the accuracy of CAP scores to predict this outcome (see **Fig. 1**, point 11). Nonetheless, the quality of the patient's life becomes increasingly important. For example, underlying comorbidities may be accelerated because of the pneumonia even if the patient is cured. This may lead to a decrease in quality of life for years after the initial episode of pneumonia, regardless of the timing of clinical cure.

Long-Term Outcomes

Quality of life at 1 or 5 years

Similar to the quality of life at 30 days, no studies have evaluated the long-term quality of life prediction of various CAP scores (see **Fig. 1**, point 12). However, some data are available to suggest that severe disease has long-term consequences for quality of life.[42] As part of the RETO study, our group is actively collecting data on the long-term quality of life of hospitalized patients with CAP and plan to report the prediction of various severity scores on this outcome.

Rehospitalization at 1 or 5 years

Data have not been reported regarding the accuracy of CAP scores to predict the need for long-term rehospitalization (see **Fig. 1**, point 13). We are collecting rehospitalization data for 6 months and 1-year postdischarge in the RETO study and will report these data as they become available.

Mortality at 1 or 5 years

Pneumonia may now be considered a chronic disease because of the long-term impact on patient survival (see **Fig. 1**, point 14).[43] However, there are still very few studies closely examining this long-term impact.[39,43–46] Understanding host/environment/pathogen factors that contribute to long-term impact is critical to ensure good patient outcomes. Moreover, predicting which patients with CAP will be more impacted in the long-term is a crucial factor for novel treatment modalities. We were not able to find data evaluating the accuracy of any available CAP score for predicting long-term mortality. As part of the RETO study, we evaluated the accuracy of the PSI and CRB-65 scores for predicting 1-year mortality (**Fig. 9**). These data suggest that the PSI and CRB-65 are not adequate for predicting 1-year mortality in hospitalized patients with CAP (AUC, 0.73 vs 0.66, respectively; $P = .083$).

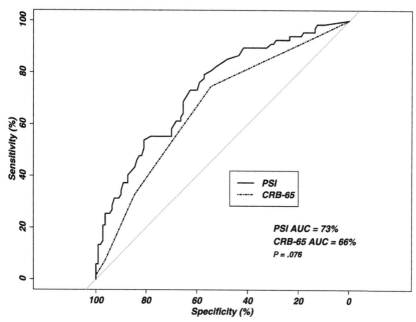

Fig. 9. Diagnostic accuracy of the PSI and the CRB-65 for the prediction of 1-year mortality in hospitalized patients with CAP.

SUMMARY

This article identifies the most critical clinical outcomes for hospitalized patients with CAP, and assesses the merits of various CAP scores for the prediction of each outcome. In regards to the best scoring tool to predict clinical response and long-term outcomes, PSI is probably more accurate score to predict a wide range of clinical outcomes. Considering the complexity of the PSI calculation and the sensitivity and specificity for any particular outcome, a great need exists for simple and more accurate scoring tools.

Currently available scores have focused on past medical history, signs and symptoms of pneumonia, and basic laboratory work-up. It is unlikely that further combinations of these variables will significantly increase the accuracy of any score. Improving these scores requires at least two areas of research. First, investigators need to incorporate biomarkers, such as proadrenumedullin, C-reactive protein, brain natriuretic peptide, and procalcitonin, which have shown promise for predicting various outcomes and enhancing currently available scoring tools.[47–49] A second area of research should focus on the identification of new biomarkers associated with early and late outcomes.

For the management of hospitalized patients with CAP, early outcomes are often considered the most important outcomes. There are currently very few accurate, validated scores to assist physicians in the prediction of any clinical outcomes.

REFERENCES

1. Fine MJ, Hough LJ, Medsger AR, et al. The hospital admission decision for patients with community-acquired pneumonia. Results from the pneumonia patient outcomes research team cohort study. Arch Intern Med 1997;157(1):36–44.

2. Fine MJ, Auble TE, Yealy DM, et al. A prediction rule to identify low-risk patients with community-acquired pneumonia. N Engl J Med 1997;336(4):243–50.

3. Lim WS, van der Eerden MM, Laing R, et al. Defining community acquired pneumonia severity on presentation to hospital: an international derivation and validation study. Thorax 2003;58(5):377–82.

4. Charles PG, Wolfe R, Whitby M, et al. SMART-COP: a tool for predicting the need for intensive respiratory or vasopressor support in community-acquired pneumonia. Clin Infect Dis 2008;47(3):375–84.

5. Espana PP, Capelastegui A, Gorordo I, et al. Development and validation of a clinical prediction rule for severe community-acquired pneumonia. Am J Respir Crit Care Med 2006;174(11):1249–56.

6. Aliberti S, Amir A, Peyrani P, et al. Incidence, etiology, timing, and risk factors for clinical failure in hospitalized patients with community-acquired pneumonia. Chest 2008;134(5):955–62.

7. Hoogewerf M, Oosterheert JJ, Hak E, et al. Prognostic factors for early clinical failure in patients with severe community-acquired pneumonia. Clin Microbiol Infect 2006;12(11):1097–104.

8. Roson B, Carratala J, Fernandez-Sabe N, et al. Causes and factors associated with early failure in hospitalized patients with community-acquired pneumonia. Arch Intern Med 2004;164(5):502–8.

9. Menendez R, Torres A, Zalacain R, et al. Risk factors of treatment failure in community acquired pneumonia: implications for disease outcome. Thorax 2004;59(11):960–5.

10. Genne D, Sommer R, Kaiser L, et al. Analysis of factors that contribute to treatment failure in patients with community-acquired pneumonia. Eur J Clin Microbiol Infect Dis 2006;25(3):159–66.

11. Genne D, Kaiser L, Kinge TN, et al. Community-acquired pneumonia: causes of treatment failure in patients enrolled in clinical trials. Clin Microbiol Infect 2003; 9(9):949–54.

12. Arancibia F, Ewig S, Martinez JA, et al. Antimicrobial treatment failures in patients with community-acquired pneumonia: causes and prognostic implications. Am J Respir Crit Care Med 2000;162(1):154–60.

13. Aliberti S, Blasi F. Clinical stability versus clinical failure in patients with community-acquired pneumonia. Semin Respir Crit Care Med 2012;33(3): 284–91.

14. Yandiola PP, Capelastegui A, Quintana J, et al. Prospective comparison of severity scores for predicting clinically relevant outcomes for patients hospitalized with community-acquired pneumonia. Chest 2009;135(6):1572–9.

15. Ramirez JA. Fostering international multicenter collaborative research: the CAPO Project. Int J Tuberc Lung Dis 2007;11(10):1062–5.

16. Ramirez JA. Worldwide perspective of the quality of care provided to hospitalized patients with community-acquired pneumonia: results from the CAPO international cohort study. Semin Respir Crit Care Med 2005;26(6):543–52.

17. Fukuyama H, Ishida T, Tachibana H, et al. Validation of scoring systems for predicting severe community-acquired pneumonia. Intern Med 2011;50(18): 1917–22.

18. Labarere J, Schuetz P, Renaud B, et al. Validation of a clinical prediction model for early admission to the intensive care unit of patients with pneumonia. Acad Emerg Med 2012;19(9):993–1003 [in Spanish].

19. Marti C, Garin N, Grosgurin O, et al. Prediction of severe community acquired pneumonia: a systematic review and meta-analysis. Crit Care 2012;16(4):R141.

20. Ewig S, Bauer T, Richter K, et al. Prediction of in-hospital death from community-acquired pneumonia by varying CRB-age groups. Eur Respir J 2012. [Epub ahead of print].
21. Richards G, Levy H, Laterre PF, et al. CURB-65, PSI, and APACHE II to assess mortality risk in patients with severe sepsis and community acquired pneumonia in PROWESS. J Intensive Care Med 2011;26(1):34–40.
22. Karmakar G, Wilsher M. Use of the 'CURB 65' score in hospital practice. Intern Med J 2010;40(12):828–32.
23. Riquelme R, Jimenez P, Videla AJ, et al. Predicting mortality in hospitalized patients with 2009 H1N1 influenza pneumonia. Int J Tuberc Lung Dis 2011;15(4):542–6.
24. Ahkee S, Smith S, Newman D, et al. Early switch from intravenous to oral antibiotics in hospitalized patients with infections: a 6-month prospective study. Pharmacotherapy 1997;17(3):569–75.
25. Ramirez JA, Srinath L, Ahkee S, et al. Early switch from intravenous to oral cephalosporins in the treatment of hospitalized patients with community-acquired pneumonia. Arch Intern Med 1995;155(12):1273–6.
26. Niederman MS, Mandell LA, Anzueto A, et al. Guidelines for the management of adults with community-acquired pneumonia. Diagnosis, assessment of severity, antimicrobial therapy, and prevention. Am J Respir Crit Care Med 2001;163(7):1730–54.
27. Halm EA, Fine MJ, Marrie TJ, et al. Time to clinical stability in patients hospitalized with community-acquired pneumonia: implications for practice guidelines. JAMA 1998;279(18):1452–7.
28. Mandell LA, Wunderink RG, Anzueto A, et al. Infectious Diseases Society of America/American Thoracic Society consensus guidelines on the management of community-acquired pneumonia in adults. Clin Infect Dis 2007;44(Suppl 2):S27–72.
29. Arnold F, LaJoie A, Marrie T, et al. The pneumonia severity index predicts time to clinical stability in patients with community-acquired pneumonia. Int J Tuberc Lung Dis 2006;10(7):739–43.
30. Arnold FW, Brock GN, Peyrani P, et al. Predictive accuracy of the pneumonia severity index vs CRB-65 for time to clinical stability: results from the Community-Acquired Pneumonia Organization (CAPO) International Cohort Study. Respir Med 2010;104(11):1736–43.
31. Menendez R, Torres A, Rodriguez de Castro F, et al. Reaching stability in community-acquired pneumonia: the effects of the severity of disease, treatment, and the characteristics of patients. Clin Infect Dis 2004;39(12):1783–90.
32. Salomoni G, Aliberti S, Travierso C. Incidence, risk factors and outcomes of non-resolving pneumonia. Presented at the European Respiratory Society Annual Congress. Barcelona, September 18–22, 2010.
33. Kyprianou A, Hall CS, Shah R, et al. The challenge of nonresolving pneumonia. Knowing the norms of radiographic resolution is key. Postgrad Med 2003; 113(1):79–82.
34. Ware JE Jr, Sherbourne CD. The MOS 36-item short-form health survey (SF-36). I. Conceptual framework and item selection. Med Care 1992;30(6):473–83.
35. El Moussaoui R, Opmeer BC, de Borgie CA, et al. Long-term symptom recovery and health-related quality of life in patients with mild-to-moderate-severe community-acquired pneumonia. Chest 2006;130(4):1165–72.
36. Medicare Payment Advisory Commission. A path to bundled payment around a rehospitalization. In: Commission MPA, editor. A report to the congress: reforming the delivery system. Washington, DC: Medicare Payment Advisory Commission; 2005. p. 83–103. Available at: http://www.medpac.gov/documents/Jun08_EntireReport.pdf.

37. Jencks SF, Williams MV, Coleman EA. Rehospitalizations among patients in the Medicare fee-for-service program. N Engl J Med 2009;360(14):1418–28.

38. Mortensen EM, Coley CM, Singer DE, et al. Causes of death for patients with community-acquired pneumonia: results from the Pneumonia Patient Outcomes Research Team cohort study. Arch Intern Med 2002;162(9):1059–64.

39. Mortensen EM, Kapoor WN, Chang CC, et al. Assessment of mortality after long-term follow-up of patients with community-acquired pneumonia. Clin Infect Dis 2003;37(12):1617–24.

40. Chalmers JD, Mandal P, Singanayagam A, et al. Severity assessment tools to guide ICU admission in community-acquired pneumonia: systematic review and meta-analysis. Intensive Care Med 2011;37(9):1409–20.

41. Flanders WD, Tucker G, Krishnadasan A, et al. Validation of the pneumonia severity index. Importance of study-specific recalibration. J Gen Intern Med 1999;14(6):333–40.

42. Lettinga KD, Verbon A, Nieuwkerk PT, et al. Health-related quality of life and post-traumatic stress disorder among survivors of an outbreak of Legionnaires disease. Clin Infect Dis 2002;35(1):11–7.

43. Bordon J, Wiemken T, Peyrani P, et al. Decrease in long-term survival for hospitalized patients with community-acquired pneumonia. Chest 2010;138(2):279–83.

44. Kaplan V, Clermont G, Griffin MF, et al. Pneumonia: still the old man's friend? Arch Intern Med 2003;163(3):317–23.

45. Koivula I, Sten M, Makela PH. Prognosis after community-acquired pneumonia in the elderly: a population-based 12-year follow-up study. Arch Intern Med 1999;159(14):1550–5.

46. Waterer GW, Kessler LA, Wunderink RG. Medium-term survival after hospitalization with community-acquired pneumonia. Am J Respir Crit Care Med 2004;169(8):910–4.

47. Courtais C, Kuster N, Dupuy AM, et al. Proadrenomedullin, a useful tool for risk stratification in high Pneumonia Severity Index score community acquired pneumonia. Am J Emerg Med 2012. http://dx.doi.org/10.1016/j.ajem.2012.07.017.

48. Espana PP, Capelastegui A, Bilbao A, et al. Utility of two biomarkers for directing care among patients with non-severe community-acquired pneumonia. Eur J Clin Microbiol Infect Dis 2012;31(12):3397–405.

49. Kolditz M, Ewig S, Hoffken G. Management-based risk prediction in community-acquired pneumonia by scores and biomarkers. Eur Respir J 2012. [Epub ahead of print].

What Is the Role of Newer Molecular Tests in the Management of CAP?

Charlotte A. Gaydos, MS, MPH, DrPH

KEYWORDS

- Community-acquired pneumonia • Diagnosis • Influenza • Respiratory viruses
- Respiratory bacteria • PCR • Point-of-care tests

KEY POINTS

- The successful management CAP requires rapid and accurate diagnosis of the etiologic agent of CAP.
- Correct diagnosis enhances the appropriate use of antiviral agents and prevents overuse of antibiotics.
- Pathogen-directed therapy requires the use of an assay that is FDA-cleared, is highly accurate, and can be completed in a timely manner.
- New tools are becoming available and include assays that are highly accurate, especially ones that use amplified technology.

INTRODUCTION

Community-acquired pneumonia (CAP) is one of the most important infectious disease problems in the United States today and accounts for major morbidity and mortality.[1] There were approximately 4.5 million ambulatory care visits in 2007 in the United States[1] and an estimated 1.1 million hospitalizations for pneumonia, with an average length of stay of 5 days.[2] CAP accounts for enormous health care costs, with an estimated $17 billion price tag annually in the United States.[3]

Unfortunately, in the past 20 to 25 years, with improved broad-spectrum antibiotics, the implementation of diagnostic studies has declined and most patients do not have an etiologic pathogen of CAP identified.[1,4,5] This has been partially because of the advance of antimicrobial agents to treat CAP, resulting in a lack of the perceived need to know the etiologic pathogen, unless the patient does not respond to empiric therapy.[1] An important consideration of the diagnosis of CAP is the age and immune

Division of Infectious Diseases, Department of Medicine, Johns Hopkins University, 530 Rangos Building, 800 North Wolfe Street, Baltimore, MD 21205, USA
E-mail address: cgaydos@jhmi.edu

Infect Dis Clin N Am 27 (2013) 49–69
http://dx.doi.org/10.1016/j.idc.2012.11.012
0891-5520/13/$ – see front matter © 2013 Elsevier Inc. All rights reserved.

id.theclinics.com

state of the patient. Severe and fatal disease can occur in the elderly, the immunocompromised, the very young, and those individuals with conditions that affect cardiopulmonary function, and these syndromes can be caused by multiple types of organisms, which may be etiologically indistinguishable on presentation.[6] The elderly represent an important factor in rapid diagnosis of CAP especially because this older generation is increasing in the United States. The Centers for Disease Control and Prevention (CDC) statistics indicate that, although pneumonia rates have been decreasing, hospitalization for the age group older than 85 years still represents the most vulnerable population (**Fig. 1**).[7] From 2000 to 2010, the hospitalization rate for pneumonia per 100,000 population decreased by 20% for the total population. The rate decreased 30% among those aged 65 to 74 years, 31% among those aged 75 to 84 years, and 33% among those aged 85 years and older. However, throughout the period, the rate of hospitalization for 85 years and older was the highest, whereas the younger than 65 years age group was substantially lower than the rate for any other age group. Thus, accurate and rapid diagnosis of CAP is important for appropriate patient management, especially in the elderly.

The diagnosis of the etiologic agent of CAP depends on the use of rapid assays. Sensitive, specific, and rapid identification of viruses and bacteria that cause CAP

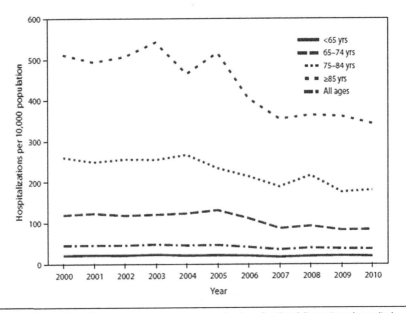

Per 10,000 population. Hospitalization for pneumonia is defined as a first-listed diagnosis on the medical record of 480-486, as coded according to the International Classification of Diseases, Ninth Revision, Clinical Modification. Rates were calculated using U.S. Census Bureau 2000-based postcensal civilian population estimates. Source: National Hospital Discharge Survey, 2000–2010. Available at http://www.cdc.gov/nchs/nhds.htm.

From 2000 to 2010, the hospitalization rate for pneumonia decreased by 20% for the total population. The rate decreased 30% among those aged 65–74 years, 31% among those aged 75–84 years, and 33% among those aged ≥85 years. Throughout the period, the rate of hospitalization for the <65 years age group was substantially lower than the rate for any other age group.

Fig. 1. Rate* of hospitalization for pneumonia, by age group. National hospital discharge survey, United States, 2000–2010. * - Rate per 10,000 population.

can enhance the appropriate use of antiviral agents and prevent overuse of antibiotics. Thus, being able to diagnose respiratory viruses and bacterial pathogens is an integral part of patient management today in the era of cost containment and antibiotic-sparing paradigms for CAP and other respiratory infections that are not of a bacterial origin. Several new molecular platforms exist today for identification of respiratory viruses, and some new broad-based platforms are on the horizon for the diagnosis of viruses, bacteria, and fungi.[8,9] Although accurate diagnosis is highly desirable, perhaps more important is the rapid diagnosis of an etiologic agent of CAP, which can affect immediate patient management. Such rapid identification of a viral agent can prevent the use of unnecessary antibiotics; reduce costs; facilitate timely, effective use of antiviral drugs for viral etiologies, such as influenza; and ultimately may shorten hospital stays.

Because a variety of viruses and bacteria can be responsible for CAP, having a platform that can accurately identify multiple agents is ideal. Additionally, having a single point-of-care (POC) molecular assay that can rapidly rule in or rule out the most common agents, such as influenza or *Streptococcus pneumoniae*, is also desirable for the immediate management of CAP.

The Diagnostic Problem

The real question for optimal and rapid patient care, however, is whether the etiologic agent of CAP is bacterial or viral, and if it is bacterial, whether it is gram-positive or gram-negative. Answers in real time can direct agent-specific therapy and avoid overuse of precious broad-spectrum antibiotics. Polymerase chain reaction (PCR) and molecular tests, which have been developed for the past 20 years and have been coexisting with routine microbiology culture, have not been widely adopted, contributing little to rapid decision making for patient care, especially for bacteria, because many of them are laboratory-developed tests (LDTs), which are not Food and Drug Administration (FDA) cleared or commercially available. Urinary pathogen nonmolecular FDA-cleared diagnostic assays for *S pneumonia* and *Legionella* are an exception, because their results are rapidly available.[10,11]

With single-pathogen molecular tests, each test requires the suspicion of a particular pathogen, but with the development of multiple-pathogen molecular assays, particularly for viruses, the tools to advance pathogen-directed therapy may now exist.[12] This article focuses on recently developed molecular multiplex diagnostic assays and platforms, many of which are FDA-cleared, and how their use can enhance and improve the management of CAP. It provides an overview of the FDA-cleared rapid nonmolecular tests compared with the new rapid molecular tests for the diagnosis of influenza, other respiratory viruses, and bacteria, with less emphasis on those molecular tests that are not FDA-cleared, because they offer clinicians less acute medical management tools, except in research studies. Many of these FDA-cleared and noncleared assays have also been recently reviewed in great detail elsewhere.[6,12–14]

Requirements of Molecular Assays that can Affect Patient Care

Advances in molecular diagnostic methods, which can improve management of CAP, dictate that the result be (1) rapid, (2) accurate, and (3) have the capability to detect multiple pathogens in one assay or a minimum of assays. Rapid POC assays are especially attractive and almost imperative because Infectious Diseases Society of America/American Thoracic Society guidelines recommend that it is very important that therapy for hospitalized patients be as soon as possible and that the first antibiotic dose be given in the emergency department (ED).[15,16] These guidelines drive how rapidly a molecular test can be performed and returned to the clinician in the ED.

Even if a molecular test is not available in time for initial therapy, a definitive diagnosis of an etiologic agent by a molecular test can promote quickly switching to pathogen-directed antibiotic or antiviral therapy, while cultures still may not be completed.

Accuracy is imperative because this is required before FDA clearance can be achieved.[17] FDA-cleared assays have a great advantage over LDTs because they have undergone extensive clinical and analytical validations, their performance characteristics are well documented, and the reagents are standardized. Their use engenders confidence in the quality assurance and accuracy of results.[18]

The ability to detect multiple pathogens simultaneously in one assay should have a major impact on management of CAP because the menu of etiologic agents has grown with newly recognized organisms and newly emerging agents, such as severe acute respiratory syndrome, human metapneumonvirus (hMPV), *Bordetella pertussis*, and new variants of influenza. Even the combination of several rapid tests can have a major impact on the type of therapy instituted (narrow agent-directed antibiotic therapy, such as for *S pneumoniae*, in the case of a positive urinary antigen test, or antiviral therapy for the influenza virus as diagnosed by a POC rapid test).

Consideration of the Diagnostic Test

Historically, in addition to the traditional Gram stain and bacterial culture of sputum or nasopharyngeal swabs for the diagnosis of CAP, there are nonmolecular and molecular assays. Before the molecular assays, there was the development of several rapid nonmolecular methods called rapid antigen direct tests (RADTs) for the detection of influenza. Additionally, the nonmolecular assay, the direct fluorescent antibody (DFA) test using monoclonal antibodies on direct patient viral transport culture sediments, has been used for rapid identification of influenza and other viruses and is still popular. The molecular tests for influenza and viruses are used the most and are FDA-cleared and have been the subject of the most advancement in diagnoses, with the exception of several newer ones for *Mycobacterium tuberculosis*,[19,20] including the recently FDA-cleared FilmArray (Idaho Technology, Salt Lake City, UT) for *Mycoplasma pneumoniae*, *Chlamydia pneumoniae*, and *B pertussis*.[21] There are many non-FDA cleared assays (LDTs), but their use has been mostly limited to research studies.[22,23] For actual use for the management of CAP, nonmolecular and molecular FDA-cleared assays are the ones most valuable for patient care.

DIAGNOSTIC TESTS FOR VIRAL INFECTIONS
Nonmolecular, Nonamplified FDA-cleared Diagnostic POC Tests for Viral Respiratory Infections

RADTs for influenza are FDA-cleared. RADTs have highly variable sensitivities (10%–75%) and specificities (50%–100%) depending on the viral target, age of the patient, sample collection, and duration of symptoms before testing. In general, RADTs perform better when testing pediatric samples, because children shed higher titers of virus and for longer time periods than adults. RADTs also perform better during periods of high prevalence (influenza seasons). They did not perform well for the detection of pandemic swine H1N1 viruses.[14,24–26] Chartrand and colleagues[14] recently provided an excellent meta-analysis their performance from 159 studies and reported a pooled sensitivity of 62.3% and a specificity of 98.2%. Performance was better for influenza A (64.6%) than influenza B (52.2%). There are 14 FDA-cleared RADTs available commercially, of which five are Clinical Laboratory Improvement Amendments (CLIA) waived; two of these can detect and distinguish between influenza A and B.[26] Development of more CLIA-waived assays with increased accuracy and better ability to accurately differentiate influenza types and subtypes will improve use and clinical management decisions in CAP.[26,27]

Direct fluorescent antibody

Rapid DFA testing of centrifuged sediments nasopharyngeal swabs of viral transport media can readily detect seven of the common respiratory viruses (adenovirus; influenza A and B; parainfluenza virus [PIV] 1, 2, and 3; and respiratory syncytial virus [RSV]). In addition, DFA testing can detect hMPV. The specificity of DFA testing is high, but the sensitivities can vary from a low of 50% to 80% when compared with nucleic acid amplification tests (NAATs). Because DFA testing can be performed in as little as 30 to 60 minutes, its use is ideal for POC tests if the laboratory is located near the clinic ordering the test, but a skilled microscopist is required and thus use is limited to performance in a clinical laboratory. Although the seven viruses are responsible for a large number of respiratory tract infections, other viruses are also important causes of respiratory disease. These include bocavirus, selected coronaviruses (229E, OC43, NL63, and HKU-1), PIV 4, and rhinovirus. They are only detected using PCR or NAATs.[25]

Types of DFA The Diagnostic Hybrid method (Diagnostic Hybrids, Athens, OH) consists of staining a cell pellet from a respiratory sample, such as a nasopharyngeal swab sample, in liquid transport media after centrifugation with a monoclonal antibody mixture, which is a pool of antibodies for seven viruses (influenza A and B, RSV, PIV 1 to 3, and adenovirus). Another cell spot is stained with a monoclonal for hMPV. If the pool stains positive by fluorescent microscopy, the cell pellet is stained individually with each monoclonal to determine which virus is staining in the pool. This is a very efficient, rapid ($\sim$2–4 hours), and cost-effective method to screen respiratory samples because about 90% are negative. The disadvantage is that a fluorescent microscope and a skilled microscopist are required. Sensitivity is approximately 80% to 85% and specificity is excellent in a skilled laboratory. An advantage is that all the negative samples can be screened in one pool with a single microscopic visual screen with the pool reagent. It is difficult to use as a POC test unless the laboratory is in very close proximity to the ED or clinic.

There is a liquid DFA test available called Fastpoint (Quidel, Athens, OH). It uses three monoclonal antibodies cocktails to detect eight viruses. This method requires reading three cell spots with two filters each for each sample. This takes longer than screening one pool. A disadvantage is that the PIV are not distinguished from each other. All PIV (1–3) are labeled with phycoerythrin.

FDA-Cleared Molecular Diagnostic Tests for Viral Respiratory Infections

Non-POC FDA-cleared molecular assays

Multiplex PCR assays There are five FDA-cleared multiplex real-time reverse transcriptase (RT) PCR assays (Gen-probe; Prodesse, Madison, WI) for the qualitative detection and identification of the respiratory viruses, influenza, hMPV, PIV, and adenoviruses (**Table 1**). These assays are intended for use in only CLIA high-complexity laboratories.

1. The ProFlu+ assay targets the matrix gene for influenza A, nonstructural genes NS-1 and NS-2 for influenza B, and the polymerase gene for RSV A and RSV B.
2. The ProFAST+ assay subtypes influenza A samples as H1N1-p, H1N1-s, or H3N2. It is a qualitative multiplex real-time RT-PCR assay that targets the nucleoprotein gene of 2009 influenza A H1N1, the specific hemagglutinin genes of seasonal influenza A/H1 and seasonal influenza A/H3, and an internal control (MS2 phage).

Table 1
Food and Drug Administration cleared molecular assays for the detection of respiratory viruses

Manufacturer and Test Name	Time	Test Method	Instrument	Specimen Type	Virus Target
Gen-Probe/Prodesse ProFlu+	3–3.5 h	Real-time RT-PCR	Cepheid SmartCycler	Nasopharyngeal swab in VTM	RSV, influenza A, influenza B
Gen-Probe/Prodesse Pro hMPV	4.5–5.5 h	Real-time RT- PCR	Cepheid SmartCycler	Nasopharyngeal swab in VTM	hMPV
Gen-Probe/Prodesse ProParaFlu+ and Adenovirus+	4.5–5.5 h	Real-time RT-PCR	Cepheid SmartCycler	Nasopharyngeal swab in VTM	PIV 1–3 Adenovirus A-F
Luminex xTAG Respiratory Virus Panel	8–10 h	RT-PCR, TSPE, bead hybridization	Luminex xMap 100/200	Nasopharyngeal swab in VTM	Influenza A, influenza B, hMPV, RSV, PIV 1–3, adenovirus, rhinovirus
Nanosphere Verigene	3–3.5 h	RT-PCR, gold nanoparticle hybridization	Verigene Processor, Verigene Reader	Nasopharyngeal swab in VTM	Influenza A, influenza B, RSV
FilmArray Idaho Technology	1 h	Nested PCR, melt curve analysis	FilmArray Instrument	Nasopharyngeal swab in VTM	Adenoviruses, bocaviruses, coronaviruses, influenza A/B, A subtypes, hMPV, PIV 1–4, RSV, rhinoviruses

Abbreviations: hMPV, human metapneumovirus; PIV 1–3, parainfluenza virus types 1, 2, and 3; RSV, respiratory syncytial virus; RT-PCR, reverse-transcription polymerase chain reaction; VTM, viral transport medium.

3. The Pro hMPV+ assay targets highly conserved regions of the nucleocapsid (N) gene for hMPV and a transcript derived from *Escherichia coli* bacteriophage MS2 A-protein gene (internal control).
4. The ProParaflu+ assay targets conserved regions of the hemagglutinin-neuraminidase gene for PIV 1 to 3 and a transcript derived from *E coli* bacteriophage MS2 A-protein gene (internal control).
5. ProAdeno+ assay targets the hexon gene and detects adenovirus subtypes A to F.

All five assays are approved for testing nasopharyngeal swab specimens obtained from symptomatic persons. Nucleic acids are extracted using a MagNA Pure LC Instrument (Roche Diagnostics, Indianapolis, Indiana) and the MagNA Pure Total Nucleic Acid Isolation Kit (Roche) or a NucliSENS easyMAG System and the Automated Magnetic Extraction Reagents (bioMérieux, Marcy, France). The purified nucleic acids are amplified by means of RT-PCR using target-specific oligonucleotide primers and Taqman probes complementary to highly conserved regions of the target gene. During each PCR cycle, the fluorescent intensity is monitored by the real-time instrument, the SmartCycler II (Cepheid, Sunnyvale CA).

The time to results, including extraction, is 3 to 3.5 hours for each test run. ProFlu+ sensitivities and specificities for the detection of influenza A were 100% and 92.6%, respectively; for influenza B they were 97.8% and 98.6%, respectively; and for RSV they were 89.5% and 94.9%, respectively.[25] In pediatric nasopharyngeal samples, results were 97% to 100% for ProFlu-1 and it detected respiratory viruses in 9% of specimens that were negative by conventional methods.[28] It has been compared with the FilmArray Respiratory Panel.[21]

The Pro hMPV+ assay was shown to be 94.1% sensitive and 99.3% specific compared with xTAG (Luminex Molecular Diagnostics, Austin, TX) respiratory virus panel (RVP) assay.[25] The Pro hMPV+ assay sensitivities were demonstrated to range from 88.9%, 96.3%, and 97.3% for PIV 1, PIV 2, and PIV 3, respectively, during clinical trials and the specificities were all higher than 99%.[25]

xTAG RVP The xTAG RVP was the first multiplex NAAT to receive clearance by the FDA, in January 2009. The original FDA-approved version of RVP detected adenovirus, influenza A (with subtyping of seasonal influenza A/H1 and seasonal influenza A/H3), influenza B, PIV 1 to 3, hMPV, rhinovirus, RSV A and B, and was approved for use with nasopharyngeal swabs from symptomatic persons.[29,30]

Currently, the RVP is an FDA-approved, multiplexed RT-PCR assay manufactured by Luminex (Toronto, Canada) for the detection of 12 viral targets in a single specimen: influenza A; influenza A, subtype H1; influenza A, subtype H3; influenza B; RSV A and B; PIV 1 to 3; hMPV; rhinovirus; and adenovirus. It is FDA-cleared for nasopharyngeal swabs, nasal washes, or bronchoalveolar lavage samples. It requires roughly 8 to 10 hours processing and running the assay. There is a second-generation assay called RVP FAST (Luminex) only available in Europe (not FDA-cleared in the United States) that reduces the number of steps and the time to results by 3 to 4 hours. This assay is intended for use in only CLIA high-complexity laboratories. It has been shown to be highly sensitive and specific for respiratory viruses.[31] It has been compared with the FilmArray respiratory panel.[32]

Respiratory virus plus, Verigene Respiratory Virus Nucleic Acid Test The first-generation Verigene Respiratory Virus Nucleic Acid Test (Nanosphere, Northbrook, IL) was cleared by the FDA in May 2009. This test was replaced by the automated Verigene Respiratory Virus Nucleic Acid Test$_{SP}$, a CLIA moderately complex test microarray-based sample-to-result that is FDA-cleared for the identification of influenza A, influenza

B (types A, Flu An H1, Flu A-2009 H1N1 Flu A-H3, and B inclusive) and RSV (A and B) from nasopharyngeal swab specimens placed in viral transport media. The Verigene System consists of two instruments (the fully automated Verigene Processor and the Verigene Reader) and single-use test cartridges, random access work flow. The entire test process only requires one user pipetting step, less than 5 minutes of technical hands-on time, and a sample-to-result turnaround time of about 2.5 hours. Test sensitivities and specificities for the detection of influenza A were 100% and 99.8%, respectively; for influenza B they were 100% and 99.1%, respectively; and for RSV they were 95.7% and 98.2%, respectively. This assay is CLIA moderate complexity, and a trained laboratory technician must perform the test. It is adequate for small- to medium-sized laboratories. Limitations of the assay include the single-test format that requires a dedicated processor for each sample for 3 to 3.5 hours.[33] The H275Y mutation for oseltamivir resistance panel is only available outside the United States.

Amplified molecular diagnostic POC tests for viral respiratory infections
The ideal influenza POC diagnostic would of necessity combine the sensitivity and specificity of RT-PCR (which are very high complexity, require experienced and highly skilled staff, and are batched, lowering clinical use) with the rapidity and simplicity of the rapid antigen test.

There are only two FDA-cleared amplified molecular assays that can be considered true POC, in that they each require approximately 1 hour to perform and thus could potentially be used for initial patient management decisions in concert with other diagnostic tests. Although FilmArray can test for 15 viruses and several bacterial pathogens, the GeneXpert System only detects influenza virus.

FilmArray technology The FilmArray system combines nucleic acid extraction, nested PCR detection, and data analysis in a single-use pouch. The automated system enables the detection of numerous viral and bacterial respiratory pathogens in a single test. The required reagents for the assay are enclosed in the single-use pouch. Water is added to hydrate the lyophilized reagents and the respiratory specimen is added. The pouch is loaded into the FilmArray instrument, and the remainder of the test is completely automated. After extraction of nucleic acid, a nested PCR reaction is performed within the pouch in an entirely closed system. The first-step PCR is a multiplexed reaction containing primers for all of the viral and bacterial targets; the amplicons from the first PCR are then diluted, and a second round of PCR reactions is performed in a multiwell array, each well containing a single primer set targeting a specific pathogen. Both amplification and melt curve analysis allow the FilmArray software to generate a result for each target.[34] The system is very robust, detecting a low concentration of pathogen in the presence of a high concentration of a second pathogen, with results available in 1 hour. The respiratory panel detects 15 respiratory viruses and B pertussis, C pneumoniae, and M pneumoniae. Originally only the viral panel was FDA-cleared, but the bacterial targets were cleared in the summer of 2012.

Several evaluations of the FilmArray platform for viral pathogens have been published. The FDA-cleared version includes the following targets: adenovirus; coronaviruses HKU1 and NL63; hMPV; influenza A virus (to type level only); influenza An H1 seasonal virus; influenza An H3 seasonal virus; influenza A virus H1-2009; influenza B virus; PIV 1 to 4; RSV; and rhinovirus/enterovirus (no differentiation).

Loeffelholtz and colleagues[21] compared the assay with Prodesse ProFlu+, Pro-FAST+, ProParaflu+, Pro hMPV+, and ProAdeno+ real-time PCR assays on 192 nasopharyngeal-secretion specimens collected from 81 children younger than 1 year of age with upper respiratory tract symptoms. FilmArray and Prodesse assays showed good overall agreement (181 [94.3%] of 192; kappa = 0.87; 95% confidence interval [CI], 0.79–0.94). FilmArray RP detected more PIV 1 and 3 than ProParaflu+ (18 vs 13), whereas ProAdeno+ detected more adenoviruses (11 vs 6), but these differences were not statistically significant. FilmArray and Prodesse assays showed good overall agreement (181 [94.3%] of 192; kappa = 0.87; 95% CI, 0.79–0.94). FilmArray RP detected more PIV 1 and 3 than ProParaflu+ (18 vs 13), whereas ProAdeno+ detected more adenoviruses (11 vs 6), but these differences were not statistically significant. Additionally, FilmArray RP detected 138 pathogens (confirmed as true-positives) not included in the Prodesse assays (rhinovirus/enterovirus, 118; bocavirus, 8; coronavirus, 7; PIV 4; *M pneumoniae*, 1).

When compared with laboratory-developed real-time PCR assays for the detection of various respiratory viruses and certain bacterial pathogens on a total of 215 frozen archived pediatric respiratory specimens previously characterized as either negative or positive for one or more pathogens by real-time PCR examined using the FilmArray RP system, the overall agreement between the FilmArray RP and corresponding real-time PCR assays for shared analytes was 98.6% (kappa = 0.92; 95% CI, 0.89–0.94).[35]

Rand and colleagues[32] compared FilmArray RP and the xTAG RVP multiplex respiratory virus PCR methods for the detection of respiratory viruses in a set of 200 patient specimens frozen at −70°C after standard viral culture and antigen detection methods had been performed. Both systems detected between 40% and 50% more viruses than traditional methods, which were mostly rhinoviruses and hMPV. The FilmArray RP detected significantly more total viruses either alone or as part of mixed infections than the xTAG RVP, and an additional 21.6% more RSVs. The xTAG RVP required 5 to 6 hours with 2.5 to 3 hours of hands-on time, whereas the FilmArray RP took about an hour with 3 to 5 minutes of hands-on time.

Fifteen viruses can be detected and differentiated including H1N1/2009/pdm influenza. Sensitivity ranged from 88.9% for adenovirus to 100% for many of the viruses with nearly perfect specificity. The ability to detect multiple pathogens in 1 hour with a simple set-up and fully automated system offers a significant benefit. It is user friendly, with about 3 to 5 minutes of labor involved, and could eventually allow POC testing in the ED or an outpatient clinic by minimally trained health care workers especially if the assay becomes CLIA waived. The time of the assay is 1 hour test time, which is a great advance.

The test is limited to a single patient test per run. Thus, its low throughput could be a significant drawback for laboratories receiving large numbers of specimens, because only a single sample can be processed at a time with one instrument.

GeneXpert system The Cepheid GeneXpert System platform for influenza is an on-demand molecular diagnostics assay that is a fully integrated system. The rapid, sophisticated genetic testing for organisms and genetic-based diseases automates otherwise complex manual laboratory procedures. The easy-to-use system integrates several complicated and time-intensive steps, including sample preparation, DNA amplification, and detection, which enable the analysis of influenza samples in a single proprietary test cartridge. It is a closed, self-contained, cartridge-based, random access assay for performing nucleic acid extraction, PCR amplification, and real-time detection of PCR products with no intermediate sample-handling steps. It is an automated platform that represents a paradigm shift in the automation of molecular analysis, producing accurate results in a timely manner with minimal risk of contamination.

The assay was first released under the FDA Emergency Use Authorization Rule during the 2009 pandemic for detection of influenza A, including 2009 H1N1 pdm.

The GeneXpert Emergency Use Authorization assay demonstrated 91% sensitivity for influenza A compared with the CDC rRT-PCR assay.[36]

Compared with the Luminex xTAG Respiratory Virus rRT-PCR Panel, the GeneXpert was 91.2% sensitive for detection of influenza A; additionally, it demonstrated a 92.1% sensitivity for the detection of 2009 H1N1 compared with the Focus Diagnostics Influenza A/H1N1 (2009) rRT-PCR assay.[37]

A newer version of the Xpert Flu (second generation) was developed subsequently with an identification for 2009 H1N1 pdm. This assay cartridge demonstrated 93% overall sensitivity for detection of influenza A and B in one study and 100% and 80.8% sensitivity for 88 influenza A and B, respectively, in another when compared with laboratory-developed rRT-PCR assays.[38] Tested against a laboratory-developed rRT-PCR assay Xpert Flu showed a sensitivity of 78.8% for influenza A and 76.5% for influenza B.[39] In contrast, the second-generation Xpert Flu test showed excellent sensitivities (98.1% and 93.8% sensitivity for influenza A and B, respectively) compared with commercially available and FDA-cleared Gen-Probe ProFlu+ rRT-PCR.[40]

DiMaio and colleagues[41] compared the X-pert Flu rapid nucleic acid testing assay with other rapid POC antigen tests for the diagnosis of influenza A. Influenza A sensitivity was 97.3% for Xpert Flu, 95.9% for DFA testing, 62.2% for BinaxNOW, and 71.6% for BD Directigen. Influenza B sensitivity was 100% for Xpert Flu and DFA testing, 54.5% for BinaxNOW, and 48.5% for BD Directigen. Specificity for influenza A was 100% for Xpert Flu, BinaxNOW, and BD Directigen, and 99.2% for DFA testing. All methods demonstrated 100% specificity for influenza B (**Table 2**).

Test performance uses three easy steps: (1) transfer 300 μl of prepared sample into the large cartridge opening, (2) dispense elution reagent into the small opening, and (3) insert cartridge and start assay. The advantage is that it is FDA-cleared and can meet the requirements for an accurate POC test for influenza for a POC assay for a clinic or ED or out-patient setting. The POC assay could eventually allow POC testing in clinics by minimally trained health care workers, if the assay becomes CLIA waived. Pandemic 2009 influenza A virus and H3N2 (including H2N2v), seasonal H1N1, and influenza B can be identified. One, or two, four 16, samples, can be run simultaneously; or 64 samples can be run if larger random access equipment is used. The test time is approximately 1 hour. The disadvantage is that only influenza A and B are identified and differentiated. No other viruses are identified.

The GeneXpert System combines on-board sample preparation with real-time PCR amplification and detection functions for fully integrated and automated nucleic acid

Table 2
Gen Xpert Fu amplified assay compared with rapid influenza tests

	Influenza A % Sensitivity	Influenza A % Specificity	Influenza B % Sensitivity	Influenza B % Specificity
Xpert Flu	97.3	100	100	100
Direct Fluorescent Antibody	95.9	99.2	100	100
Binax NOW	62.2	100	54.5	100
BD Directogen	71.6	100	48.5	100

Sensitivity and specificity were calculated using rRT-PCR as the comparator standard.
Data from DiMaio MA, Sahoo MK, Waggomer J, et al. Comparison of Xpert Flu rapid nucleic acid testing with rapid antigen testing for the diagnosis of influenza A and B. J Virol Methods 2012; 86(1–2):137–40.

analysis. The system is designed to purify, concentrate, detect, and identify targeted nucleic acid sequences thereby delivering answers directly from unprocessed samples. Modular in design, the GeneXpert System has a variety of configurations from a single test format to a random access 64-test sample robot to meet the broad range of testing demands of any clinical environment. More studies are required to determine its use in various testing algorithms, and the cost-effectiveness of allowing a more rapid, accurate diagnosis and treatment of influenza-infected patients at the POC setting.

Non–FDA-cleared Molecular Diagnostic Tests for Viral Respiratory Infections

This field is rapidly emerging and mostly involves assays that are multiplexed. These assays were recently reviewed in detail by Caliendo.[42] They may soon achieve FDA clearance and should be evaluated for their advantages on the management of CAP.

Multiplex PCR-electrospray ionization mass spectrometry platform for viruses

A novel molecular approach to the identification of nearly all human respiratory viral pathogens directly from clinical patient specimens, PCR-electrospray ionization mass spectrometry (Ibis Biosciences, Carlsbad, CA; Abbott Molecular, DesPlains, IL) has the potential to revolutionize diagnostic virology, but is not yet FDA-cleared.[43] The platform involves the nucleic acid extraction, rt-PCR, or PCR using sets of primers targeting highly conserved genes that flank variable genomic regions, and then followed by injection of amplicons into an electrospray ionization time-of-flight mass spectrometer, where the mass and number of each nucleic is measured. An excellent review of the literature that discusses the advantages and limitations of the relatively new platform has been published.[12] Thus far, several publications point to its usability for identification of a broad range of viral respiratory pathogens.[44–46] Several formats are available, in addition to the one for common respiratory viruses, including specifically for rapid influenza typing of all H and N types.[47–51] This platform was instrumental in identifying and characterizing the H1N1 2009 influenza strain.[52] FDA clearance may be coming soon for influenza typing.

ResPlex technology

ResPlex Technology (QIAplex Technology; Qiagen, Gaithersburg, MD) uses PCR of extracted nucleic acid followed by a liquid-phase bead-based array technology.[53] There is now a second-generation of the assay called ResPlex II and it detects more than 15 viruses; it was compared with conventional virology and the PCR-electrospray ionization mass spectrometry assay in which both assays performed well, detecting more viruses than conventional virology.[46,54] It is a highly complex assay with multiple steps including postamplification handling of samples, which can increase the potential for contamination.[42]

Infiniti system

This system (AutoGenomics) uses multiplex RT-PCR primers for more than 20 viruses with automated microarray hybridization, requiring 3.5 to 4 hours for first result for 24 specimens.[42] One evaluation comparing it to single real-time virus-specific demonstrated an overall concordance of 94.1%.[55]

Jaguar system

This system (Handy Lab, acquired with Becton Dickinson Diagnostics, Becton Dickinson, Sparks, MD) uses automated nucleic acid extraction with real-time PCR for multiple respiratory pathogens, requiring 3.5 hours for 24 samples.[42] For the detection of influenza A/B and RSV, it demonstrated sensitivities of 100%, 90%, and 100%, respectively.[56]

MOLECULAR DIAGNOSTIC TESTS FOR BACTERIAL INFECTIONS

Although most of the advances in molecular diagnosis of CAP, such as PCR, have been in the area of viral infections, and there has been less development in assays for bacterial infections that are FDA-cleared and commercially available, there have been some outstanding ones, mostly for tuberculosis.[19] However, in the area of non–FDA-cleared research studies, there have been many assays developed, especially for pneumococcus, and some are in use in laboratories, such as LDTs. However, the LDTs are not widely available and are less useful to practicing clinicians until they become commercially available.[6,57]

FDA-Cleared Molecular Amplification Assays for Bacteria

The commercialization and FDA clearance of molecular amplified assays for bacteria is rapidly taking place and more of these assays will soon be available for the practicing clinician for the management of CAP.

Mycobacterium tuberculosis

One of the most outstanding success stories in molecular amplification for an important worldwide respiratory pathogen had been for mycobacteria. In view of the lack of poor sensitivity (45%–80%) of acid-fact smear results and expensive and complex culture methods, which can take 1 to 4 weeks for identification, the development of FDA-cleared molecular tests had played an important role in improved patient outcomes.[25]

The CDC recommends that NAATs be used for at least one respiratory sample from patients suspected of having M tuberculosis.[19] There are now several FDA-cleared assays to choose from: (1) Amplicor Mycobacterium tuberculosis Test (Amplicor; Roche Diagnostics)[58]; (2) Amplified Mycobacterium tuberculosis Direct Test (Gen-Probe, San Diego, CA)[59]; and (3) the Xpert MTB/RIF (Cepheid, Sunneyvale, CA), which detects M tuberculosis and rifampin resistance directly from clinical specimens in approximately 2 hours, allows nucleic acid extraction within the cartridge, has low complexity, and demonstrates high sensitivity compared with standard methodologies (**Table 3**).[20,60,61]

Mycoplasma pneumoniae, Chlamydia pneumoniae, and Bordetella pertussis

M pneumoniae, C pneumoniae, and B pertussis have been recently FDA-cleared (FilmArray).[21] Only one published article mentions the detection of one M pneumoniae organism in its evaluation of viral pathogens.[21] It is expected that the FDA clearance for these organisms will greatly enhance the understanding of the role they each play in CAP in the near future (**Table 4**).

Staphylococcus aureus

Although S aureus was usually considered to be mostly a hospital-acquired cause of pneumonia, it is now recognized as a more common cause of CAP, especially methicillin-resistant S aureus (MRSA).[62] The FDA has cleared several PCR tests for the detection of MRSA in nasal swab specimens; however, there are no cleared assays to detect MRSA or methicillin-sensitive S aureus as agents of CAP.[62] Several POC assays that are cleared for screening using nasal/nares swabs have sensitivities from 95% to 100% sensitivity and provide results in less than 2 hours.[63,64] It has also been evaluated in skin and soft tissue and blood cultures.[65]

Gram-positive bacteria Verigene platform

The FDA cleared the Verigene platform (Verigene GP Blood Culture Nucleic Acid Test) in June 2012 for the identification of gram-positive bacteria from positive blood culture

Table 3
FDA-cleared assays for the detection of tuberculosis bacterial agents in community-acquired pneumonia and lower respiratory infections

Manufacturer and Test Name	Test Method	Instrument	Specimen Type	Gene Target	Turnaround Time
Gen-Probe Amplified *Mycobacterium tuberculosis* Direct Test	TMA, HPA	Gen-Probe Leader 50	AFB smear-positive and smear-negative respiratory specimens	*M tuberculosis* complex rRNA	2.5–3.5 h
Roche Amplicor *Mycobacterium tuberculosis* Direct Test	PCR, colorimetric detection	Thermocycler EIA reader	AFB smear-positive respiratory specimens	*M tuberculosis* complex DNA	6.5 h
Cepheid Xpert *Mycobacterium tuberculosis*	PCR	Cepheid SmartCycler	Respiratory specimens	*M tuberculosis*, rifampin resistance	<2 h

Abbreviations: AFB, acid-fast bacilli; EIA, enzyme immunoassay; HPA, hybridization protection assay; TMA, transcription mediated amplification.

Table 4
FDA-cleared assays for the detection of bacterial agents in community acquired pneumonia and lower respiratory infections

	Assay	Manufacturer	Date Cleared	Turnaround Time
Chlamydia pneumoniae	FilmArray	Idaho Technology	2012	1 h
Mycoplasma pneumoniae	FilmArray	Idaho Technology	2012	1 h
Bordetella pertusis	FilmArray	Idaho Technology	2012	1 h

bottles. The targets identified include staphylococci (including MRSA), streptococci, Enterococcus (including vancomycin-resistant Enterococcus), and Listeria spp.

Non–FDA-Cleared Molecular Assays for Bacteria

The advance in the development of NAATs, such as PCR, in the last two decades has offered a huge understanding of the diagnostic capability of such assays for the management of CAP. The development of research assays has paved the way for commercialization and FDA clearance rapidly taking place today.

Notably, these non-FDA cleared assays include the ones for atypical agents, such as C pneumoniae, M pneumoniae, and Legionella pneumophilia.[66–71]

Chlamydia pneumoniae

Multiple in-house nucleic acid amplification (PCR) methodologies have been published, but the literature has been confounded by lack of standardization and validation.[72,73] The CDC workshop identified a few assays that were considered to be "validated" enough to be used for research studies; others have been developed and used.[66,74–82]

The advantages of these assays are their sensitivity, decreased possibility of contamination, and ability to quantify DNA. A PCR assay has recently been used to identify an outbreak of CAP among navy SEALs.[83] More research using FDA-cleared assays is necessary to further understand the role that C pneumoniae has in CAP. An extensive study of real-time PCR in a CAP study tested 355 samples and compared them with nested PCR, and touchdown enzyme time-released PCR[79] demonstrated increased sensitivity compared with traditional PCR methods.[82]

There has previously never been a commercially available NAAT assay developed, until recently (FilmArray). A LCx research-use-only PCR developed by Abbott Laboratories was used in a multicenter study for comparison with PCR results using in-house PCRs from five different laboratories, which performed very well but it was never taken to a trial.[84] Becton Dickinson performed a clinical trial for a strand displacement amplification assay (SDA), but it was not cleared by the FDA.

Mycoplasma pneumoniae

Many assays have been developed for the detection of Mycoplasma and have been reported to work very well, especially in outbreak situations.[67,71,85] Becton Dickinson performed a clinical trial for SDA, but it was not cleared by the FDA. There has previously never been an FDA-cleared commercially available NAAT assay developed, until recently (FilmArray).

Legionella pneumophilia

Several PCR assays have been published and are reviewed by Murdoch.[68] Becton Dickinson performed a clinical trial for SDA, which was cleared by the FDA, but never commercialized.

Streptococcus pneumoniae

Many research assays have been developed for the PCR amplification of the pneumo-coccus, but thus far none are FDA-cleared.[22,86,87] One of the main problems for using these assays on sputa, nasopharyngeal swabs, and oropharyngeal swabs is how to interpret the result, because a very sensitive assay can also detect pneumococcal carriage and serious infection. The evolution of the noncleared PCR assays and the challenges in the interpretation of these assays are discussed in an excellent review by Blaschke.[23] Early assays targeted the pneumolysin gene, but showed rather poor sensitivity and specificity because of cross-reactivity with viridians strepto-cocci.[88] A comparison of several genes as targets for PCR indicted that the autolysis (lyt) gene was the most specific target.[89] Sheppard and colleagues[90] demonstrated the specificity of this target in clinical samples. Progress is being made with regard to distinguishing carriage or colonization from pneumonia by detecting the coloniza-tion density using real-time PCR.[91]

Multiplex PCR-electrospray ionization mass spectrometry platform for bacteria

A novel approach to the identification of nearly all human bacterial pathogens directly from clinical patient specimens has the potential for revolutionize diagnostic bacteri-ology, but is not yet FDA-cleared. An excellent review of the literature that discusses the advantages and limitations of the relatively new platform, and that covers thou-sands of bacteria and does not require the designation of a specific agent for the test target, has been recently published.[12]

OTHER TESTS THAT ARE NOT DIAGNOSTIC

A newly recognized biomarker assay that is neither diagnostic nor molecular deserves mentioning in consideration of CAP, and this is the procalcitonin test.[92] The blood level of procalcitonin is elevated in patients who have a bacterial infection, who have sepsis with a bacterial agent, or who are in shock.[92] Although a thorough discussion is beyond the scope of this article, it needs to be mentioned as a new tool in the consid-eration of other rapid diagnostic tests in making decisions regarding the diagnosis of possible bacterial cause versus a viral cause of CAP. There is only one FDA-cleared assay at this time (Biomerieux), and it is a 20-minute assay, making it a valuable adjunct in clinical management of CAP when other rapid diagnostic tests are available. The potential use of this assay has been reviewed recently and clinicians will want to evaluate its use in future study of CAP.[6,92,93]

Recommendations for Use of Molecular Assays Based on Present Evidence

For optimal patient care and management of CAP, clinicians require an accurate test that is available in real time, so that decisions about pathogen-directed antimi-crobial therapy or antiviral therapy can be instituted rapidly. Antivirals should be prescribed when the etiologic agent is influenza.[94,95] Presently, pathogen-directed therapy requires the use of an assay that is FDA-cleared, is highly accurate, and can be completed in a timely manner. The last 20 years have greatly advanced the molecular and nonmolecular diagnostic assays for routine care of patients with CAP, and the clinician now has assays that can meet these requirements. Some of these include:

- Rapid influenza tests that are highly accurate, especially ones that use amplified technology
- Rapid molecular tests for M tuberculosis, especially ones that can be completed in a few hours

- Accurate and rapid tests for most other common respiratory viruses that can cause CAP and lower respiratory infections
- Rapid assays that have the ability to accurately detect atypical pathogens, such as *M pneumoniae*, *C pneumoniae*, *Legionella* spp, and *B pertussis*

Future Molecular Studies Needed to Assist Clinicians in the Medical Management of CAP

More research is required before accurate and rapid assays are available, especially for the FDA clinical trials clearing them for routine use, and comparisons involving the newer POC molecular assays, which now have the potential to influence immediate management decisions for CAP. The Infectious Diseases Society of America has stated that "Better, rapid molecular diagnostic tests are an unmet need for respiratory tract infections."[57] FDA-cleared assays are especially needed for the rapid diagnosis of *S pneumoniae*. More research is required to ascertain the ability of rapid molecular identification of genetic markers to predict antibiotic and antiviral resistance, which may be the next generation of new assays. More research is needed to define the role of highly multiplexed assays that can identify hundreds of organisms to know how they can be implemented, especially in light of cost-containment issues in medicine. Lastly, clinicians have to consider the role of antimicrobial stewardship in improving outcomes of patients with CAP (eg, changing, de-escalation, and duration of antimicrobials) and whether molecular diagnostic tools play a role in changing therapy when the etiologic agent is identified.[96]

SUMMARY

Although clinicians have many new and sometimes rapid molecular diagnostic tools that are the result of the explosion of new assays, and need to be using the ones that are available, future research will advance the field such that etiologic agent identification for agents of CAP will be the routine[97] rather than the exception.

REFERENCES

1. Bartlett J. Diagnostic tests for agents of community-acquired pneumonia. Clin Infect Dis 2011;52(Suppl 4):S296–304.
2. Hall MJ, DeFrances CJ, Williams SN, et al. National hospital discharge survey: 2007 summary. Natl Health Stat Report 2010;(29):1–20 Hyattsville (MD).
3. File TM, Marrie TJ. Burden of community-acquired pneumonia in North American adults. Postgrad Med 2010;122:130–41.
4. Bartlett J. Diagnostic test for etiologic agent of community-acquired pneumonia. Infect Dis Clin North Am 2004;18:809–27.
5. Bartlett JG. Decline in microbial studies for patients with pulmonary infections. Clin Infect Dis 2004;39:170–2.
6. File T Jr. New diagnostic tests for pneumonia: what is their role in clinical practice? Clin Chest Med 2011;32:417–30.
7. Centers for Disease Control and Prevention. Rate of hospitalization for pneumonia, by age group. National Hospital Discharge Survey, United States, 2000-2012. MMWR Morb Mortal Wkly Rep 2012;61:657.
8. Ecker DJ, Sampath R, Blyn LB, et al. Rapid identification and strain-typing of respiratory pathogens for epidemic surveillance. Proc Natl Acad Sci U S A 2005;102:8012–7.

9. Ecker DJ, Sampath R, Willett P, et al. The microbial Rosetta Stone database: a compilation of global and emerging infectious microorganisms and bioterrorist threat agents. BMC Microbiol 2005;5:19.

10. Selickman P, Paxos M, File TM Jr, et al. Performance measure of urinary antigen in patients with *Streptococcus pneumoniae* bacteremia. Diagn Microbiol Infect Dis 2010;67:129–33.

11. Shimada T, Noguchi Y, Jackson JL, et al. Systematic review and meta-analysis: urinary antigen tests for legionellosis. Chest 2009;136:1576–85.

12. Wolk DM, Kaleta EJ, Wysocki VH. PCR-electrospray ionization mass spectrometry. J Mol Diagn 2012;14:295–304.

13. Bhat N, O'Brien KL, Karron RA, et al. Use and evaluation of molecular diagnostics for pneumonia etiology studies. Clin Infect Dis 2012;54(Suppl 2):S153–8.

14. Chartrand C, Leeflang MM, Minion J, et al. Accuracy of rapid influenza diagnostic tests: a meta-analysis. Ann Intern Med 2012;156(7):500–11.

15. Lindenauer PK, Remus DW, Roman S, et al. Public reporting and pay for performance in hospital quality improvement. N Engl J Med 2007;356:486–96.

16. Houck PM, Bratzler DW, Nsa W, et al. Timing of antibiotic administration and outcomes for Medicare patients hospitalized with community-acquired pneumonia. Arch Intern Med 2004;164:637–44.

17. Russek-Cohen E, Feldblyum T, Whitaker KB, et al. FDA perspectives on diagnostic device clinical studies for respiratory infections. Clin Infect Dis 2011; 52(Suppl 4):S305–11.

18. Ginocchio CC. Quality assurance in clinical virology. In: Specter S, Hodinka R, Young SA, et al, editors. Clinical virology manual. 4th edition. Washington, DC: ASM Press; 2009. p. 3–17.

19. Centers for Disease Control and Prevention. Updated guidelines for the use of nucleic acid amplification tests in the diagnosis of tuberculosis. MMWR Morb Mortal Wkly Rep 2009;58:7–10.

20. Van Rie A, Page-Shipp L, Sanne I, et al. Xpert M tuberculosis RIF for point-of-care diagnosis of TB in high-HIV-burden, resource limited countries: hype or hope? Rev Molecular Diagnosis 2010;10:937–46.

21. Loeffelholtz M, Pong D, Pyles R, et al. Comparison of the filmarray respiratory panel and Prodesse real-time PCR assays for detection of respiratory pathogens. J Clin Microbiol 2011;49:4083–8.

22. Yang S, Shin L, Khalil A, et al. Quantitative PCR assay using sputum samples for rapid diagnosis of pneumococcal pneumonia in adult emergency department patients. J Clin Microbiol 2005;43:3221–6.

23. Blaschke AJ. Interpreting assays for the detection of *Streptococcus pneumoniae*. Clin Infect Dis 2011;52(Suppl 4):S331–7.

24. Babin SM, Hsieh YH, Rothman RE, et al. Meta-analysis of point-of-care laboratory tests in the diagnosis of novel 2009 swine-lineage pandemic influenza A(H1N1). Diagn Microbiol Infect Dis 2011;69:410–8.

25. Ginocchio CC. Strengths and weaknesses of FDA-approved/cleared diagnostic devices for the molecular detection of respiratory pathogens. Clin Infect Dis 2011;52(Suppl):S312–25.

26. Kumar S, Henrickson KJ. Update on influenza diagnostics: lessons from the novel H1N1 influenza A pandemic. Clin Microbiol Rev 2012;25:361.

27. Lee CK, Cho HC, Woo MK, et al. Evaluation of Sofia fluorescent immunoassay analyzer for influenza A/B virus. J Clin Virol 2012;55(3):239–43.

28. LeGoff J, Kara R, Moulin F, et al. Evaluation of the one-step multiplex real-time reverse transcriptase-PCR ProFlu-1 assay for the detection of influenza A and

influenza B viruses and respiratory syncytial viruses in children. J Clin Microbiol 2008;46:789–91.

29. Mahony J, Chong S, Erante F, et al. Development of a respiratory virus panel test for detection of twenty human respiratory viruses by use of a multiplex PCR and a fluid mirco-bead-based assay. J Clin Microbiol 2007;45:2965–70.

30. Merante F, Yaghoubian S, Janeczko R. Principles of the xTAG respiratory viral panel (RVP assay). J Clin Virol 2007;40:S31–5.

31. Pabbaraju K, Tokaryk KL, Wong S, et al. Comparison of the Luminex xTAG respiratory panel with in-house nucleic acid amplification tests for diagnosis of respiratory virus infections. J Clin Microbiol 2008;49:3056–62.

32. Rand KH, Rampersaud H, Houck H. Comparison of two multiplex methods for detection of respiratory viruses: filmarray RP and xTAG RVP. J Clin Microbiol 2011;49:2449.

33. Jannetto PJ, Buchan BW, Vaughan KA, et al. Real-time detection of influenza a, influenza B, and respiratory syncytial virus a and B in respiratory specimens by use of nanoparticle probes. J Clin Microbiol 2011;48:3997–4002.

34. Poritz M, Blaschke A, Byington C, et al. FilmArray, an automated nested multiplex PCR system for multi-pathogen detection: development and application to respiratory tract infection. PLoS One 2011;6:e26047.

35. Pierce V, Elkan M, Leet M, et al. Comparison of the Idaho Technology FilmArray system to real-time PCR for detection of respiratory pathogens in children. J Clin Microbiol 2012;50:364–71.

36. Miller S, Moayeri M, Wright C, et al. Comparison of GeneXpert FluA PCR to direct fluorescent antibody and respiratory viral panel PCR assays for detection of 2009 novel H1N1 influenza virus. J Clin Microbiol 2010;48:4684–5.

37. Sambol AR, Iwen PC, Pieretti M, et al. Validation of the Cepheid Xpert Flu A real time RT-PCR detection panel for emergency use authorization. J Clin Virol 2010; 48:234–8.

38. Popowitch EB, Rogers E, Miller MB. Retrospective and prospective verification of the cepheid Xpert influenza virus assay. J Clin Microbiol 2011;49:3368–9.

39. Li M, Brenwald N, Bonigal S, et al. Rapid diagnosis of influenza: an evaluation of two commercially available RT-PCR assays. J Infect 2012;65:60–3.

40. Novak-Weekley SM, Marlowe EM, Poulter M, et al. Evaluation of the Cepheid Xpert Flu Assay for rapid identification and differentiation of influenza A, influenza A 2009 H1N1, and influenza B viruses. J Clin Microbiol 2012;50:1704–10.

41. DiMaio MA, Sahoo MK, Waggomer J, et al. Comparison of Xpert Flu rapid nucleic acid testing with rapid antigen testing for the diagnosis of influenza A and B. J Virol Methods 2012;86(1–2):137–40. http://dx.doi.org/10.1016/j.jviromet.2012.07.023.

42. Caliendo AM. Multiplex PCR and emerging technologies for the detection of respiratory pathogens. Clin Infect Dis 2011;52(Suppl 4):S326–30.

43. Ecker DJ, Sampath R, Massire C, et al. Ibis T5000: a universal biosensor approach for microbiology. Nat Rev Microbiol 2008;6:553–8.

44. Chen KF, Rothman RE, Ramachandron P, et al. Rapid identification of viruses from nasal pharyngeal aspirates in acute viral respiratory infections by RT-PCR and electrospray ionization mass spectrometry. J Virol Methods 2011;173:60–6.

45. Chen KF, Blyn L, Rothman RE, et al. Reverse transcriptase polymerase chain reaction and electrospray ionization mass spectrometry for identifying acute viral upper respiratory tract infections. Diagn Microbiol Infect Dis 2011;69:179–86.

46. Forman MS, Advani S, Newman C, et al. Diagnostic performance of two highly multiplexed respiratory virus assays in a pediatric cohort. J Clin Virol 2012; 55(2):168–72.

47. Sampath R, Russell KL, Massire C, et al. Global surveillance of emerging influenza viruses genotypes by mass spectrometry. PLoS One 2007;2:2489.
48. Deyde VM, Sampath R, Garten RJ, et al. Genomic signature-based identification of influenza A viruses using RT=PCR/electrospray ionization mass spectrometry (ESI-MS) technology. PLoS One 2010;5:e13293.
49. Deyde VM, Sampath R, Gubareva LV. RT-PCR/electrospray ionization mass spectrometry approach in detection and characterization of influenza viruses. Expert Rev Mol Diagn 2011;11:41–52.
50. Jeng K, Massire C, Zembower TR, et al. Monitoring seasonal influenza A evolution: Rapid 2009 pandemic H1N1 surveillance with a reverse transcription-polymerase chain reaction/electrospray ionization mass spectrometry assay. J Clin Virol 2012. http://dx.doi.org/10.1016/j.jcv.2012.05.002.
51. Tang YW, Lowery K, Valsamakis A, et al. Evaluation of a PLEX-ID flu assay for simultaneous detection and identification of influenza viruses A and B. J Clin Microbiol 2013;51. [Epub ahead of print].
52. Metzgar D, Baynes D, Myers CA, et al. Initial identification and characterization of an emerging zoonotic influenza virus prior to pandemic spread. J Clin Microbiol 2010;48:4228–34.
53. Benson R, Tondella ML, Bhatnagar J, et al. Development and evaluation of a novel multiplex PCR technology for molecular differential detection of bacterial respiratory disease pathogens. J Clin Microbiol 2008;46:2074–7.
54. Balada-Llasat JM, LaRue H, Kelly C, et al. Evaluation of commercial ResPlex II v2.0, Multicode-PLx and xTAG respiratory viral panels for the diagnosis of respiratory viral infections in adults. J Clin Virol 2011;50:42–5.
55. Raymond F, Carbonneau J, Boucher N, et al. Comparison of automated microarray detection with real-time PCR assays for detection of respiratory viruses in specimens obtained from children. J Clin Microbiol 2009;47:743–50.
56. Beck ET, Jurgens LA, Ehl SC, et al. Development of a rapid automated influenza A, influenza B, and respiratory syncytial virus A/B multiplex real-time RT-PCR assay and its use during the 2009 H1N1 swine-origin influenza virus epidemic in Milwaukee, Wisconsin. J Mol Diagn 2010;12:74–81.
57. Infectious Diseases Society of America. An unmet medical need: rapid molecular diagnostics tests for respiratory tract infections. Clin Infect Dis 2011;52(Suppl 4):S384–95.
58. D'Amato RF, Wallman AA, Hochstein LH, et al. Rapid diagnosis of pulmonary tuberculosis by using the Roche AMPLICOR *Mycobacterium tuberculosis* PCR test. J Clin Microbiol 1995;33:1832–4.
59. Lemaitre N, Armand S, Vachee A, et al. comparison of the real-time PCR method and the gen-probe amplified *Mycobacterium tuberculosis* direct test for detection of *Mycobacterium tuberculosis* in pulmonary and nonpulmonary specimens. J Clin Microbiol 2004;42:4307–9.
60. Dorman SE, Chihota VN, Ewis JJ, et al. Performance characteristics of the Cepheid Xpert MTB/RIF test in a tuberculosis prevalence survey. PLoS One 2012;7(8):e43307.
61. Scott LE, McCarthy K, Gous N, et al. Comparison of Xpert MTB/RIF with other nucleic acid technologies for diagnosing pulmonary tuberculosis in a high HIV prevalence setting: a prospective study. PLoS Med 2011;8(7):e1001061.
62. Peterson LR. Molecular laboratory tests for the diagnosis of respiratory tract infection due to *Staphylococcus aureus*. Clin Infect Dis 2011;52(Suppl 4):S361–6.
63. Paule SM, Hacek DM, Kufner B, et al. Performance of the BDGeneOhm methicillin-resistant *Staphylococcus aureus* test before and during high-volume clinical use. J Clin Microbiol 2007;45:2993–8.

64. Wolk DM, Picton E, Johnson D, et al. Multicenter evaluation of the Cepheid Xpert methicillin-resistant *Staphylococcus aureus* (MRSA) test as a rapid screening method for detection of MRSA in nares. J Clin Microbiol 2009;47:758–64.

65. Wolk DM, Struelens MJ, Pancholi P, et al. Rapid detection of *Staphylococcus aureus* and methicillin *S. aureus* in wound specimens and blood cultures: multicenter preclinical evaluation of the Cepheid Xpert MRSA/SA skin and soft tissue and blood culture assays. J Clin Microbiol 2009;47:823–6.

66. Kumar S, Hammerschlag MR. Acute respiratory infection due to *Chlamydia pneumoniae*: current status of diagnostic methods. Clin Infect Dis 2007;44:568–76.

67. Loens K, Goossens H, Ieven M. Acute respiratory infections due to *Mycoplasma pneumoniae*: current status of diagnostic methods. Eur J Clin Microbiol Infect Dis 2010;29:1055–69.

68. Murdoch DR. Diagnosis of *Legionella* infection. Clin Infect Dis 2003;36:64–9.

69. Cloud JL, Carroll KC, Pixton P, et al. *Legionella* species in respiratory specimens using PCR with sequencing confirmation. J Clin Microbiol 2000;33:1709–12.

70. Diederen BM, Van Der Eerden MM, Viaspolder F, et al. Detection of respiratory viruses and *Legionella* spp. by real-time polymerase chain reaction in patients with community acquired pneumonia. Scand J Infect Dis 2009;41:45–50.

71. Liu FC, Chen PY, Huang FL, et al. Rapid diagnosis of *Mycoplasma pneumoniae* infection in children by polymerase chain reaction. J Microbiol Immunol Infect 2007;40:507–12.

72. Apfalter P, Blasi F, Boman J, et al. Multicenter comparison trial of DNA extraction methods and PCR assays for detection of *Chlamydia pneumoniae* in endarterectomy specimens. J Clin Microbiol 2001;39:519–24.

73. Dowell SF, Peeling RW, Boman J, et al. Standardizing chlamydia pneumoniae assays: recommendations from the Centers of Disease Control and Prevention (USA) and the Laboratory Centre for Disease Control (Canada). Clin Infect Dis 2001;33:492–503.

74. Gaydos CA, Quinn TC, Eiden JJ. Identification of *Chlamydia pneumoniae* by DNA amplification of the 16S rRNA gene. J Clin Microbiol 1992;30:796–800.

75. Gaydos CA, Roblin PM, Hammerschlag MR, et al. Diagnostic utility of PCR-enzyme immunoassay, culture, and serology for detection of *Chlamydia pneumoniae* in symptomatic and asymptomatic patients. J Clin Microbiol 1994;32:903–5.

76. Gaydos CA, Fowler CL, Gill VJ, et al. Detection of *Chlamydia pneumoniae* by polymerase chain reaction-enzyme immunoassay in an immunocompromised population. Clin Infect Dis 1993;17:718–23.

77. Gaydos CA, Eiden JJ, Oldach D, et al. Diagnosis of *Chlamydia pneumoniae* infection in patients with community acquired pneumonia by polymerase chain reaction enzyme immunoassay. Clin Infect Dis 1994;19:157–60.

78. Boman J, Allard A, Person K, et al. Rapid diagnosis of respiratory *Chlamydia pneumoniae* infection by nested touchdown polymerase chain reaction compared with culture and antigen detection by EIA. J Infect Dis 1997;175:1523–6.

79. Madico G, Quinn T, Boman J, et al. Touchdown enzyme time release-PCR for detection and identification of *C. trachomatis*, *C. pneumoniae*, and *C. psittaci* using the 16S and 16S-23S spacer rRNA genes. J Clin Microbiol 2000;38:1085–93.

80. Tondella ML, Talkington DF, Holloway BP, et al. Development and evaluation of real-time PCR-based fluorescence assays for the detection of *Chlamydia pneumoniae*. J Clin Microbiol 2002;40:575–83.

81. Apfalter P, Barousch W, Nehr M, et al. Comparison of a new quantitative ompA-based real-Time PCR TaqMan assay for detection of *Chlamydia pneumoniae*

DNA in respiratory specimens with four conventional PCR assays. J Clin Microbiol 2003;41:592–600.

82. Hardick J, Maldeis N, Theodore M, et al. Real-Time PCR for *Chlamydia pneumoniae* utilizing the Roche Lightcycler and a 16S rRNA gene target. J Mol Diagn 2004;6:132–6.

83. Coon RG, Balansay MS, Faix DJ, et al. *Chlamydophilia pneumoniae* infection among basis underwater demolition/SEALS (BUD/S) candidates, Coronado, California, July 2008. Mil Med 2011;176:320–3.

84. Chernesky MS, Schachter J, Summersgill J, et al. Comparison of an industry derived LCx *Chlamydia pneumoniae* PCR research kit to in-house assays performed in five laboratories. J Clin Microbiol 2002;40:2357–62.

85. Morozumi M, Ito A, Murayama SY, et al. Assessment of real-time PCR for diagnosis of *Mycoplasma pneumoniae* in pediatric patients. Can J Microbiol 2006; 52:125–9.

86. Avni T, Mansur N, Leibovici L, et al. PCR using blood for diagnosis of invasive pneumococcal disease: systematic review and meta-analysis. J Clin Microbiol 2010;48: 489–96.

87. Smith MD, Sheppard CL, Hogan A, et al. Diagnosis of *Streptococcus pneumoniae* infections in adults with bacteremia and community-acquired pneumonia: clinical comparison of pneumococcal PCR and urinary antigen detection. J Clin Microbiol 2009;47:1046–9.

88. Murdock DR, Anderson TP, Beynon KA, et al. Evaluation of a PCR assay for detection of *Streptococcus pneumoniae* in respiratory and nonrespiratory samples from adults with community-acquired pneumonia. J Clin Microbiol 2003;41:63–6.

89. Carvalho Mda MG, Tondella ML, Mc Caustland K, et al. Evaluation and improvement of real-time PCR assays targeting lytA., ply, and psaA genes for detection for pneumococcal DNA. J Clin Microbiol 2007;45:2460–6.

90. Sheppard CL, Harrison TG, Morris R, et al. Autolysin-targeted LightCycler assay including internal process control for detection of *Streptococcus pneumoniae* DNA in clinical samples. J Med Microbiol 2004;53:189–95.

91. Albrich WC, Madhi SA, Adrian PV, et al. Use of a rapid test of pneumococcal colonization density to diagnose pneumococcal pneumonia. Clin Infect Dis 2012;54: 601–9.

92. Gilbert DN. Procalcitonin as a biomarker in respiratory tract infection. Clin Infect Dis 2011;52(Suppl 4):S346–50.

93. Fowler CL. Procalcitonin for triage of patients with respiratory tract symptoms: a case study in the trial design process for approval of a new diagnostic test for lower respiratory tract infections. Clin Infect Dis 2011;52(Suppl 4):S351–6.

94. Jain S, Benoit SR, Skarbinski J, et al. Influenza-associated pneumonia among hospitalized patients with 2009 pandemic influenza A (H1N1)—United States, 2009. Clin Infect Dis 2012;54:1221–9.

95. Harper SA, Bradley JS, Englund JA, et al. Seasonal influenza in adults and children: diagnosis, treatment chemoprophylaxis, and institutional outbreak management: clinical practice guidelines of the Infectious Diseases Society of America. Clin Infect Dis 2009;48:1003–32.

96. Avdic E, Cushinotto LA, Hughes AH, et al. Impact of an antimicrobial stewardship intervention on shortening the duration of therapy for community-acquired pneumonia. Clin Infect Dis 2012;54:1581–7.

97. Johansson N, Kalin M, Tiveijung-Lindell A, et al. Etiology of community-acquired pneumonia: increased microbiological yeils with new diagnostic methods. Clin Infect Dis 2010;50:202–9.

Guidelines and Quality Measures
Do They Improve Outcomes of Patients with Community-Acquired Pneumonia?

Jennie Johnstone, MD, FRCPC[a,b], Lionel Mandell, MD, FRCPC[a],*

KEYWORDS

- Community-acquired pneumonia • Guidelines • Outcome measures
- Quality indicators • Quality measures • Pay for performance

KEY POINTS

- Community-acquired pneumonia (CAP) has a significant impact in terms of morbidity, mortality, and cost of care.
- Guidelines play an important role in the management of this disease.
- Many of the current CAP quality indicators have only low-quality evidence supporting their use.
- Future CAP quality indicators should be based on evidence-based interventions.
- Pay-for-performance quality-improvement measures do not appear to improve clinically important outcomes.

PNEUMONIA

Pneumonia represents an infection of the pulmonary parenchyma, and is currently classified according to where it is acquired. Three categories now exist: community-acquired pneumonia (CAP), health care–acquired pneumonia (HCAP), and hospital-acquired/ventilator-acquired pneumonia (HAP/VAP). In general, as one moves from CAP to HCAP to HAP/VAP there is an increase in multidrug-resistant pathogens and mortality.

The focus of this article is on the influence of guidelines and quality measures on CAP outcomes in adults. In the United States there are more than 5.6 million cases of CAP annually,[1,2] of which approximately 80% are managed on an outpatient basis and 20% are treated in a hospital setting. The majority of this latter group is handled outside the intensive care unit (ICU) setting, but approximately 10% of those admitted to hospital require admission to an ICU. The overall annual rate in the United States is

[a] Department of Medicine, McMaster University, 1200, Main Street, West Hamilton, Ontario L8N 3Z5, Canada; [b] Institute for Infectious Disease Research, McMaster University, 1200, Main Street, West Hamilton, Ontario L8N 3Z5, Canada
* Corresponding author. 11 Old Park Road, Toronto, Ontario M6C 3H4, Canada.
E-mail address: lmandell@mcmaster.ca

Infect Dis Clin N Am 27 (2013) 71–86
http://dx.doi.org/10.1016/j.idc.2012.11.001
0891-5520/13/$ – see front matter © 2013 Elsevier Inc. All rights reserved.

12 cases per 1000 persons, but jumps to 20 per 1000 persons for those older than 60 years. It is estimated that more than 900,000 episodes of CAP occur annually in the United States in adults 65 years of age or older.

The impact of CAP is very significant because annually it results in more than 64 million days of restricted activity, and carries an age-adjusted mortality rate of up to 22%.[3] The associated costs are more than $10 billion, and in Europe costs are estimated at around €10.1 billion with indirect costs attributable to lost work time of €3.6 billion.[4]

When faced with a patient with possible pneumonia, the physician must try to determine if in fact the clinical entity is pneumonia rather than some other clinical problem. If it is pneumonia, one must then try to ascertain the etiologic pathogen. In the outpatient setting both of these tasks can be difficult, particularly determination of etiology. The diagnosis in most cases is made based on a careful history and physical examination plus chest radiographic data whenever possible. Often, laboratory-based tests are either not done or provide data too late to be of use in determining initial treatment. Recognition of this problem was one of the driving forces behind the development of guidelines to help in the management of CAP.

GUIDELINES

Each year more than $50 billion are spent on biomedical research and more than 15,000 trials are reported, often with a bias against reporting results with negative findings. It can be difficult enough for the average physician to deal with patients, let alone to stay abreast of new information. Guidelines provide a relatively efficient means of evaluating and reporting a body of evidence dealing with a specific clinical issue such as CAP. When compiled carefully, they represent the essential essence of an evidence-based approach to a clinical problem.

With CAP, the aim of guidelines is to improve patient management and outcomes while controlling costs and informing physicians about advances and controversies in the management of this problem. Perhaps just as importantly, they provide a standard against which care can be evaluated and highlight gaps in knowledge, thereby helping to direct future research.

Evaluating the impact of guidelines on CAP is not as straightforward as one might imagine. Different outcome measures can be identified, and methods assessing the effect of guidelines vary. Typical outcome measures include mortality, length of stay, and cost. Although the ideal evaluation process of guidelines themselves would be a randomized controlled trial comparing patients managed according to a predetermined set of guidelines with individual physician judgment, there are potential ethical issues associated with such an approach, and to date no such study has been performed that the authors are aware of. Typically data are analyzed retrospectively, usually using a before-and-after event design.

Outcomes such as mortality, length of stay, and cost are, to a significant extent, functions of severity of illness, and this ultimately is often related to the site of care. For this reason it seems easier and more logical to look at the impact of guidelines according to where patient care is administered, namely the outpatient setting, the hospitalized non-ICU setting, and the ICU itself.

Outpatient Management

Of the 3 settings referred to, this is perhaps the hardest to evaluate because length of stay does not apply and overall mortality rates are generally less than 1%. Any differences among various treatment approaches would be exceedingly difficult to detect.

One of the earliest studies to address this problem compared medical outcomes and antimicrobial costs in patients whose treatment regimens were concordant with or different from the American Thoracic Society (ATS) CAP guidelines.[5] Threefold lower costs were found in those 60 years or younger without comorbidity given therapy consistent with the guidelines, but no significant differences in medical outcomes were found. A later study found that by following the ATS recommendations of 1993, hospital admission rates for CAP patients seen at urgent care clinics decreased.[6,7] **Table 1** lists references of relevant studies examining the effects of guidelines on various outcome measures.

A Cochrane review in 2009 failed to find evidence supporting any one particular antibiotic regimen.[8] Six randomized controlled trials involving 1857 patients aged 12 years and older with CAP were reviewed. Five antibiotic pairs were examined: Erythromycin versus clarithromycin, azithromycin versus levofloxacin, azithromycin versus clarithromycin, telithromycin versus levofloxacin, and telithromycin versus clarithromycin. The investigators concluded that there were insufficient data to recommend one antibiotic as superior to another for the treatment of CAP in the outpatient setting.

This finding is not surprising, as these drugs generally provide coverage for the usual pathogens of concern in ambulatory CAP patients. Atypicals such as *Mycoplasma pneumoniae*, *Chlamydophila pneumoniae*, and *Streptococcus pneumoniae* are each covered. It would be far more meaningful to compare antibiotic regimens that do or do not cover the atypicals as well as *S pneumoniae*, for example, a macrolide or a fluoroquinolone versus a β-lactam.

A study in Utah that focused on the effects of guideline implementation on mortality also reported that lower hospital admission rates were found for the outpatients included in the trial, although the reduction did not reach statistical significance.[9]

Hospitalized Patients (Non-ICU)

For those patients requiring admission to hospital for the management of CAP there is substantially more information regarding the impact of guidelines on outcomes. Several end points have been studied, including mortality, length of stay, costs,

Table 1
Outcome measures and their references

	References
Outpatients	
Mortality	8
Costs	5
Hospitalization rates	6,8,9
Hospitalized Patients (Non-ICU)	
Mortality	9,11–16,18–20,24,25,27
Length of stay/costs	12–14,18–20,24,27,29,31–34,37
Time to clinical stability	14,20,27,38
Readmission rates	15,24
Hospitalized Patients (ICU)	
Mortality	37,44,47
Duration of MV	45
Length of stay	37

Abbreviations: ICU, intensive care unit; MV, mechanical ventilation.

time to clinical stability, duration of parenteral treatments, and readmission rates. This greater detail is to be expected, as the patients are more closely followed and the outcome measures more easily discernible and measurable. For the purposes of this article, the sections dealing with hospitalized patients are further subdivided according to the relevant outcomes and the published studies reviewed in chronologic order.

Mortality

Unlike cost of care, which is inextricably related to length of stay, mortality is certainly easy to define and identify, but even here there is some room for debate. All-cause mortality and attributable mortality are ultimately two sides of the same coin, and certainly not all articles have looked at this. In light of data linking pneumonia and particularly pneumococcal pneumonia with events such as myocardial infarction and stroke, this may not be of paramount importance.[10]

In a nonrandomized observational study involving 2963 eligible hospitalized CAP patients, Dudas and colleagues[11] examined the empiric antimicrobial treatment of presumed CAP in 72 nonteaching United States hospitals, compliance with ATS guidelines, and the impact of such treatment on mortality and length of stay. Using multivariate logistic regression analysis they found that use of a second-generation or third-generation cephalosporin or a β-lactam β-lactamase inhibitor plus a macrolide, as recommended in the guidelines, was independently associated with reduced mortality. The next year Dean and colleagues[7,9] published a study specifically focusing on the impact of guidelines on mortality. A CAP guideline was developed at Intermountain Healthcare in Utah based on the 1993 ATS guidelines, and 30-day mortality rates before and after implementation of the guidelines determined. In total 28,661 CAP cases were assessed, including 7719 that were hospitalized. A reduction in mortality was found among hospitalized patients after the introduction of guidelines. Further support of the impact of guidelines on mortality was furnished by Menendez and colleagues[12] in a Spanish study involving 295 consecutively admitted CAP patients. The effects of compliance with Spanish and United States (ATS) guidelines were assessed, whereby mortality in severe CAP (Fine class 5) was found to be significantly higher in patients given discordant therapy from the guidelines. A multivariate analysis also showed that compliance with the ATS guidelines was independently associated with decreased mortality after adjusting for the Fine score. Additional data from Spain further bolstered the concept of guidelines and their positive impact on mortality.[13] Using a before-and-after approach in a controlled fashion, outcome measures were examined in one hospital before and after the introduction of guidelines, and compared with outcomes for control hospitals where guidelines were not used during both time periods. Use of guidelines resulted in a reduction in 30-day mortality and in-hospital mortality.

Frei and colleagues[14] retrospectively reviewed data on 631 patients with CAP managed on the wards of 5 hospitals over a 6-month period. Guideline-concordant therapy was associated with improved survival. In a follow-up to an earlier study, Dean and colleagues[9,15] reviewed 17,728 CAP patients. Patients with respiratory failure and sepsis cases resulting from pneumonia were included, and once again use of guidelines was associated with lower mortality. The investigators concluded that these data validated their local CAP guidelines, which in turn were based on ATS guidelines.[7]

Mortensen and colleagues[16] looked at mortality from a slightly different perspective and assessed the impact of guideline-concordant therapy on mortality at 48 hours as opposed to the usual end point of 30 days. This retrospective study was of a cohort of 787 CAP patients at two teaching hospitals using a multivariable logistic regression model to evaluate any association, adjusting for potential confounders. Adherence to guidelines resulted in a significant reduction in mortality at the 48-hour point after admission. A criticism of the study, and one acknowledged by the investigators themselves, is that in the first 48 hours the mortality rate was only 2.5%. Patients were assessed in terms of severity at presentation using the Pneumonia Severity Index (PSI) whereby 53% were low risk (class 1–3), 33% were of moderate risk (class 4), and only 14% were high risk (class 5). It is not surprising, therefore, that the mortality rate was so low because generally for patients of class 1 to 3 these rates are less than 1%.[17]

Calzada and colleagues[18] evaluated 425 CAP patients hospitalized on a ward in a prospective multicenter study. Using the Spanish guidelines as the basis for therapy, they found that not adhering to the recommended regimens was associated with greater mortality. A 1-year retrospective multicenter study involving 3233 hospitalized CAP patients found that treatment according to guidelines as well as positive blood cultures and establishment of an etiologic diagnosis were associated with reductions in late and global mortality.[19] The investigators concluded that compliance with appropriate therapeutic guidelines has a significant influence on outcome.

Although not specifically evaluating guidelines per se, Arnold and colleagues[7,20–23] assessed the effect of atypical pathogen coverage on CAP outcomes and thereby essentially validated one of the key themes of CAP guidelines from Canada, the United States, Japan, and Germany. Using international databases, several outcomes including mortality were compared between patients treated with and without atypical antimicrobial coverage. Better outcomes were reported with regimens providing atypical coverage.

A prospective cohort study of 271 hospitalized CAP patients focused on a cost-effectiveness analysis of CAP treatment.[24] Outcome measures were mortality and readmission at 30 days, and the former was significantly reduced for those patients treated according to the Spanish guidelines. Blasi and colleagues[25] performed a multicenter interventional trial before and after study of the impact of compliance with Italian guidelines on mortality. Reduced mortality was found with concordant therapy such as a cephalosporin and macrolide combination or levofloxacin alone, as opposed to monotherapy with a cephalosporin. Arnold and colleagues[20,26] examined the effect of adherence to the Infectious Disease Society of America (IDSA)/ATS guidelines on outcomes in elderly CAP patients requiring hospitalization. Using the CAPO (Community-Acquired Pneumonia Organization) International Study Database, they evaluated the impact on 1725 patients aged 65 years or older and found that the use of guidelines improved several outcomes, including mortality. McCabe and colleagues,[27] using a database with 54,619 non-ICU hospitalized CAP patients at 113 community hospitals and tertiary care centers, also found that guideline-concordant treatment was associated with decreased in-hospital mortality.

Length of stay and costs

Because cost of care is so closely tied to length of stay, these two outcomes are dealt with together. Prolonged length of stay is the result of several factors including severity, comorbid conditions and, as the data strongly suggest, inappropriate or guideline-discordant antimicrobial treatment. A total of 17 articles were found to deal with these end points, many of which have already been mentioned because they also included mortality. Although the study by Stahl and colleagues[28] did not examine guidelines specifically, they did find that of 76 hospitalized CAP patients, length of stay was almost 50% shorter (2.75 vs 5.3 days) for patients given a macrolide in the first 24 hours. Like the Arnold study, it too validated one of the key tenets of CAP guidelines from several countries.[20] Analysis of a best-practice model developed at the University of Kentucky Medical Center focused on the efficiency of managing patients with CAP.[29] Guidelines for the management of CAP patients were developed locally based on IDSA recommendations, and the treatment regimen associated with the best cost-effective relationship was found to be the one based on the guidelines.[29,30] Like several other investigators, Dudas and colleagues[11] found that addition of a macrolide to a cephalosporin or β-lactam/β-lactamase inhibitor was associated with decreased length of stay and mortality. Two subsequent studies published within a year of each other found positive impacts on costs and length of stay.[31,32] Marrie and colleagues[31] performed a multicenter controlled trial to determine whether a critical pathway improves the efficiency of CAP treatment without compromising patient well-being. The study reported that implementation of such a pathway reduced the use of institutional resources as measured by the number of bed days per patient managed. Meehan and colleagues[32] reported a reduction in length of stay from 7 to 5 days following a statewide initiative based on an evidence-based critical pathway of pneumonia. An assessment by Menendez and colleagues[12] of adherence to Spanish or ATS CAP guidelines found no significant differences in duration of hospitalization between adherent and nonadherent regimens, whereas Battleman and colleagues[30,33] found that appropriateness of antibiotic selection as defined by the IDSA CAP guidelines has a significant association with shorter length of stay.

Capelastegui and colleagues[13] found that in a hospital where guidelines were implemented, the percentage of appropriate treatment given was increased and length of stay was reduced compared with control hospitals. A multicenter observational study involving only 99 patients was performed by Orrick and colleagues[30,34] and found, as did others, that compliance with guidelines (in this case the 1998 IDSA version) resulted in a shorter mean length of hospital stay, a lower total cost of hospitalization, and lower costs of antibacterial therapy. A retrospective cohort study by Frei and colleagues[14] studied 631 CAP patients and also found that guideline-concordant therapy was associated with several improved outcomes, including length of stay. These data were based on the 2001 ATS and 2003 IDSA CAP guidelines.[35,36]

Calzada and colleagues,[18] in a study of adherence to Spanish guidelines, found that whereas concordant therapy was associated with reduced mortality and β-lactam monotherapy was an independent risk factor for readmission, length of stay was independently associated with the admitting hospital and not with antibiotics. In 2008, Garau and colleagues[19] looked at factors influencing length of stay and mortality. Treatment according to guidelines was associated with reduced mortality but not length of stay. PSI classes 4 and 5, positive blood cultures, admission to an ICU, multilobar involvement, and alcohol ingestion were the variables independently associated with length of stay.[19]

In contrast to the Calzada and Garau articles, two other studies in 2007 found different results. Arnold and colleagues[20] reported that patients receiving coverage for atypical pathogens had better outcomes, which included reduced length of stay, and Menendez and colleagues,[24] using a cost-effectiveness ratio, found that guideline-adherent treatment saved €1121 per patient cured compared with nonadherent treatment.

Over the next 2 years, 3 additional studies generated data supporting the use of CAP guidelines as a means of reducing length of stay. Dambrava and colleagues[37] studied 780 CAP patients consecutively admitted to hospital, and showed a reduction in length of stay from 10.4 to 7.6 days with nonadherent versus adherent treatment. Using an international CAP cohort study database, Arnold and colleagues[20] focused on the elderly and found that concordance with the IDSA CAP guidelines was associated with shorter length of stay.[26] In one of the largest studies, McCabe and colleagues[27] reported on 54,619 non-ICU hospitalized CAP patients in whom decreased length of stay was associated with guideline-adherent antimicrobial therapy.

Time to clinical stability

A study of 1424 hospitalized CAP patients in Spain used a Cox proportional-hazard model to identify independent variables associated with time to clinical stability. Adherence to the Spanish CAP guidelines was one such variable.[38] The Frei study[14] evaluated several outcome measures including time to clinical stability and time to switch therapy, and found that using the ATS and IDSA CAP guidelines to guide initial antibiotic treatment was associated with all the outcomes measured. The importance of providing coverage that includes the atypical pathogens was emphasized by the Arnold study,[20] which showed a positive correlation between the use of such drugs and a reduction in time to clinical stability. Arnold and colleagues[20] went on to show that implementation of the latest iteration of the IDSA/ATS CAP guidelines reduced time to clinical stability in the elderly.

Although not a direct measure of time to clinical stability, the duration of parenteral therapy provides some glimpse into the clinical status of the patient. McCabe and colleagues[27] reported that guideline-concordant treatment was associated, among other improvements, with a statistically significant reduction in duration of parenteral therapy.

Readmission rates

In one of the two studies by Dean's group already referred to, the use of CAP guidelines was associated with a reduction in readmission rates.[15] Menendez and colleagues[24] reported the same findings using the Spanish CAP guidelines.

Hospitalized Patients (ICU)

From the perspective of patient management, severe CAP is probably best defined as CAP requiring admission to an ICU.[26] Rates of severe illness among hospitalized CAP patients vary from 6.6% to 16.7% and mortality rates range from 20% to 50%.[39–42] Major and minor criteria suggested by the IDSA/ATS CAP guidelines appear helpful in selecting patients for ICU care and, as stated in a review of the topic by Rello, "the introduction of IDSA/ATS guidelines for antibiotic administration also represents a step forward in patient management."[43]

Several studies have addressed a variety of issues concerning CAP patients in the ICU and their management and, as with the non-ICU hospitalized cohort, the data strongly support the use of guidelines. Of the studies examined, articles are included here only if it is clear from the methods described that patients had actually been admitted to an ICU. Simply listing patients as Fine class 5 without further elaboration regarding the site of in-hospital care was considered inadequate.

Five such studies were published between 2005 and 2010. Bodi and colleagues[44] performed a prospective multicenter study involving 529 CAP patients admitted to ICUs in 33 hospitals, and found a significantly higher mortality in those not treated according to IDSA recommendations (33.2% vs 24.2%, $P = .05$). A retrospective analysis of a multicenter registry of patients with severe CAP by Shorr and colleagues[45] showed that of 199 subjects, the duration of mechanical ventilation in a patient cohort given IDSA-concordant treatment was shorter by 3 days than in a cohort given discordant treatment.

Dambrava and colleagues[37] did a prospective observational study of 642 CAP patients admitted to an 800-bed hospital over a 1-year period. Seventy-one patients (9%) were admitted to the ICU and were retrospectively classified into ATS risk groups based on the 2001 ATS CAP guidelines and PSI classes.[17,35] Overall adherence to guideline recommendations was relatively low among ICU patients (52%), and no significant differences were found between adherent and nonadherent groups in terms of mortality and length of stay. Given the small numbers, however, this may simply represent a type II statistical error.

A study by Martin-Loeches and colleagues[46] using a prospective observational approach reported on outcomes for 218 CAP patients managed in 27 ICUs in 9 European countries. The objective of the study was not to compare guideline-based therapy with non-guideline therapy but instead to examine the impact of a macrolide-based regimen on mortality. Based on level 1 evidence, the 2007 IDSA/ATS CAP guidelines recommend a β-lactam such as ceftriaxone plus either azithromycin or a respiratory fluoroquinolone.[26] These agents can be modified if *Pseudomonas aeruginosa* is a consideration. A Cox regression analysis adjusted by etiology and severity showed that mortality was significantly lower when a macrolide was used as opposed to a fluoroquinolone (hazard ratio 0.48, 95% confidence interval [CI] 0.23–0.97, $P = .04$).

Frei and colleagues[26,47] reported a retrospective cohort study of 129 CAP patients admitted to 5 community hospital ICUs based on the 2007 IDSA/ATS guidelines. Overall mortality was 19%, but nonadherent treatment was associated with an inpatient mortality of 25% versus 11% for adherent therapy (odds ratio [OR] 2.99, 95% CI 1.08–9.54).

QUALITY-IMPROVEMENT MEASURES

As discussed in detail in the foregoing sections, adherence to CAP guidelines improves outcomes. Despite this, however, compliance with guidelines is suboptimal.[44,48,49] In an effort to monitor and ultimately improve quality of care by organizations, several quality measures have been created for various clinical conditions.[50] Perhaps the most well-known quality measures are those developed by the Joint Commission and the Centers for Medicare and Medicaid Services (CMS), which includes CAP as one of the targeted clinical conditions. Data on adherence and nonadherence to the measures are collected and publicly reported. Since their inception, several quality measures have been used including pneumococcal vaccination, smoking cessation, blood cultures, antibiotics within 6 hours, guideline-compliant antibiotics, influenza vaccination, and measures of oxygen levels.[50]

Evidence for Use of Quality Measures

Pneumococcal vaccination

One of the most serious sequelae of CAP is invasive pneumococcal disease (IPD).[51] Pneumococcal vaccination with the 23-valent pneumococcal polysaccharide vaccine (PPV-23) is currently recommended for all adults 65 years or older and others at increased risk of IPD.[52,53] This recommendation is based on prior research suggesting that the vaccine prevents IPD.[26] The pneumococcal vaccination performance measure determines the proportion of patients aged 65 years and older, hospitalized with CAP, who were screened for pneumococcal vaccine status and then vaccinated before discharge, if indicated.[54]

However, there is ongoing controversy over the efficacy of this vaccine, and there have been at least 12 meta-analyses attempting to determine its benefit.[55] In a Cochrane review, both randomized controlled trials (RCTs) and non-RCTs provided strong and consistent evidence of the effectiveness of the polysaccharide vaccine against IPD (OR 0.26, 95% CI 0.15–0.46), but efficacy against all-cause pneumonia was inconclusive.[56]

A systematic review of the evidence underlying performance measures for CAP found similar results; in addition, the investigators concluded that the quality of evidence supporting the use of the polysaccharide vaccine in adults 65 years or older for all outcomes studied (mortality due to pneumonia, pneumococcal pneumonia, and IPD) was very low.[54] Despite the fact that 15 RCTs met their study criteria, the RCT results were inconsistent and the generalizability of the RCTs to the patients targeted by the quality measure was questionable. In general, the RCTs did not include patients hospitalized or recovering from CAP; many patients in the trials were younger than 65 years and many did not have patients with comorbidities.[54]

The pneumococcal conjugate vaccine 13 (PCV13) was recently licensed for use in North America for adults 50 years or older, although its efficacy in the elderly is not yet clear.[57] A placebo-controlled trial of PCV13 in patients 65 years or older is currently under way in the Netherlands and is likely to provide more information about the protective effect of PCV13 against pneumococcal pneumonia in adults, but the results are not expected to be available until 2013.[58] For a more in-depth review of the value of the pneumococcal vaccine, refer to the article by Musher and colleagues elsewhere in this issue.

Smoking cessation

Smoking is an established risk factor for CAP, thereby making smoking cessation an appealing quality measure for patients with CAP.[59] The smoking-cessation performance measure determines the proportion of adult patients with CAP and a history of smoking any time during the past year who were given smoking-cessation advice or counseling during their hospitalization.[54] A 2012 Cochrane review of 50 RCTs or quasi-RCTs evaluating behavioral, pharmacologic, or multicomponent interventions in hospitalized patients to help them stop smoking found increased smoking cessation with interventions that began during the hospital stay and continued for at least 1 month after discharge (risk ratio [RR] 1.37, 95% CI 1.27–1.48).[60] However, no significant benefit was found for less intensive or shorter-duration counseling interventions.[60] The systematic review of the evidence underlying performance measures for CAP found similar results; inpatient smoking-cessation advice without outpatient follow-up did not improve smoking quit rate (relative risk [RR] 1.05, 95% CI 0.90–1.22).[54] Thus the results of the meta-analyses conflict with the recommended performance measure.[54,60]

Blood cultures

Guidelines recommend obtaining blood cultures in selected populations, including those who are critically ill.[26] The quality measure determines the proportion of adult ICU patients transferred or admitted to the ICU within 24 hours of hospital arrival with CAP, who had blood cultures performed within 24 hours before or after hospital arrival.[54] Systematic review of the evidence underlying performance measures for CAP found few data to support this quality measure. No RCTs were identified and only 2 retrospective cohort studies met inclusion criteria.[54,61,62] Blood cultures were associated with an increased likelihood of being clinically stable at 48 hours in the one study that evaluated this outcome (adjusted OR 1.62; 95% CI 1.33–2.33).[54,61] Point estimates in both included studies found an associated reduction in the relative risk of mortality among patients who had blood cultures performed; however, neither met statistical significance (adjusted OR 0.86, 95% CI 0.36–2.07[61]; and adjusted OR 0.90, 95% CI 0.81–1.0[62]). The evidence supporting this quality measure was very low for both outcomes.[54]

Antibiotics within 6 hours

The antibiotic-timing performance measure determines the proportion of adult patients with CAP who received their first dose of antibiotic(s) within 6 hours of hospital arrival.[54] Systematic review of the evidence underlying performance measures for CAP found 2 retrospective cohort studies evaluating the relationship between initial antibiotic use and risk of mortality, and 1 retrospective cohort study describing the relationship between initial antibiotic use and length of hospital stay beyond 9 days.[54] Of the studies evaluating mortality as an outcome, one showed associated benefit in adjusted analyses (adjusted OR 0.84, 95% CI 0.73–0.95)[63] and the other point estimate was associated with benefit but did not reach statistical significance (adjusted OR 0.93, 95% CI 0.85–1.02).[62] The quality of evidence was very low, as there was a serious risk of bias and imprecise estimates.[54] The one study looking at length of stay as outcome showed that patients given antibiotics within 6 hours had a lower likelihood of a prolonged length of stay (>9 days) (RR 0.31, 95% CI 0.19–0.48),[33] and the investigators concluded that this was low-quality evidence; it was an observational study with a large effect but serious risk of bias.[54] This quality measure is no longer used.

Guideline-compliant antibiotics

The antibiotic-selection performance measure determines the proportion of adult patients with CAP who received an initial antibiotic regimen consistent with current guidelines during the first 24 hours of their hospitalization.[54] As reviewed in the foregoing sections, numerous observational studies consistently show that guideline-compliant antibiotic regimens are associated with decreased mortality. Systematic review of the evidence underlying performance measures for CAP concluded that there was a moderate quality of evidence for this quality measure given the multiple observational studies, strengthened by a large effect.[54]

Influenza vaccination

Influenza is the most common viral cause of CAP,[64] therefore vaccination of elderly individuals is recommended worldwide as people aged 65 years and older are at a higher risk of complications, hospitalization, and death from influenza.[65] The influenza-vaccination performance measure determines the proportion of patients aged 50 years and older hospitalized with CAP during the months of October through March who were screened for influenza-vaccine status and then vaccinated before discharge.[54]

Cochrane systematic reviews have separated the vaccine evaluation into two separate reviews; vaccines for the prevention of influenza in healthy adults (age 16–65 years)[66] and vaccines for the prevention of influenza in the elderly (age >65 years).[65] The Cochrane systematic review summarizing influenza vaccines for the prevention of influenza in healthy adults included 50 trials.[66] When the vaccine matched the circulating viral strain, 4% of unvaccinated people versus 1% of vaccinated people developed influenza symptoms (risk difference [RD] 3%, 95% CI 2%–5%).[66] When there was a poor match between the vaccine and the circulating strain, 2% of unvaccinated people versus 1% of vaccinated people developed influenza (RD 1, 95% CI 0%–3%).[66] There was no evidence that the influenza vaccine affected complications such as pneumonia or transmission.[66]

The Cochrane systematic review summarizing influenza vaccines for the prevention of influenza in the elderly included 75 studies, but only one RCT assessed the currently available vaccines and reached satisfactory completion[65,67]; the remainder of the studies were observational. In the one RCT the incidences of clinical influenza were 2% in the vaccinated group and 3% in the unvaccinated group (RR 0.53, 95% CI 0.39–0.73).[67] The Cochrane review concluded that the available evidence is of poor quality and provides no guidance regarding the safety, efficacy, or effectiveness of influenza vaccines for people aged 65 years or older.[65] It is thought that the relative ineffectiveness of inactivated influenza vaccine in an elderly population is due to immunosenescence.[68]

The systematic review of the evidence underlying performance measures for CAP identified 26 RCTs that compared influenza vaccination with no influenza vaccination, and measured patient-important outcomes.[54] Meta-analysis of the RCTs found that influenza vaccination decreased the incidence of both laboratory-confirmed cases of symptomatic influenza (RR 0.30, 95% CI 0.22–0.40) and influenza-like illness (RR 0.74, 95% CI 0.67–0.82). The investigators concluded that the performance measures provided high-quality evidence for laboratory-confirmed cases of symptomatic influenza, because of the numerous RCTs with large effect, but only moderate-quality evidence for influenza-like illness because of the inconsistent results associated with the RCTs.[54] Of note, the investigators did not comment on the generalizability of the RCTs despite the fact that many of them included healthy adults younger than 50 years, and in general the RCTs did not include hospitalized acutely ill patients.

Oxygen

The initial Joint Commission and CMS quality measures included measures of blood oxygen levels, as hypoxemia is common among patients with severe pneumonia and is associated with risk of mortality.[26] However, as of 2006 compliance with this measure was reported as 99%, thus it is no longer included as a quality measure.[69]

Summary of CAP quality indicators

Of the CAP quality indicators, influenza vaccination and guideline-compliant antibiotics have the highest quality of evidence to support them. In the 2012 version of the Joint Commission and CMS quality indicators, the CAP quality indicators included obtaining blood cultures and guideline-compliant antibiotic use. Smoking cessation and use of influenza and pneumococcal vaccination are now part of the core measure set for all inpatient admissions, not just CAP.[50] Although it is unknown whether the process of simply implementing such indicators improves outcomes given that all hospitals in the United States are required to report on the quality indicators, it would be ideal if future CAP quality indicators were based on sound evidence.

Does Pay for Performance Using Quality Indicators Improve Outcomes?

In an effort to accelerate hospitals' quality-improvement outcomes, the idea of tying financial incentives to outcomes has gained acceptance as an approach to improving the quality of health care in the United States.[70] Several quality measures have been used by CMS to determine reimbursement eligibility including CAP quality indicators.[69] Studies evaluating the effect of pay-for-performance measures on process-based quality have been mixed. An initial study evaluated quality-improvement scores in 613 hospitals over a period of 2 years.[71] The study compared results between 207 facilities that participated in pay for performance and 406 hospitals that did not. After adjustments were made for differences in baseline performance and other hospital characteristics, pay for performance was associated with improvements ranging from 2.6% to 4.1%.[71] However, a follow-up study showed that although there was initial improvement, after 5 years there was no difference in quality-improvement scores between hospitals who did or did not participate in pay-for-performance measures.[72] Neither study considered clinically important outcomes.

A recently published study sought to determine whether pay-for-performance measures between 2002 and 2009 improved the clinically important outcome, 30-day mortality.[70] The study compared the effect of the addition of pay for performance to public reporting with public reporting alone. At baseline the 30-day mortality was similar between the two groups (12.33% for pay-for-performance hospitals and 12.40% for non–pay-for-performance hospitals, difference of −0.07%, 95% CI −0.40 to 0.26). Mortality rates remained similar after 6 years under the pay-for-performance system (11.82% for pay-for-performance hospitals and 11.74% for non–pay-for-performance hospitals, difference of 0.08%, 95% CI −0.30 to 0.46). The effects of pay for performance did not differ significantly among conditions for which outcomes were explicitly linked to incentives including CAP. At the end of the study period, 30-day mortality for patients with CAP was 11.71% for pay-for-performance hospitals and 11.85% for non–pay-for-performance hospitals (difference of −0.14%, 95% CI −0.67 to 0.38).[70]

SUMMARY

Taken as a whole, the body of evidence supporting the positive effects of guidelines on outcomes in patients with CAP is extraordinary. Particularly for those ill enough to require hospitalization, the data appear to be compelling. A recent meta-analysis dealing with mortality in hospitalized CAP patients concluded that "guideline concordance is more important than choice of antibiotics when treating CAP."[73] By contrast, the evidence supporting many of the CAP quality indicators is low, and pay-for-performance measures do not seem to influence clinically important outcomes. Future CAP quality indicators should incorporate evidence-based interventions.

REFERENCES

1. Brar NK, Niederman MS. Management of community-acquired pneumonia: a review and update. Ther Adv Respir Dis 2011;5(1):61–78.
2. Jackson ML, Neuzil KM, Thompson WW, et al. The burden of community-acquired pneumonia in seniors: results of a population-based study. Clin Infect Dis 2004;39:1642–50.
3. Nazarian D, Eddy OL, Lukens TW, et al. Clinical policy: critical issues in the management of adult patients presenting to the emergency department with community-acquired pneumonia. Ann Emerg Med 2005;54(5):704–31.
4. European Respiratory Society. Pneumonia. In: Loddenhempe R, editor. European lung white book. Lausane. European Respiratory Society; 2003. p. 55–65.
5. Gleason PP, Kapoor WN, Stone RA, et al. Medical outcomes and antimicrobial costs with the use of the American Thoracic Society guidelines for outpatients with community-acquired pneumonia. JAMA 1997;278:32–9.
6. Suchyta MR, Dean NC, Narus S, et al. Effects of a practice guideline for community-acquired pneumonia in an outpatient setting. Am J Med 2001;110: 306–9.
7. Niederman MS, Bass JB, Campbell GD, et al. Guidelines for the initial management of adults with community-acquired pneumonia: diagnosis, assessment of severity, and initial antimicrobial therapy. American Thoracic Society. Medical Section of the American Lung Association. Am Rev Respir Dis 1993;148:1418–26.
8. Bjerre LM, Verheij TJ, Kochen MM. Antibiotics for community acquired pneumonia in adult outpatients. Cochrane Database Syst Rev 2009;(4):CD002109.

9. Dean NC, Silver MP, Bateman KA, et al. Decreased mortality after implementation of a treatment guideline for community-acquired pneumonia. Am J Med 2001; 110:451–7.
10. Musher DM, Rueda AM, Kaka AS, et al. The association between pneumococcal pneumonia and acute cardiac events. Clin Infect Dis 2007;45(2):158–65.
11. Dudas V, Hopefl A, Jacobs R, et al. Antimicrobial selection for hospitalized patients with presumed community-acquired pneumonia: a survey of non-teaching US community hospitals. Ann Pharmacother 2000;34:446–52.
12. Menendez R, Ferrando D, Valles JM, et al. Influence of deviation from guidelines on the outcome of community-acquired pneumonia. Chest 2002;122:612–7.
13. Capelastegui A, Espana PP, Quintana JM, et al. Improvement of process-of-care and outcomes after implementing a guideline for the management of community-acquired pneumonia: a controlled before-and-after design study. Clin Infect Dis 2004;39:955–63.
14. Frei CR, Restrepo MI, Mortensen EM, et al. Impact of guideline-concordant empiric antibiotic therapy in community-acquired pneumonia. Am J Med 2006; 119:865–71.
15. Dean NC, Bateman KA, Donnelly SM, et al. Improved clinical outcomes with utilization of a community-acquired pneumonia guideline. Chest 2006;130:794–9.
16. Mortensen EM, Restrepo MI, Anzueto A, et al. Antibiotic therapy and 48-hour mortality for patients with pneumonia. Am J Med 2006;119:859–64.
17. Fine MJ, Auble TE, Yealy DM, et al. A prediction rule to identify low risk patients with community-acquired pneumonia. N Engl J Med 1997;336(4):243–50.
18. Calzada RS, Martinez Tomas R, Cremades Romero MJ, et al. Empiric treatment in hospitalized community-acquired pneumonia. Impact on mortality, length of stay and re-admission. Respir Med 2007;101(9):1909–15.
19. Garau J, Baquero F, Perez-Trallero E, et al. Factors impacting on length of stay and mortality of community-acquired pneumonia. Clin Microbiol Infect 2008;14:322–9.
20. Arnold FW, Summersgill JT, Lajoie AS, et al, Community-Acquired Pneumonia Organization (CAPO) Investigators. A worldwide perspective of atypical pathogens in community-acquired pneumonia. Am J Respir Crit Care Med 2007; 175(10):1086–93.
21. Mandell LA, Marrie TJ, Grossman RF, et al. Canadian guidelines for the initial management of community-acquired pneumonia: an evidence-based update by the Canadian Infectious Diseases Society and the Canadian Thoracic Society. The Canadian Community-Acquired Pneumonia Working Group. Clin Infect Dis 2000;31(2):383–421.
22. Yanagihara K, Kohno S, Matsusima T. Japanese guidelines for the management of community-acquired pneumonia [review]. Int J Antimicrob Agents 2001; 18(Suppl 1):S45–8.
23. Vogel F, Worth H, Adam D, et al, For the Paul Ehrlich Society for Chemotherapy and the German Respiratory Association. Rational treatment of bacterial respiratory tract infections. Chemotherapie Journal 2000;1:3–23 [in German].
24. Menendez R, Reyes S, Martinez R, et al. Economic evaluation of adherence to treatment guidelines in non-intensive care pneumonia. Eur Respir J 2007;29: 751–6.
25. Blasi F, Iori I, Bulfoni A, et al. Can CAP guideline adherence improve patient outcome in internal medicine departments? Eur Respir J 2008;32:902–10.
26. Mandell LA, Wunderink RG, Anzueto A, et al. IDSA/ATS consensus guidelines on the management of community-acquired pneumonia. Clin Infect Dis 2007;44: S27–72.

27. McCabe C, Kirchner C, Zhang H, et al. Guideline-concordant therapy and reduced mortality and length of stay in adults with community-acquired pneumonia: playing by the rules. Arch Intern Med 2009;169(16):1525–31.
28. Stahl JE, Barza M, DesJardin J, et al. Effect of macrolides as part of initial empiric therapy on length of stay in patients hospitalized with community-acquired pneumonia. Arch Intern Med 1999;159:2576–80.
29. Gora-Harper ML, Rapp RP, Finney JP. Development of a best-practice model at a university hospital to increase efficiency in the management of patients with community-acquired pneumonia. Am J Health Syst Pharm 2000;57(Suppl 3):S6–9.
30. Bartlett JG, Breiman RF, Mandell LA, et al. Community-acquired pneumonia in adults: guidelines for management. The Infectious Diseases Society of America. Clin Infect Dis 1998;26(4):811–38.
31. Marrie TJ, Lau CY, Wheeler SL, et al. A controlled trial of a critical pathway for treatment of community-acquired pneumonia. Capital Study Investigators. Community-acquired pneumonia intervention trial assessing levofloxacin. JAMA 2000;283:749–55.
32. Meehan TP, Weingarten SR, Holmboe ES, et al. A statewide initiative to improve the care of hospitalized pneumonia patients: the Connecticut Pneumonia Pathway Project. Am J Med 2001;111:203–10.
33. Battleman DS, Callahan M, Thaler HT. Rapid antibiotic delivery and appropriate antibiotic selection reduce length of hospital stay of patients with community-acquired pneumonia: link between quality of care and resource utilization. Arch Intern Med 2002;162:682–8.
34. Orrick JJ, Segal R, Johns TE, et al. Resource use and cost of care for patients hospitalised with community acquired pneumonia: impact of adherence to Infectious Diseases Society of America guidelines. Pharmacoeconomics 2004;22: 751–7.
35. Niederman MS, Mandell LA, Anzueto A, et al. Guidelines for the management of adults with community-acquired pneumonia. Diagnosis, assessment of severity, antimicrobial therapy, and prevention. American Thoracic Society. Am J Respir Crit Care Med 2001;163(7):1730–54.
36. Mandell LA, Bartlett JG, Dowell SF, et al. Update of practice guidelines for the management of community-acquired pneumonia in immunocompetent adults. Infectious Diseases Society of America. Clin Infect Dis 2003;37(11):1405–33.
37. Dambrava PG, Torres A, Valles X, et al. Adherence to guidelines' empirical antibiotic recommendations and community-acquired pneumonia outcome. Eur Respir J 2008;32:892–901.
38. Menendez R, Torres A, Rodriguez de Castro F, et al. Reaching stability in community-acquired pneumonia: the effects of the severity of disease, treatment, and the characteristics of patients. Clin Infect Dis 2004;39:1783–90.
39. Marrie TJ, Shariatzadeh MR. Community-acquired pneumonia requiring admission to an intensive care unit: a descriptive study. Medicine (Baltimore) 2007; 86:103–11.
40. Riley PD, Aronsky D, Dean NC. Validation of the 2001 American Thoracic Society criteria for severe community-acquired pneumonia. Crit Care Med 2004;32: 2398–402.
41. Woodhead MA, Macfarlane JT, Rodgers FG, et al. Aetiology and outcome of severe community-acquired pneumonia. J Infect 1985;10:204–10.
42. Leroy O, Saux P, Bedos JP, et al. Comparison of levofloxacin and cefotaxime combined with ofloxacin for ICU patients with community-acquired pneumonia who do not require vasopressors. Chest 2005;128:172–83.

43. Rello J. Demographics, guidelines, and clinical experience in severe community-acquired pneumonia. Crit Care 2008;12(Suppl 6):S2.
44. Bodí M, Rodríguez A, Solé-Violán J, et al. Community-acquired pneumonia intensive care units (CAPUCI) study investigators. Antibiotic prescription for community-acquired pneumonia in the intensive care unit: impact of adherence to Infectious Diseases Society of America guidelines on survival. Clin Infect Dis 2005;41(12):1709–16.
45. Shorr AF, Bodi M, Rodriguez A, et al, CAPUCI Study Investigators. Impact of antibiotic guideline compliance on duration of mechanical ventilation in critically ill patients with community-acquired pneumonia. Chest 2006;130(1):93–100.
46. Martin-Loeches I, Lisboa T, Rodriguez A, et al. Combination antibiotic therapy with macrolides improves survival in intubated patients with community-acquired pneumonia. Intensive Care Med 2010;36(4):612–20.
47. Frei CR, Attridge RT, Mortensen EM, et al. Guideline-concordant antibiotic use and survival among patients with community-acquired pneumonia admitted to the intensive care unit. Clin Ther 2010;32(2):293–9.
48. Wu J, Howard D, McGowan J Jr, et al. Adherence to Infectious Diseases Society of America guidelines for empiric therapy for patients with community acquired pneumonia in a commercially insured cohort. Clin Ther 2006;28:141–1461.
49. Menendez R, Torres A, Zalacain R, et al. Guidelines for the treatment of community-acquired pneumonia: predictors of adherence and outcome. Am J Respir Crit Care Med 2005;172:757–62.
50. Centers for Medicare and Medicaid Services, the Joint Commission. Specification manual for national hospital quality measures. Available at: http://www.jointcommission.org/specifications_manual_for_national_hospital_inpatient_quality_measures.aspx. Accessed August 31, 2012.
51. Feikin DR, Schuchat A, Kolczak M, et al. Mortality from invasive pneumococcal pneumonia in the era of antibiotic resistance, 1995-1997. Am J Public Health 2000;90(2):223–9.
52. Centers for Disease Control and Prevention. Updated recommendations for prevention of invasive pneumococcal disease among adults using the 23-valent pneumococcal polysaccharide vaccine (PPSV23). MMWR Morb Mortal Wkly Rep 2010;59(34):1102–6.
53. Pneumococcal vaccination. In: Public Health Agency of Canada. Canadian immunization guide. 7th edition. Ottawa (Canada): Public Health Agency of Canada; 2006. p. 267–76.
54. Wilson K, Schunemann H. An appraisal of the evidence underlying performance measures for community acquired pneumonia. Am J Respir Crit Care Med 2011;183:1454–62.
55. Andrews R, Moberley A. The controversy over the efficacy of pneumococcal vaccine. CMAJ 2009;180:18–9.
56. Moberley S, Holden J, Tatham DP, et al. Vaccines for preventing pneumococcal infection in adults. Cochrane Database Syst Rev 2008;(1):CD000422.
57. Centers for Disease Control and Prevention. Licensure of 13-valent pneumococcal conjugate vaccine for adults aged 50 years and older. MMWR Morb Mortal Wkly Rep 2012;61:394–5.
58. Hak E, Grobbee DE, Sanders EA, et al. Rationale and design of CAPITA: a RCT of 13-valent conjugated pneumococcal vaccine efficacy among older adults. Neth J Med 2008;66(9):378–83.
59. Nuorti J, Butler J, Farley M, et al. Cigarette smoking and invasive pneumococcal disease. Active Bacterial Core Surveillance Team. N Engl J Med 2000;342:681–9.

60. Rigotti N, Clair C, Munafo M, et al. Interventions for smoking cessation in hospitalized patients. Cochrane Database Syst Rev 2012;(5):CD001837.
61. Dedier J, Singer D, Chang Y, et al. Processes of care, illness severity, and outcomes in the management of community-acquired pneumonia at academic hospitals. Arch Intern Med 2001;161:2099–104.
62. Meehan T, Fine M, Krumholz H, et al. Quality of care process and outcomes in elderly patients with pneumonia. JAMA 1997;278:2080–4.
63. Houck P, Bratzler D, Nsa W, et al. Timing of antibiotic administration and outcomes for Medicare patients hospitalized with community-acquired pneumonia. Arch Intern Med 2004;164:637–44.
64. Falsey AR, Walsh EE. Viral pneumonia in older adults. Clin Infect Dis 2006;42:518–24.
65. Jefferson T, Di Pietrantonj C, Al-Ansary LA, et al. Vaccines for preventing influenza in the elderly. Cochrane Database Syst Rev 2010;(2):CD004876.
66. Jefferson T, Di Pietrantonj C, Rivetti A, et al. Vaccines for preventing influenza in healthy adults. Cochrane Database Syst Rev 2010;(7):CD001269.
67. Govaert TM, Thijs CT, Masurel N, et al. The efficacy of influenza vaccination in elderly individuals. A randomized double-blind placebo-controlled trial. JAMA 1994;272:1661–5.
68. Fulop T, Pawelec G, Castle S, et al. Immunosenescence and vaccination in nursing home residents. Clin Infect Dis 2009;48:443–8.
69. Shorr A, Owens R Jr. Guidelines and quality for community-acquired pneumonia: measures from the Joint Commission and the Centers for Medicare and Medicaid Services. Am J Health Syst Pharm 2009;66:S2–7.
70. Jha A, Joynt K, Orav J, et al. The long-term effect of premier pay for performance on patient outcomes. N Engl J Med 2012;366:1606–15.
71. Lindenauer P, Remus D, Roman S, et al. Public reporting and pay for performance in hospital quality improvement. N Engl J Med 2007;356:486–96.
72. Werner R, Kolstad J, Stuart E, et al. The effect of pay-for-performance in hospitals: lessons for quality improvement. Health Aff (Millwood) 2011;30:690–8.
73. Asadi L, Sligl WI, Eurich DT, et al. Macrolide based regimens and mortality in hospitalized patients with community-acquired pneumonia: a systematic review and meta-analysis. Clin Infect Dis 2012;55(3):371–8.

What Is the Relevance of Antimicrobial Resistance on the Outcome of Community-Acquired Pneumonia Caused by *Streptococcus pneumoniae*? (Should Macrolide Monotherapy Be Used for Mild Pneumonia?)

Donald E. Low, MD, FRCP(C)

KEYWORDS

- Community-acquired pneumonia • *Streptococcus pneumoniae*
- Antimicrobial resistance • Resistance paradox • Pollyanna phenomenon
- Macrolides • β-lactams • Fluoroquinolones

KEY POINTS

- The prevalence and degree of antimicrobial-resistant *Streptococcus pneumoniae* continue to increase worldwide.
- Many practitioners believe in what has been promulgated by some as the resistance paradox: in vivo susceptibility in the face of in vitro resistance.
- Although there is a need for high-quality evidence to define the level of resistance that is relevant, the complexity and cost of such studies make this unlikely to occur.
- There is also a need to define the prevalence of resistance at which changes in recommendations for empirical therapy are warranted.
- In the face of increasing rates of macrolide-resistant pneumococci and evidence that both low-level and high-level macrolide resistance are associated with clinical failures, it is no longer prudent to recommend macrolides for the monotherapy for CAP.

INTRODUCTION

Community-acquired pneumonia (CAP) is a common clinical disease with considerable morbidity and mortality. *Streptococcus pneumoniae* is the leading cause of CAP across all severities of illness. It accounts for approximately two-thirds of cases

Department of Microbiology, Mount Sinai Hospital/University Health Network and University of Toronto, 600 University Avenue, Room 1487, Toronto, Ontario M5G 1X5, Canada
E-mail address: delow@mtsinai.on.ca

Infect Dis Clin N Am 27 (2013) 87–97
http://dx.doi.org/10.1016/j.idc.2012.11.013
0891-5520/13/$ – see front matter © 2013 Elsevier Inc. All rights reserved.

id.theclinics.com

in which an etiologic diagnosis has been made, as well as for two-thirds of the cases of bacteremia.[1] The frequency of other agents, especially those designated atypical pathogens (*Legionella pneumophila*, *Mycoplasma pneumoniae* and *Chlamydophila pneumoniae*), varies with season, geographic area, age groups, and diagnostic means available and these agents more typically cause mild to moderate severity of illness. The advent of antibiotics was a transforming intervention for the treatment of pneumococcal pneumonia. However, the emergence and dissemination of resistance in *S pneumoniae* have caused considerable concern in the infectious diseases community and confusion amongst medical practitioners. The concern is that we are losing some of our most safe and effective antimicrobials for the treatment of this important infection. The confusion amongst practitioners is a result of being warned about the problem of emerging resistance but failing to see its consequences in their clinical practice. This belief has been promulgated by some as the resistance paradox.

THE ROOT OF THE PROBLEM

Antimicrobial resistance among *S pneumoniae* continues to increase in prevalence, especially for the frequently used β-lactams, macrolides, and fluoroquinolones.[2] Modified antimicrobial use, the introduction of the 7-valent and 13-valent pneumococcal conjugate vaccines (PCV-7 and PCV-13), changing in vitro antimicrobial susceptibility criteria, as well as other variables, have altered antimicrobial resistance patterns among pneumococci (**Fig. 1**).[2]

β-lactams

Breakpoints are minimum inhibitory concentrations (MICs), which define bacteria as susceptible (treatable), intermediate (possibly treatable with higher doses), and resistant (not treatable) to certain antimicrobials. In January, 2008, the Clinical and

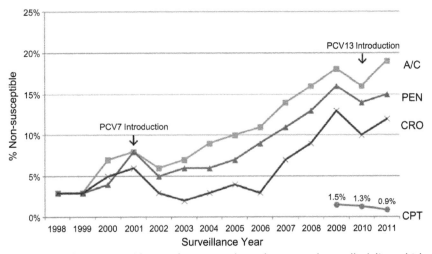

Fig. 1. Profile of nonsusceptible rates for commonly used parenteral or orally delivered β-lactams tested against 18,911 *S pneumoniae* isolates from the US SENTRY Program (1998–2011). A/C, amoxicillin/clavulanate; PEN, penicillin, high-dose; CRO, ceftriaxone; CPT, ceftaroline. (*Reprinted from* Jones RN, Sader HS, Mendes RE, et al. Update on antimicrobial susceptibility trends among *Streptococcus pneumoniae* in the United States: report of ceftaroline activity from the SENTRY Antimicrobial Surveillance Program (1998–2011). Diagn Microbiol Infect Dis 2012; doi:10.1016/j.diagmicrobio.2012.08.024; with permission.)

Laboratory Standards Institute (CLSI) published new *S pneumoniae* break points for penicillin.[3] Previously, susceptibility breakpoints were based on MIC distributions, the severity of the infection that an organism may cause, and anecdotal case reports. For *Pneumococcus*, it also included attainable concentrations of penicillin in cerebrospinal fluid and the MIC at which meningitis treatment was believed to fail. The result was overly conservative breakpoints for nonmeningeal infections, with the susceptible category defined as 0.06 μg/mL or less. However, published studies evaluating penicillin as monotherapy for treatment during the first 48 hours of nonmeningitis pneumococcal infections have not shown increased case-fatality rates associated with penicillin MICs of 2 μg/mL or less.[4–6] These studies provided evidence that the original breakpoints for penicillin underestimated the clinical usefulness of that agent for intravenous therapy for nonmeningitis pneumococcal infections. This information, in addition to pharmacokinetic (PK) and pharmacodynamic (PD) data resulted in a significant change in breakpoints for *S pneumoniae*. Under the former criteria, susceptible, intermediate, and resistant MIC breakpoints for penicillin were 0.06 or less, 0.12 to 1, and 2 μg/mL or greater, respectively, for all pneumococcal isolates, regardless of clinical syndrome or route of penicillin administration. Those breakpoints remain unchanged for patients without meningitis who can be treated with oral penicillin. However, for patients without meningitis who are treated with intravenous penicillin, the new breakpoints are 2 or less, 4, and 8 μg/mL or greater, respectively. In addition, isolates from patients with meningitis are now categorized as either susceptible or resistant, with intravenous penicillin breakpoints of 0.06 or less or 0.12 μg/mL or greater, respectively.

To assess the potential effects of the new breakpoints on susceptibility categorization, the Centers for Disease Control and Prevention applied them to MICs of invasive pneumococcal disease isolates collected by the Active Bacterial Core surveillance system at sites in 10 states during 2006 to 2007. The percentage of invasive pneumococcal disease nonmeningitis *S pneumoniae* isolates categorized as susceptible, intermediate, and resistant to penicillin changed from 75%, 15%, and 10% under the former breakpoints to 93%, 6%, and 1.2%, respectively, under the new breakpoints (**Fig. 2**).[7] The hope is that this categorization results in the increased use of

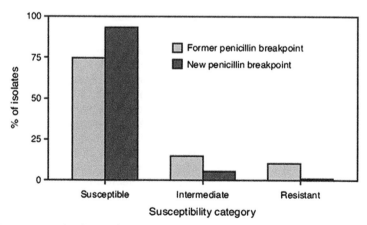

Fig. 2. Percentage of isolates of *S pneumoniae* that were categorized as susceptible, intermediate, or resistant under former and new penicillin breakpoints. (*From* Centers for Disease Control and Prevention (CDC). Effects of new penicillin susceptibility breakpoints for Streptococcus pneumoniae–United States, 2006–2007. MMWR Morb Mortal Wkly Rep 2008; 57:1353–5.)

penicillin for the treatment of pneumococcal infections. However, there is concern, and some evidence for this, that the inconvenience of intravenous penicillin may limit its use, despite a reduction in numbers of infections considered resistant.[8]

Macrolides

Macrolide resistance has emerged worldwide.[2,9–11] A global international surveillance project found that the overall rate of erythromycin resistance was 37%, although significant geographic differences in these rates were observed. In North America, resistant rates hover at about 45%,[2] whereas in Asia, they are greater than 80%.[11] Macrolide resistance in *S pneumoniae* is mediated mainly by 2 major mechanisms; target site modification encoded by the *erm*(B) gene (resulting in high-level resistance; MIC, ≥ 16 µg/mL) and an efflux pump encoded by *mef* genes (resulting in low-level resistance; MIC <16 µg/mL).

Despite the high prevalence of macrolide resistance, macrolides continue to be recommended as monotherapy for CAP in the outpatient setting for patients who have been previously healthy and have no risk factors for drug-resistant pneumococcal infection. The Infectious Diseases Society of America (IDSA) and the American Thoracic Society (ATS) Consensus Guidelines on the management of CAP have considered only a macrolide MIC of 16 µg/mL or greater as the breakpoint for resistance.[12] Only in regions with a high rate (>25%) of infection with high-level macrolide-resistant *S pneumoniae*, have they suggested the use of alternative agents.

WHY THE CONFUSION?

In most infections, the patient presents with a clinical illness, a pathogen is identified, antimicrobial susceptibility testing is performed to determine if the organism is susceptible, the patient is treated, and the response to therapy can be observe. If discordant therapy results in clinical or bacteriologic failures and exceeds an agreed failure rate, alternative antimicrobials can be recommended for empirical therapy. Urethritis caused by *Neisseria gonorrhoeae* is 1 example in which the relevance of a decrease in the activity of an antimicrobial can be determined, and guidelines exist that inform us when to change empirical therapy.

So why is the process of dealing with emerging resistance not so straightforward in CAP? There are several reasons:

1. The Pollyanna phenomenon, or false optimism, that is experienced when, despite the use of an antibiotic for which high levels of resistance exist, few if any clinical failures are seen.[13] The patient presenting to a health care setting with lower respiratory tract symptoms is not infrequently diagnosed with CAP, but does not meet diagnostic criteria for CAP.[14] Most CAP is managed in primary care, where access to rapid chest radiography is limited or nonexistent. Consequently, in contrast with the hospital setting (where the diagnosis of CAP is confirmed by chest radiographic features), diagnosis in the community is often based only on the clinical features. In this setting, clinicians have to differentiate those patients presenting with CAP from most patients who have acute, nonpneumonic lower respiratory tract infections or other diagnoses. As a result, often patients are treated with antibiotics who do not have CAP or who have CAP with a nonbacterial cause, giving the physician the impression that resistance is not a concern in their patient population, because most patients' symptoms resolve.
2. In those patients who meet the diagnostic criteria for CAP in the outpatient setting, only about 20% have CAP caused by *S pneumoniae*, and of those, only 15% have an MIC greater than 2 µg/mL. Because almost all decisions regarding therapy are

empirical and because in most cases, a cause is not identified, most patients are treated with a pneumococcal antimicrobial who do not have CAP caused by a pneumococcal-resistant strain. For those patients who do fail therapy, the physician often changes therapy without further diagnostic testing.

3. Depending on the age of the patient and the presence of comorbidities, many patients with bacterial infections recover without antimicrobials. Tilghman and Finland[15] in the 1930s, even before the advent of antimicrobial therapy, showed that many patients with pneumococcal pneumonia recovered; morbidity and mortality depended on the type of *Pneumococcus* causing the infection, the age of the patient, the extent of the pulmonary involvement, alcoholism, and preexisting diseases and conditions. Evans and Gaisford[16] reported that 73 of 100 patients with untreated lobar pneumonia survived their illness.

4. The original CLSI penicillin antimicrobial susceptibility breakpoints were too conservative. Peterson[17] found in his review of the literature that documentation of failure of penicillin treatment, particularly with aminopenicillins administered at adequate dosages (eg, parenterally), was virtually nonexistent.

5. Some patients with adequately treated CAP caused by *S pneumoniae* die despite adequate therapy.[18]

6. As pointed out by Metaly and Singer,[19] drug resistance translates into clinical failures only if clinicians continue to use agents that are affected by the resistance mechanisms shown by the bacteria: discordant therapy. Recent trends in antimicrobial drug prescribing in the United States suggest that physicians move on to newer therapies soon after the emergence of resistance to older drugs, thus limiting the frequency of observable discordant therapy in most outcomes studies.

DOES RESISTANCE MATTER?

The use of antimicrobials has reduced the morbidity and mortality associated with pneumococcal pneumonia, and the emergence of resistance has resulted in clinical failures.[17] One of the first clinical trials on the treatment of pneumonia with an antimicrobial documented treatment failure in association of the emergence of resistance. Moore and Chesney[20] treated 32 cases of lobar pneumonia (31 confirmed as caused by *S pneumoniae*) with ethylhydrocuprein (optochin) for a mortality of 25%. In 1 patient who failed therapy, a strain of *Pneumococcus* obtained at autopsy, which was originally susceptible to optochin, had become fast or resistant to optochin. If antimicrobials have been responsible for such a dramatic reduction in mortality from pneumococcal pneumonia, resistance to that antimicrobial would result in clinical failure. The challenge is defining the level of resistance (MIC) that accurately defines resistance.

β-lactams

Despite the decreasing susceptibility of pneumococci to penicillin, convincing evidence that resistance has an adverse effect on clinical outcomes, particularly mortality, is lacking.[1] Tleyieh and colleagues[21] conducted a meta-analysis, including 10 prospective cohort studies, that involved 3430 patients who developed pneumococcal pneumonia between 1998 and 2001. Although the investigators concluded that there was an increased short-term risk for mortality associated with penicillin-resistant pneumococcal pneumonia, there was no difference in the outcome between patients with penicillin-resistant pneumococcal pneumonia treated concordantly (susceptible at the former MIC of ≤ 0.06 μg/mL) and those who were treated discordantly. This finding suggests that the increase in short-term mortality might be associated with factors other than discordance of therapy such as disease severity and comorbidity. Feikin and colleagues[22] examined cases of invasive pneumococcal pneumonia and found that, although the impact of penicillin resistance on overall mortality did not achieve statistical significance, when deaths within the first 4 days of hospitalization were excluded, mortality was significantly associated with isolates resistant to penicillin (MIC >4 μg/mL; odds ratio = 7). However, the data were not adjusted for severity nor was antimicrobial therapy included in this study, preventing the impact of antimicrobial discordance on mortality from being determined. A study by Turett and colleagues[23] described an association of penicillin MICs greater than 2 μg/mL with mortality, yet the study was limited in that more than half of the patients had human immunodeficiency virus (HIV) infection, making it difficult to extrapolate findings to the general population, and most patients received vancomycin or ceftriaxone, not penicillin. Thus, the prevailing view has been that current levels of penicillin resistance do not adversely affect outcomes for CAP in immunocompetent patients if the MIC is less than 4.0 mg/mL (most nonsusceptible isolates).

Macrolides

Lonks and colleagues[24] reviewed medical records of 76 patients with macrolide-resistant pneumococci in their bloodstream. These investigators found that 18 patients had received treatment with a macrolide and had developed bacteremia after 3 to 5 days of therapy. Occurrence of treatment failure was evenly divided among patients who received older and newer macrolides and patients infected with pneumococcal strains, with resistance based on either drug efflux or target mutation. Daneman and colleagues[10] reviewed 5 years of prospective surveillance data that included 1696 episodes of pneumococcal bacteremia (8.5 cases/100,000 population/y), of which 60 (3.5%) were failures of outpatient macrolide therapy. Resistant isolates were more common among cases of bacteremia after failure of macrolide therapy (64%) than among cases of bacteremia after failure of nonmacrolide antibiotics (22%) or cases of bacteremia that occurred without previous antibiotic therapy (12%). Macrolide failures were significantly more common among cases of pneumococcal bacteremia with isolates showing an erythromycin MIC of 1 μg/mL than among isolates showing MICs 0.25 μg/mL or less. Low-level resistance conferred by mefA and high-level resistance conferred by ermB were equally overrepresented among macrolide failures.

Fluoroquinolones

Ciprofloxacin, the first fluoroquinolone to be used to treat lower respiratory tract infections, shows poor potency against S pneumoniae, and its introduction was associated with the rapid emergence of resistance in pneumococci.[25] Since the late 1990s, newer fluoroquinolones with enhanced pneumococcal activity, including levofloxacin and moxifloxacin, have replaced these earlier antimicrobials as the fluoroquinolones of choice for the treatment of CAP. Despite the widespread use of these agents, fluoroquinolone-resistant pneumococci have remained less than 2% in most countries.[2,26] Several case reports of treatment failures caused by fluoroquinolone-resistant pneumococcal infections in adults with CAP have been reported.[27,28] Many of the patients described in these reports had been previously treated with fluoroquinolones.

WHAT IS THE SOLUTION?
Clinical Trials

Why have increasing rates of drug resistance among bacteria isolated from clinical infections not translated into easily recognizable rates of treatment failure with specific antibiotic drugs? The major methodological challenges underlying research in this area are summarized in **Table 1**. With so many variables that affect the outcome (age of the patient, comorbidities, dose of the antimicrobial, the level of resistance, the type of organism, the time of onset of symptoms until the diagnosis and initiation of appropriate therapy), designing and funding a clinical trial, just to clarify the level of resistance that would be relevant for 1 antimicrobial within a class, would be difficult. Therefore, we continue to have to rely on case reports and observational studies.

Breakpoints

The approach that CLSI took in reevaluating the penicillin susceptibility breakpoints for pneumococci is a model that should be used to determine breakpoints for current and new antimicrobials.[29] Three types of data sets were used: microbiologic, PK/PD, and clinical outcome.[3] The microbiologic data include MIC distributions of the relevant drug against clinical isolates from broad geographic origins, strains with known drug resistance mechanisms, analysis of cross-susceptibility or resistance with other relevant antimicrobials (eg, penicillins and cephalosporins), and correlation of results obtained with different testing methods (eg, disk diffusion vs broth dilution). PK/PD data include PK profiles of the drug in serum or plasma, the percentage of protein binding of the drug, and information linking drug exposure to killing of the organisms observed in vitro or in animal models. Clinical outcome data for new drugs usually come from controlled clinical trials. However, in the case of an older agent such as penicillin, data must be collected from a variety of sources and include dosage used, frequency of administration, and a measure of clinical response stratified by the MICs of the organisms recovered.

Diagnostic Testing

Timely knowledge as to whether or not an infection has a bacterial or viral cause is necessary for appropriate management. In recent years, procalcitonin (the prohormone of calcitonin) has emerged as a promising marker for the diagnosis of bacterial infections, because higher levels are found in severe bacterial infections but remain low in viral infections and nonspecific inflammatory diseases. Procalcitonin is released in multiple tissues in response to bacterial infections via a direct stimulation of

Table 1
Methodological challenges in assessing the impact of antibiotic resistance on medical outcomes for patients with lower respiratory tract infections

Methodological Challenge	Impact on Outcomes Studies	Solution
Antibiotic efficacy only partially determines outcomes	Decreases power of studies to detect the impact of drug resistance	Increase sample size of outcomes studies
Interpretation of in vitro levels of susceptibility not correlated with in vivo predictions of PK/PD models	Misclassification of patients as exposed to resistant infections	Apply PK/PD-predicted breakpoints to interpretation of susceptibility results
Drug resistance only affects outcomes in setting of discordant therapy	Misclassification of patients as exposed to resistant infections	Consider both treatment and pathogen susceptibility in interpreting outcomes research

Reprinted from Metlay JP and Singer DE. Outcomes in lower respiratory tract infections and the impact of antimicrobial drug resistance. Clin Microbiol Infect 2002;8(Suppl 2):1–11; with permission.

cytokines, such as interleukin 1β (IL-1β), tumor necrosis factor α, and IL-6. Conversely, procalcitonin production is blocked by interferon γ, a cytokine released in response to viral infections. Hence, procalcitonin may be used to support clinical decision making for the initiation and discontinuation of antibiotic therapy. This subject is reviewed by Niederman elsewhere in this issue.

Having the ability to identify the cause of CAP would not only assist in determining the relevance of resistance, but avoids unnecessary antimicrobial use, which is an inevitable consequence of the empirical choices based on the IDSA/ATS guidelines.[12] Although urinary antigen detection has proved to be rapid and accurate, there are only 2 pathogens that have been approved: *Legionella* and *Pneumococcus*. However, there are several new technologies that may prove useful. Two examples that are currently available are polymerase chain reaction–based technologies and matrix-assisted laser desorption ionization–time-of-flight mass spectrometry. This subject is reviewed by Gaydos elsewhere in this issue.

SHOULD WE USE MACROLIDE MONOTHERAPY FOR MILD PNEUMONIA?

Macrolides have long been recommended and commonly prescribed for the treatment of outpatients with CAP in North America, because of their activity against *S pneumoniae* and the atypical pathogens (*M pneumoniae, L pneumophilia*, and *C pneumoniae*). Numerous randomized clinical trials have documented the efficacy of clarithromycin and azithromycin as monotherapy for outpatient CAP. However, the rationale for this recommendation is waning.

1. Legionella infections typically cause more severe pneumonia than *M pneumoniae* and *C pneumoniae*, can be readily diagnosed by a urinary antigen test, and require specific therapy.
2. It is controversial whether there is benefit shown with empirical atypical coverage in hospitalized or nonhospitalized patients with CAP.[30,31] This subject is reviewed by File and Marrie elsewhere in this issue.
3. There is now evidence for the increasing prevalence of macrolide-resistant *M pneumoniae* and its clinical relevance.[32–35]
4. The prevalence of macrolide-resistant pneumococci is now greater than 40% in the United States, and there is increasing evidence that both low-level and high-level resistance are associated with clinical failures.[10,24,36]

It seems prudent not to recommend macrolide monotherapy for the management of mild pneumonia when there are effective alternative agents, including the aminopenicillins and the respiratory fluoroquinolones, for which resistance rates are lower.[2]

SUMMARY

The prevalence of multidrug-resistant *S pneumoniae* continues to increase. Confusion regarding the relevance of resistance has been mostly a result of clinicians not being able to recognize the consequence of resistance in their practice, the failure of previous in vitro penicillin breakpoints to accurately predict clinical failures for parenteral therapy for nonmeningeal infections, and the lack of clinical data to clarify the significance of low-level macrolide resistance. Ideally, prospective clinical trials should be performed to define the level of resistance that predicts clinical failure; however, this is unlikely to be either possible or practical. Rather, we will continue to have to rely on PK/PD data and observational studies. There is also a need to define at what prevalence of resistance a change in recommendations for empirical therapy is warranted. However, what does seem prudent now, in the face of increasing rates of macrolide-resistant pneumococci, is to no longer recommend macrolides for monotherapy for CAP when effective alternatives are available.

REFERENCES

1. File TM Jr, Tan JS, Boex JR. The clinical relevance of penicillin-resistant *Streptococcus pneumoniae*: a new perspective. Clin Infect Dis 2006;42:798–800.
2. Jones RN, Sader HS, Mendes RE, et al. Update on antimicrobial susceptibility trends among *Streptococcus pneumoniae* in the United States: report of ceftaroline activity from the SENTRY Antimicrobial Surveillance Program (1998-2011). Diagn Microbiol Infect Dis 2012. http://dx.doi.org/10.1016/j.diagmicrobio.2012.08.024.
3. Clinical and Laboratory Standards Institute. Performance standards for antimicrobial susceptibility testing: eighteenth informational supplement. CLSI document M100–S18. Wayne (PA): Clinical and Laboratory Standards Institute; 2008.
4. Pallares R, Linares J, Vadillo M, et al. Resistance to penicillin and cephalosporin and mortality from severe pneumococcal pneumonia in Barcelona, Spain [see comments] [published erratum appears in N Engl J Med 1995;333(24):1655]. N Engl J Med 1995;333:474–80.
5. Yu VL, Chiou CC, Feldman C, et al. An international prospective study of pneumococcal bacteremia: correlation with in vitro resistance, antibiotics administered, and clinical outcome. Clin Infect Dis 2003;37:230–7.
6. Song JH, Jung SI, Ki HK, et al. Clinical outcomes of pneumococcal pneumonia caused by antibiotic-resistant strains in Asian countries: a study by the Asian Network for Surveillance of Resistant Pathogens. Clin Infect Dis 2004;38:1570–8.
7. Centers for Disease Control and Prevention (CDC). Effects of new penicillin susceptibility breakpoints for *Streptococcus pneumoniae*–United States, 2006-2007. MMWR Morb Mortal Wkly Rep 2008;57:1353–5.
8. Rosen J, Beekmann S, Polgreen P, et al. Barriers to intravenous penicillin use for treatment of nonmeningitis pneumococcal disease. J Clin Microbiol 2010;48: 3372–4.
9. Klugman KP, Lonks JR. Hidden epidemic of macrolide-resistant pneumococci. Emerg Infect Dis 2005;11:802–7.
10. Daneman N, McGeer A, Green K, et al. Macrolide resistance in bacteremic pneumococcal disease: implications for patient management. Clin Infect Dis 2006;43: 432–8.
11. Farrell DJ, Couturier C, Hryniewicz W. Distribution and antibacterial susceptibility of macrolide resistance genotypes in *Streptococcus pneumoniae*: PROTEKT Year 5 (2003-2004). Int J Antimicrob Agents 2008;31:245–9.
12. Mandell LA, Wunderink RG, Anzueto A, et al. Infectious Diseases Society of America/American Thoracic Society consensus guidelines on the management of community-acquired pneumonia in adults. Clin Infect Dis 2007;44(Suppl 2): S27–72.
13. Marchant CD, Carlin SA, Johnson CE, et al. Measuring the comparative efficacy of antibacterial agents for acute otitis media: the "Pollyanna phenomenon". J Pediatr 1992;120:72–7.
14. Levy ML, Le JI, Woodhead MA, et al. Primary care summary of the British Thoracic Society Guidelines for the management of community acquired pneumonia in adults: 2009 update. Endorsed by the Royal College of General Practitioners and the Primary Care Respiratory Society UK. Prim Care Respir J 2010;19:21–7.
15. Tilghman RC, Finland M. Clinical significance of bacteremia in pneumococcic pneumonia. Arch Intern Med 1937;59:602–19.

16. Evans GM, Gaisford WF. Treatment of pneumonia with 2-(p-aminobenzenesul-phonamido) pyridine. Lancet 1938;2:14–9.
17. Peterson LR. Penicillins for treatment of pneumococcal pneumonia: does in vitro resistance really matter? Clin Infect Dis 2006;42:224–33.
18. Austrian R, Gold J. Pneumococcal bacteremia with especial reference to bacteremic pneumococcal pneumonia. Ann Intern Med 1964;60:759–70.
19. Metlay JP, Singer DE. Outcomes in lower respiratory tract infections and the impact of antimicrobial drug resistance. Clin Microbiol Infect 2002;8(Suppl 2):1–11.
20. Moore HF, Chesney AN. A study of ethylhydrocuprein (Optochin) in the treatment of acute lobar pneumonia. Arch Intern Med 1917;19:611–82.
21. Tleyjeh IM, Tlaygeh HM, Hejal R, et al. The impact of penicillin resistance on short-term mortality in hospitalized adults with pneumococcal pneumonia: a systematic review and meta-analysis. Clin Infect Dis 2006;42:788–97.
22. Feikin DR, Schuchat A, Kolczak M, et al. Mortality from invasive pneumococcal pneumonia in the era of antibiotic resistance, 1995-1997. Am J Public Health 2000;90:223–9.
23. Turett GS, Blum S, Fazal BA, et al. Penicillin resistance and other predictors of mortality in pneumococcal bacteremia in a population with high human immunodeficiency virus seroprevalence. Clin Infect Dis 1999;29:321–7.
24. Lonks JR, Garau J, Gomez L, et al. Failure of macrolide antibiotic treatment in patients with bacteremia due to erythromycin-resistant *Streptococcus pneumoniae*. Clin Infect Dis 2002;35:556–64.
25. Chen D, McGeer A, de Azavedo JC, et al. The Canadian Bacterial Surveillance Network. Decreased susceptibility of *Streptococcus pneumoniae* to fluoroquinolones in Canada. N Engl J Med 1999;341:233–9.
26. Patel SN, McGeer A, Melano R, et al. Susceptibility of *Streptococcus pneumoniae* to fluoroquinolones in Canada. Antimicrob Agents Chemother 2011;55:3703–8.
27. Davidson R, Cavalcanti R, Brunton JL, et al. Resistance to levofloxacin and failure of treatment of pneumococcal pneumonia. N Engl J Med 2002;346:747–50.
28. Anderson KB, Tan JS, File TM Jr, et al. Emergence of levofloxacin-resistant pneumococci in immunocompromised adults after therapy for community-acquired pneumonia. Clin Infect Dis 2003;37:376–81.
29. Weinstein MP, Klugman KP, Jones RN. Rationale for revised penicillin susceptibility breakpoints versus *Streptococcus pneumoniae*: coping with antimicrobial susceptibility in an era of resistance. Clin Infect Dis 2009;48:1596–600.
30. Eliakim-Raz N, Robenshtok E, Shefet D, et al. Empiric antibiotic coverage of atypical pathogens for community-acquired pneumonia in hospitalized adults. Cochrane Database Syst Rev 2012;9:CD004418.
31. Mills GD, Oehley MR, Arrol B. Effectiveness of beta lactam antibiotics compared with antibiotics active against atypical pathogens in non-severe community acquired pneumonia: meta-analysis. BMJ 2005;330:456.
32. Bebear C, Pereyre S, Peuchant O. *Mycoplasma pneumoniae*: susceptibility and resistance to antibiotics. Future Microbiol 2011;6:423–31.
33. Yamada M, Buller R, Bledsoe S, et al. Rising rates of macrolide-resistant *Mycoplasma pneumoniae* in the central United States. Pediatr Infect Dis J 2012;31:409–11.
34. Centers for Disease Control and Prevention. Health hazards associated with laundry detergent pods–United States, May–June 2012. MMWR Morb Mortal Wkly Rep 2012;61:825–9.
35. Watanabe A, Yanagihara K, Matsumoto T, et al. Nationwide surveillance of bacterial respiratory pathogens conducted by the Surveillance Committee of Japanese

Society of Chemotherapy, Japanese Association for Infectious Diseases, and Japanese Society for Clinical Microbiology in 2009: general view of the pathogens' antibacterial susceptibility. J Infect Chemother 2012;18(5):609–20.

36. Daneman N, Low DE, McGeer A, et al. At the threshold: defining clinically meaningful resistance thresholds for antibiotic choice in community-acquired pneumonia. Clin Infect Dis 2008;46:1131–8.

Does Empiric Therapy for Atypical Pathogens Improve Outcomes for Patients with CAP?

Thomas M. File Jr, MD, MSc[a,b],*, Thomas J. Marrie, MD[c]

KEYWORDS

- Community-acquired pneumonia • Atypical • Mycoplasma • Chlamydophila
- Legionella • Treatment • Empiric

KEY POINTS

- The "atypical pneumonia" field is compromised by virtue of controversy related to terminology, suboptimal diagnostics methods, and studies that have failed to resolve key questions, and hence aggregating them into meta-analysis does not improve understanding.
- The self-limited nature of infections caused by *Mycoplasma* and *Chlamydophila* further complicates the issue.
- Outcome assessment of clinical trials at an early time point (eg, 3–5 days) rather than a later test of cure evaluation may better identify differential effects of treatments for community-acquired pneumonia caused by atypical pathogens.

INTRODUCTION: NATURE OF THE CONTROVERSY

Including coverage of atypical bacteria in the spectrum of empiric treatment of community-acquired pneumonia (CAP) is controversial.[1–5] This controversy is related to several issues, including relevance of terminology, pathogen awareness, imprecision of present diagnostic methods, and perceived contradictory results of published evidence (**Box 1**).

Although the original classification of atypical and typical pneumonia arose from the observation that the clinical presentation of these two groups of patients was different, recent studies have shown that there is considerable overlap of the clinical manifestations of these two categories of pneumonia such that empiric therapeutic decisions cannot be made solely on this basis.[2–4] Thus, the designation of atypical pneumonia is controversial in relation to scientific and clinical merit, and many authorities have

[a] Infectious Disease Section, Department of Internal Medicine, Northeast Ohio Medical University, PO Box 95, Rootstown, OH 44272, USA; [b] Infectious Disease Division, Summa Health System, 75 Arch St. Suite 506, Akron, OH 44304, USA; [c] Dalhousie University, Clinical Research Centre, Room C-205, 5849 University Ave., Halifax, Nova Scotia, B3H 4H7, Canada
* Corresponding author. 75 Arch Street, Suite 506, Akron, OH 44304.
E-mail address: filet@summahealth.org

Infect Dis Clin N Am 27 (2013) 99–114
http://dx.doi.org/10.1016/j.idc.2012.11.005
0891-5520/13/$ – see front matter © 2013 Elsevier Inc. All rights reserved.

Box 1
Issues of controversy regarding significance of atypical pathogens

- The clinical relevance of terminology
- Awareness of such pathogens
- Diagnostic testing
- Debate as to the clinical impact of treating these infections
- Perceived contradictory results of published evidence

---

suggested that the term "atypical" be discontinued. However, the term remains popular among clinicians and investigators and remains prevalent in recent literature regardless of its clinical value. Moreover, options for appropriate antimicrobial therapy for the most common causes of atypical pneumonia are similar, which is considered justification by some to lump these together. This article focuses on three causes of atypical pneumonia because much of the published reports on the effects of therapy are based on these pathogens: (1) *Mycoplasma pneumoniae*, (2) *Chlamydophila pneumoniae*, and (3) *Legionella* spp (with acknowledgment of many other possible causes of this syndrome, such as *Coxiella burnetii*, *Chlamydophila psittaci*, and viruses).

The diagnostic accuracy for *M pneumoniae*, *C pneumoniae*, and *Legionella* is variable, because of the diversity of and variations in the quality of the tests used. Thus, many of these infections are unrecognized. The quality of the various diagnostic tests is generally good for *Legionella* spp, is variable for *M pneumoniae*, and is poor for *C pneumoniae*.[6,7] Because accurate and rapid diagnostic methods are not presently readily available to the practicing clinician, the microbiologic diagnosis at the point of initial care is unknown and initial antibiotic treatment of CAP is largely empiric. However, several studies using available tests have found atypical pathogens, primarily *M pneumoniae*, *C pneumoniae*, and *Legionella* spp as common causes of CAP, of ambulatory patients or those requiring hospitalization, and represent 10% to 30% of cases depending on the population studied.[8–11] Recent advances in molecular testing methods should improve the diagnosis and awareness of these pathogens.[12]

Although there is little debate regarding the importance of treating *Legionnella*, therapy for *Mycoplasma* and *Chlamydophila* has been the subject of some conjecture. A common view is that it really does not matter whether antibiotics are given for most of these infections because the mortality is low, these infections are often self-limiting, and there may be ambiguity of diagnosis (especially for *C pneumoniae*). Most often *Mycoplasma* and *Chlamydophila* infections are unrecognized and recovery uneventful; however, such infections may occasionally cause rapidly progressive pneumonia for which appropriate antimicrobial therapy is needed for optimal outcomes.

Differences in approaches to empiric therapy are illustrated by the recommendations in North American and many international guidelines, especially for nonsevere CAP.[13,14] North American guidelines for management of CAP acknowledge the significance of these pathogens by suggesting the need for empiric therapy that is active against these organisms.[15] The North American approach is to use initial antimicrobial therapy that provides coverage for *S pneumoniae* plus atypical pathogens (particularly *M pneumoniae* or *C pneumoniae*, which are common causes of outpatient CAP). In contrast, many international guidelines place less significance than the North American approach on the need to treat the atypical pathogens empirically except for severe CAP. The British Thoracic Society approach for initial empiric therapy recommends that coverage for *M pneumoniae* is considered unnecessary, because the pathogen exhibits epidemic periodicity every 4 to 5 years and largely affects younger persons.[16]

EVIDENCE AGAINST EMPIRIC TREATMENT OF ATYPICAL PATHOGENS

There have been several systematic reviews of randomized clinical trials performed within the past decade to address this issue.[17–20] Overall these reviews concluded there was no significant difference between the outcomes for the groups receiving an agent active against atypical pathogens and the groups receiving β-lactams, in terms of survival or clinical efficacy.

In 2003, Oosterheert and colleagues[17] evaluated eight relevant studies of patients admitted to the hospital for CAP to assess whether guideline-recommended treatment to cover atypical pathogens with empiric therapy of a β-lactam plus macrolide or quinolone monotherapy is superior to β-lactam treatment alone. Although they found six studies that resulted in reduction in mortality, the authors concluded the design of the studies may have resulted in confounding that influenced these results and inferred that the addition of a macrolide or monotherapy with a fluoroquinolone could not be supported as a standard of care of patients admitted to the hospital with CAP.

In 2005, two systematic reviews were published. Both used a similar study format with a review of comparative trials of agents showing activity against atypical pathogens (macrolides, fluoroquinolones, or tetracyclines) versus β-lactams. Mills and colleagues[18] evaluated 18 trials totaling 6749 patients with nonsevere CAP. The summary relative risk for treatment failure or mortality in all-cause CAP showed no advantage of antibiotics active against atypical pathogens over β-lactam therapy **(Table 1)**. However, in a subgroup analysis they found a significant benefit for *Legionella* infections. Of note, however, only 501 patients (7%) were diagnosed as having atypical pneumonia based on serologic methods. Shefet and colleagues[19] reported from a Cochrane Library Report a review of 24 randomized clinical trials encompassing 5015 patients and found similar results **(Fig. 1)**. The primary outcome assessed was mortality. The authors did observe that regimens with coverage of atypical pathogens showed a trend toward clinical success and bacteriologic eradication; however, both disappeared when evaluating high-quality studies (ie, studies that scored A in randomization allocation) alone. There was a significant advantage for regimens with atypical coverage in clinical success for *L pneumophila*. The authors concluded there was no benefit of survival or clinical efficacy to empiric atypical coverage in

Table 1 Meta-analysis comparing antibiotic coverage with no coverage of atypical pathogens in nonsevere community-acquired pneumonia			
	No. Failing Treatment/No. Treated		Relative Risk
Treatment Group	Antimicrobials Active Against Atypicals	β-Lactam Therapy	(95% Confidence Interval)
All patients	667/3681 (18.1%)	564/3068 (18.4%)	0.97 (0.87–1.07)
Mycoplasma pneumoniae	11/152 (7.2%)	20/159 (12.6%)	0.60 (0.31–1.17)
Chlamydia pneumoniae	8/63 (12.7%)	2/52 (3.8%)	2.32 (0.67–8.03)
Legionella pneumophila	4/38 (10.5%)	15/37 (40.5%)	0.40 (0.19–0.85)[a]

[a] Statistically significant difference (all other comparisons were not statistically significant).
Data from Mills GD, Oehley MR, Arrol B. Effectiveness of β lactam antibiotics compared with antibiotics active against atypical pathogens in nonsevere community acquired pneumonia: meta-analysis. BMJ 2005;330:456–60.

Review: Empiric antibiotic coverage of atypical pathogens for community acquired pneumonia in hospitalized adults

Comparison: 01 Atypical versus non-ayptical

Outcome: 01 Mortality per Antibiotic (ABx) Treatment

Study	Atypical ABx n/N	Non-atypical ABx n/N	Relative Risk (Fixed) 95% CI	Weight (%)	Relative Risk (Fixed) 95% CI
01 Quinolone (atypical arm)					
Aubier 1998	1/159	3/170		4.1	0.36 [0.04, 3.39]
Carbon 1992	0/125	1/121		2.1	0.32 [0.01, 7.85]
x Chuard 1989	0/59	0/62		0.0	Not estimable
Feldman 2001	1/35	0/34		0.7	2.92 [0.12, 69.20]
Fournier 1986	5/20	5/20		7.0	1.00 [0.34, 2.93]
x Gleadhill 1986	0/26	0/22		0.0	Not estimable
Hirata-Dulas 1991	2/24	2/26		2.7	1.08 [0.17, 7.10]
x Kalbermatter 2000	0/28	0/56		0.0	Not estimable
Khan 1989	4/66	3/56		4.6	1.13 [0.26, 4.84]
Lephonte 2004	4/167	3/153		4.4	1.22 [0.28, 5.37]
x Miki 1984	0/73	0/72		0.0	Not estimable
Norrby 1998	21/314	22/305		31.3	0.93 [0.52, 1.65]
Peterson 1988	3/30	1/30		1.4	3.00 [0.33, 27.23]
Petitpretz 2001	3/200	4/208		5.5	0.78 [0.18, 3.44]
Rizzato 1997	7/110	5/115		6.9	1.46 [0.48, 4.47]
Tremolieres 1998	4/173	3/169		4.3	1.30 [0.30, 5.73]
x Vanderdonckt 1990	0/82	0/88		0.0	Not estimable
Vogel 1991	0/49	3/51		4.8	0.15 [0.01, 2.80]
Subtotal (95% CI)	1740	1758		79.7	0.98 [0.69, 1.41]

Total events: 55 (Atypical ABx), 55 (Non-atypical ABx)
Test for heterogeneity chi-square=5.16 df=12 p=0.95 I² =0.0%
Test for overall effect z=0.08 p=0.9

02 Macrolide (atypical arm)					
x Bohte 1995	0/36	0/30		0.0	Not estimable
Genne 1997	2/56	1/56		1.4	2.00 [0.19, 21.43]
Romanelli 2002	7/101	7/103		9.7	1.02 [0.37, 2.80]
Zeluff 1988	1/80	0/78		0.7	2.93 [0.12, 70.75]
Subtotal (95% CI)	273	267		11.8	1.25 [0.52, 3.01]

Total events: 10 (Atypical ABx), 8 (Non-atypical ABx)
Test for heterogeneity chi-square=0.58 df=2 p=0.75 I² =0.0%
Test for overall effect z=0.50 p=0.6

03 Combined quinolone and macrolide (atypical arm)					
Lode 1995	28/609	4/199		8.5	2.29 [0.81, 6.44]
Subtotal (95% CI)	609	199		8.5	2.29 [0.81, 6.44]

Total events: 28 (Atypical ABx), 4 (Non-atypical ABx)
Test for heterogeneity: not applicable
Test for overall effect z=1.57 p=0.1

| Total (95% CI) | 2622 | 2224 | | 100.0 | 1.13 [0.82, 1.54] |

Total events: 93 (Atypical ABx), 67 (Non-atypical ABx)
Test for heterogeneity chi-square=7.91 df=16 p=0.95 I² =0.0%
Test for overall effect z=0.74 p=0.5

0.1 0.2 0.5 1 2 5 10

Favours atypical   Favours non-atypical

Fig. 1. Comparison of atypical versus nonatypical coverage for empiric therapy for CAP. Mortality per antimicrobial treatment group. ABx, Antibiotic; CI, confidence interval. (*From* Shefet D, Robenshtok E, Paul M, et al. Empiric antibiotic coverage of atypical pathogens for community acquired pneumonia in hospitalized adults. Cochrane Database Syst Rev 2005;2:CD004418; with permission.)

hospitalized patients with CAP. This conclusion relates mostly to the comparison of quinolone monotherapy with nonatypical monotherapy. Furthermore, they suggested that expanding coverage to atypical pathogens is bound to increase toxicity, resistance, and cost.

The most recent report by Maimon and colleagues[20] reviewed 13 randomized, double-blind studies from 1966 through July 2007 involving 4314 outpatients greater than or equal to 18 years of age with CAP and concluded that there was no significant difference detected regarding clinical success or mortality regardless of atypical coverage advantage in otherwise healthy outpatients. The primary outcome assessed was clinical cure or improvement at a designated time point; in all studies evaluation occurred within 10 days after treatment completion. The authors acknowledged that it was not possible to address whether or not there was a difference in recovery time between regimens.

The conclusion from these reviews is that a substantial number of randomized trials have been performed and they do not provide compelling evidence of a need to treat atypical pathogens empirically, with the exception of treatment of legionnaires disease. Limitations of these studies are listed in **Box 2**.

EVIDENCE FOR EMPIRIC TREATMENT OF ATYPICAL PATHOGENS

Support for atypical coverage was implied by evaluation of a Medicare database, in which 113,000 hospitalized patients with CAP were analyzed for outcome on the basis of antibiotic selection and were stratified by severity of illness.[21] This study showed a statistically significant survival advantage with the use of a fluoroquinolone or a β-lactam plus a macrolide, compared with a β-lactam alone. This result supports the

---

Box 2
Limitations of clinical trials included in systematic reviews

- Most of the studies were registration studies and many were nonmasked.

- Most did not identify atypical pathogens. Only 501 of >6000 analyzable participants in the study by Mills and colleagues[18] study were diagnosed as having atypical pneumonia.

- Coinfection with typical pathogens may explain some of the results. In such cases, clinical response to agents without atypical coverage can be caused by the response of the coinfecting typical pathogen. Those with atypical pneumonia may have undiagnosed bacterial or aspiration pneumonia, which responds to nonatypical focused antimicrobial agents.

- Time points for assessment were variable and included end of treatment ($\leq$14 days); within 10 days of completion of treatment; or end of follow-up (which could be several weeks after end of treatment). Thus, there was an inability to distinguish a more rapid resolution of illness with atypical agent therapy if an earlier time point was used. Many atypical pneumonias (eg, *Mycoplasma*, *Chlamydophila*, and *Coxiella*) may be associated with a self-limiting illness and using late time point does not differentiate early response (discussed later).

- Serology was the basis for most of the diagnoses, which has the major drawbacks of variable sensitivity and specificity. As a result the diagnoses are uncertain, highlighting one of the reasons that the role of atypical pathogens has remained controversial.

- Most studies used mortality rate as the primary outcome; such an endpoint is unable to differentiate a treatment effect of infections with overall low mortality rate. Rapidity of clinical resolution of illness may be a better endpoint to differentiate treatment regimens for such infections.

benefit of coverage of atypical pathogens, but the conclusion is limited based on the uncertain value of these antibiotics, in terms of anti-inflammatory properties and the lack of any accompanying microbiologic data.

Subsequently, several large observational studies that assessed the use of a macrolide with a cephalosporin as part of an initial empiric regimen have suggested a benefit with a shorter length of hospital stay and lower mortality rate than was lower than with treatment with a cephalosporin alone.[22–24] These large observational studies showed benefit for atypical coverage; however, correction for the baseline differences between patients and the potential confounding effect of the immunomodulatory properties of macrolides is impossible to discern.

Additional retrospective or observational studies have suggested that benefit from combination therapy, which usually included a macrolide, may also apply to CAP associated with Streptococcus pneumoniae bacteremia.[25–31] The possible coexistence of atypical pathogens or the immunomodulating effect of the macrolides may be responsible for this finding. However, interpretation of these studies is subject to limitations inherent in their retrospective design. Furthermore, because only empiric therapy was evaluated, the findings are not necessarily applicable to pathogen-directed therapy, which is usually started 24 to 48 hours after initial therapy.

A retrospective study evaluated almost 3000 Medicare patients hospitalized from either home (75%) or a nursing home (25%, now considered "health care–associated pneumonia") with bacteremic CAP caused by one of several pathogens, with S pneumoniae the most common (38%).[28] The use of a macrolide (as part of combination therapy), but not a fluoroquinolone (usually monotherapy), was associated with a reduced 30-day mortality. There was a trend toward improved survival with longer courses of the macrolide (eg, >96 hours vs 24 hours); the authors speculated the benefit was related to the immunomodulating effect of the macrolides.

A series of studies from Edmonton, Alberta, Canada shed additional light on the impact of appropriate empiric antibiotic therapy in CAP. From 2000 to 2002 all patients with pneumonia presenting to six emergency departments in this city of 1,000,000 people were treated according to a pathway for CAP.[32] Antibiotic therapy was as according to the guidelines of the Canadian CAP working group and was slightly modified to the American Thoracic Society recommendations published in 2001.[33,34]

Asadi and colleagues[35] examined outcomes for 3203 patients who required admission to hospital for treatment of CAP and found that 321 (10%) died and 306 (10%) were admitted to intensive care unit (ICU). Treatment with guideline concordant antibiotics, cefotaxime plus azithromycin or levofloxacin monotherapy, occurred in 78.2% of the patients and was associated with a reduction in the composite endpoint of mortality or admission to ICU from 29% to14.7% (odds ratio [OR], 0.44; 95% confidence interval [CI], 0.36–054; P<.001). Macrolide/β-lactam regimens were not associated with decreases in hospital mortality or the composite endpoint. When outcomes for those treated on an ambulatory basis were examined, it was noted that for 126 of 2973 patients the antibiotic recommendations of doxycycline, clarithromycin, azithromycin, erythromycin, or levofloxacin were not followed.[36] The 30-day mortality rate was 1% for those who were treated in concordance with the guidelines and 6% for those who were not so treated (P<.007).

The same group went on to a meta-analysis of macrolide-based regimens and mortality in 135,000 hospitalized patients with CAP.[37] There was a 22% relative reduction in mortality associated with use of macrolide-based regimens compared with nonmacrolide-based regimens. The authors postulate the potential benefit of the macrolide to the immunomodulatory effect or inhibition of microbial virulence factors, such as biofilm formation or decreased mucus hypersecretion.

LESSONS FROM ATYPICAL PATHOGEN-SPECIFIC STUDIES
Studies from 1960s and 1970s for Mycoplasma

There is substantial evidence that use of an appropriate antiatypical agent does lead to better outcomes if *Mycoplasma* is identified as the cause of CAP. The data for *Chlamydophila* are sparse mostly because of the lack of adequate identification of this pathogen.

Soon after the demonstration that *M pneumoniae* was the major cause of atypical pneumonia, several studies demonstrated a benefit of erythromycin or tetracycline in illness resolution compared with no treatment or penicillin. Kingston and colleagues[38] evaluated the clinical course of marine recruits with *M pneumoniae* pneumonia based on clinical and chest radiograph findings in a double-blind study comparing demethylchlortetracycline with placebo. Infection identification was based on serologic diagnosis. Patients treated with the active agent had significantly reduced duration of fever, cough, and fatigue (**Table 2**). Similar results were reported by Rasch and Mogabgab[39] for erythromycin and tetracycline. In a placebo-controlled clinical trial of antimicrobial agents for therapy for *M pneumoniae* pneumonia, Shames and colleagues[40] studied military recruits who received one of several different regimens. Trainees with serologically identified *M pneumoniae* who received either no therapy or penicillin G served as control subjects. Erythromycin or tetracycline was given to the active treatment group. Effective antimicrobials for *Mycoplasma* (erythromycin or tetracycline) were more effective in reducing clinical illness and resolving abnormalities on chest radiograph than no therapy or penicillin (**Table 3**).

More recently Shah and colleagues[41] evaluated data from a multicenter retrospective cohort study from 36 children's hospitals to determine whether macrolide therapy is associated with improved outcomes among children hospitalized with *M pneumoniae* pneumonia. Of 690 patients assessed with a diagnosis of *M pneumoniae* pneumonia based on International Classification of Diseases-9 discharge code (validated by a single hospital confirmation based on polymerase chain reaction test of nasopharyngeal washings), 405 (58.7%) received empiric macrolide therapy, which was associated with a 32% shorter overall length of stay compared with non-macrolide therapy. Macrolide therapy was not associated with a 28-day or 15-month readmission rate.

The benefit of active anti-*Mycoplasma* therapy in patients with *M pneumoniae* infection can also be indirectly assessed by observations of therapy for macrolide-resistant strains. With the emergence of macrolide-resistant *M pneumoniae* in Asia, several reports have documented better clinical response of infection treated with a macrolide

Table 2		
Duration of manifestations of marine recruits with mycoplasma pneumonia		
Characteristic	Mean Days Treated Group (N = 59) (Demethylchlortetracycline)	Mean Days Without Antimicrobial (N = 50)
Fever (>100°F)	2.1[a]	8.1
Abnormal chest radiograph	9.5[a]	20
Rales	6.9[a]	15.5
Cough	9.7[a]	22
Fatigue, malaise	2.7[a]	8.5

[a] *P*<.01 compared with no treatment (placebo).
Data from Kingston JR, Chanock RM, Mufson MA, et al. Eaton agent pneumonia. JAMA 1961; 176;118–23.

Table 3
Duration of fever and hospital day among airmen with *Mycoplasma pneumonia*

Treatment	Number of Patients	Mean Number Days of Fever	Mean Number Days in Hospital	Mean Number Days of Abnormal Chest Radiograph
Erythromycin	76	2.4	7	7.2
Tetracycline	89	2.4	7.6	9.3
Penicillin[a]	39	4.2[b]	14.1[b]	14.8

[a] Or no antimicrobial.
[b] Statistically significant difference between penicillin and the other two agents.
  Data from Shames JM, George RB, Holliday WB, et al. Comparison of antibiotics in the treatment of mycoplasmal pneumonia. Arch Intern Med 1970;125:680–4.

for macrolide-susceptible strains compared with macrolide-resistant strains, suggesting a clinical benefit for agents effective against this common atypical pathogen.[42,43]

Legionella

Data for empiric treatment of *Legionella* sp are noncontroversial, because the need to treat infection with these species was demonstrated very early, based on anecdotal experience with antibiotics that showed a better survival rate among those patients who received agents that, in retrospect, were shown to be active against *L pneumophila*.[44,45] A delay in therapy is associated with an increased mortality rate, and treatment should be started as soon as possible.[46]

Large, Multicenter Observational Study

Arnold and colleagues[11] evaluated outcomes for hospitalized patients treated empirically with antimicrobials with and without coverage for atypical pathogens using two large international databases of CAP. The diagnosis of atypical pathogens (*Mycoplasma*, *Chlamydophila*, and *Legionella*) was determined at The University of Louisville Atypical Pathogen Reference Laboratory using a variety of techniques and reported the results for specimens obtained from 1996 to 2004 from 4337 patients in 21 countries. The results showed an incidence of 21% to 28% in adults with CAP in virtually all regions of the world. There were 2220 patients who received atypical coverage compared with 658 patients who did not. The regimens for atypical coverage were β-lactam + macrolide (51%); quinolone (31%); β-lactam + quinolone (11%); and macrolide (6%). The most common regimen for no atypical coverage was monotherapy with a β-lactam (84%). A total of 201 patients (11%) were admitted to an ICU from the group who received atypical coverage, whereas 33 patients (8%) were admitted to an ICU from the group who did not receive atypical coverage. The mean time to clinical stability was 3.2 days (standard deviation [SD], 1.7) for those who received atypical coverage (N = 1186), and 3.7 days (SD, 1.6) for those who did not receive atypical coverage (N = 272). The mean difference, 0.5 days (95% CI, 0.29–0.73), was significant ($P<.01$). The multivariate analysis for time to clinical stability is shown in **Fig. 2**. Patients with an atypical regimen reached clinical stability sooner, whereas patients with altered mental status or admission to an ICU reached clinical stability later.

  This study also indicates that, in hospitalized patients with CAP, initial empiric therapy with coverage for atypical pathogens is associated with decreased duration of hospitalization and decreased patient mortality. The authors concluded there are benefits of empiric therapy for atypical pathogens and strongly recommend that all hospitalized patients with CAP should receive empiric therapy with a regimen that

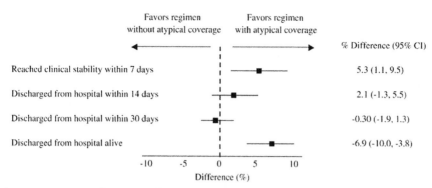

Fig. 2. Comparison of outcomes for patients who received treatment with and without coverage for atypical pathogens (from large multicenter, observational study). (*From* Arnold FW, Summersgill JT, Lajoie AS, et al. A worldwide perspective of atypical pathogens in community-acquired pneumonia. Am J Respir Crit Care Med 2007;175:1086–93; with permission.)

covers typical and atypical pathogens. The primary limitations of this study are its retrospective nature; the lack of control for unmeasured confounders; and potential nonantimicrobial, immunomodulatory effect of a macrolide.

Doxycycline Versus Macrolides for CAP

In a retrospective analysis of the comparative efficacy of two drug combinations (β-lactam plus macrolide versus β-lactam plus doxycycline) among patients recruited to a large prospective study of CAP in Australia, Teh and colleagues[47] observed similar outcomes for CAP caused by atypical pathogens (defined as *Chlamydophila*, *Legionella*, or *Mycoplasma* spp based on serologic diagnosis and urinary antigen for *Legionella*). The doxycycline-containing regimen was possibly superior in terms of reduced length of hospital stay (see **Table 4**). The authors believed either of these regimens was appropriate for empiric therapy for CAP; furthermore, they commented that doxycycline may be superior for *C psittaci*.

Table 4
Clinical features and response of CAP episodes with typical and atypical subgroups with β-lactam + macrolide or β-lactam + Doxycycline[a]

	Typical			Atypical		
Clinical Features	β-lactam + Macrolide (31)	β-lactam + Doxycycline (124)	P Value	β-lactam + Macrolide (26)	β-lactam + Doxycycline (80)	P Value
Age (mean, years)	73.6	70	0.29	49.2	53.8	0.37
Median days to clinical stability	2	2	1.00	2	2	0.12
Median days length of stay	5	6	0.64	3.5	5	<0.001

( ) Number in each group.
[a] Retrospective subanalysis from large prospective study.
Data from Teh B, Grayson ML, Jonhson PD, et al. Doxycycline versus macrolides in combination therapy for treatment of community-acquired pneumonia. Clin Microbiol Infect 2012;18:E71–3.

Subset Analysis of Prospective Randomized Trials (FOCUS Trials)

Several of the authors of the systematic reviews and observational studies reviewed previously indicate the best way to assess the need to treat for atypical pathogens for all CAP empirically is by a well-designed randomized, control trial. As stated by Shafet and colleagues, a "randomized controlled trial of BL or cephalosporin monotherapy compared with BL or cephalosporin combined with a macrolide in hospitalized patients with CAP should be performed."[19] Such a study has not been performed, but two recent studies (FOCUS trials) to evaluate the efficacy of ceftaroline for community-acquired bacterial pneumonia may shed some light.

The FOCUS trials (NCT00621504 and NCT00509106) were global, double-blind, randomized, multicenter, phase III studies in patients hospitalized for moderate to severe CAP (Patient Outcomes Research Team [PORT] risk class III or IV) requiring intravenous therapy comparing the efficacy and safety of ceftaroline fosamil with ceftriaxone.[48] Patients were randomized (1:1) to ceftaroline fosamil, 600 mg intravenous every 12 hours, or ceftriaxone, 1 g intravenous every 24 hours, for 5 to 7 days. All patients in FOCUS 1 also received two doses of oral clarithromycin, 500 mg every 12 hours, on Day 1 to provide initial atypical pathogen coverage. Atypicals were diagnosed only with serologic criteria, and subjects with a positive *Legionella* serotype based on urinary-antigen testing at baseline were excluded from enrollment. In addition to the standard Test of Cure (TOC) endpoint (8–15 days posttherapy), the US Food and Drug Administration also specified and assessed post hoc clinical stability and symptom improvement on Day 4 of study therapy. For this analysis, the Food and Drug Administration MITT population included patients who received any amount of study therapy and had a baseline pathogen identified.

The FOCUS trials were identical in design except for a 24-hour course of clarithromycin on Day 1 in FOCUS 1.[49,50] This difference offered a unique opportunity to assess the effect of a macrolide on the outcome of CAP caused by greater than or equal to one atypical pathogen. A subset analysis evaluated Day 4 clinical stability and symptom response and clinical response at TOC (7–10 days after study treatment). A differential clinical benefit was observed at Day 4 in patients with CAP caused by an atypical pathogen only (this included 130 patients and represented?10% of all the patients initially enrolled in the study despite an intention of investigations to avoid pneumonia caused by nontypical pathogens), specifically *M pneumoniae* or *C pneumoniae*, and who received 1 day of clarithromycin (76.6% vs 57.6%) (**Table 5**).[51] No difference was seen at the TOC visit, perhaps because of the self-limited course of many atypical pneumonias. The addition of a macrolide made no difference for typical pathogens, either at Day 4 or TOC. In this exploratory analysis, the estimated unadjusted OR was 2.4 (95% CI, 1.1–5.1) for the comparison between the two studies, suggesting an advantage for patients treated with 1 day of macrolide for coverage of atypical pathogens. This OR was virtually unaffected when adjusted for known risk factors measured in the study. Although not a prospective, randomized comparison, these observations suggest that outcome assessment at an early time point may better identify differential effects of two treatments than a later evaluation and that empiric atypical coverage may impact early clinical response. Recent recommendations suggest that such outcome assessment at an early time point (eg, 3–5 days) may be better to identify differential effects of two treatments.[52]

INTERPRETATION OF EVIDENCE

Although there seems to be good evidence to support the use of active antimicrobial agents for therapy for *Mycoplasma* and certainly *Legionella* to benefit patient

Table 5				
Assessment of outcomes at an early time point compared with standard test of cure identifying a differential effect of macrolide therapy on CAP caused by atypical pathogens				
	FOCUS 1[a] (Macrolide); n/N (%)		FOCUS 2[a] (no Macrolide); n/N (%)	
Subjects with	S & S Day 4	TOC (7–10 Days After Therapy)	S & S Day 4	TOC (7–10 Days After Therapy)
Typical pathogens only	105/155 (68)	126/155 (81)	114/178 (64)	138/178 (76)
Atypical pathogens only	49/64 (76.6)[b]	57/64 (89.1)	38/66 (57.6)[b]	58/66 (87.9)

[a] FOCUS 1 and 2 were randomized phase III studies in CAP comparing ceftaroline with ceftriaxone; FOCUS 1 included two doses of a macrolide (clarithromycin), whereas FOCUS 2 did not include a macrolide.
[b] Odds ratio compared with FOCUS, 2–2.5 (95% CI, 1.1–5.3); $P = 0.0219$.
Data from File T Jr, Eckburg P, Low D, et al. Assessment of outcomes at an early time point may identify a differential effect of macrolide therapy on community-acquired pneumonia due to atypical pathogens. Presented at the 22nd European Congress of Clinical Microbiology and Infectious Diseases. London, March 31, 2012, P 721.

outcomes when these infections are identified, there is no consensus based on several systematic reviews regarding the benefit of empirically treating for atypical pathogens for all patients empirically. There are several possible explanations for this:

- Most studies used mortality as an endpoint; thus the low mortality rate of most nonlegionella atypical pneumonias precludes differentiation of different therapeutic regimens on this basis
- Time of outcome assessment may not assess early outcomes of patient-relevant benefit
- Nonspecific diagnosis of atypical and bacterial cause
- Confounding effect of macrolides on bacterial pneumonia, which might preclude a benefit differentiation effect for bacterial versus atypical. The macrolide benefits bacterial (immunomodulatory effect) and atypical because of nonantimicrobial effect (immunomodulatory and virulence inhibition)

Although the clinical course of *M pneumoniae* or *C pneumoniae* infection is often self-limited, these pathogens can cause severe CAP, and appropriate treatment of even mild CAP caused by *Mycoplasma* reduces the morbidity of pneumonia and shortens the duration of symptoms. In several observational studies of patients who require hospitalization, antimicrobial regimens that have activity against atypical pathogens have been associated with better outcomes. Although these findings are not definitive, they support an important role for atypical pathogens.

RECOMMENDATION BASED ON PRESENT EVIDENCE

Despite the findings of several systematic reviews that have concluded "no benefit …was shown to empiric atypical coverage in hospitalized patients with community-acquired pneumonia," the available evidence does support the recommendations of the North American guidelines to provide such coverage. Thus, empiric therapy for atypical pathogens does improve outcomes for patients with CAP. This is based on the many limitations of the systematic reviews as indicated previously and newer information that a patient-relevant outcome, such as faster resolution of illness, is associated with appropriate therapy when an atypical pathogen is identified (even if longer-term outcomes and mortality may not be observed except for *Legionella* infection). Because many surveillance studies report the prevalence of atypical pathogens as 20% to 30% as monopathogens or copathogens, empiric use is reasonable. Effective agents include the macrolides, tetracyclines, and respiratory fluoroquinolones. The added benefit of a potential immunomodulatory and antivirulence effect of macrolides is also a consideration.

With development of newer molecular tests and potential point-of-care diagnostics for the atypical pathogens, it is quite possible that in the near future such methods may become available on a general use basis to allow pathogen-directed therapy at the time of initial administration. At such time the decision to treat for atypical or typical pathogens no longer becomes empiric.

In 1989, Kim and Gallis[53] stated that "empiric therapy at its best is set between the Scylla of unnecessary delay and the Charybdis of therapeutic voyeurism." The best approach is to treat every patient with pneumonia as an emergency, as advocated by Ewig and Torres.[54] At the time of initial assessment one should come to a conclusion about the likely cause of the pneumonia: bacterial definite or probable; atypical (*Legionella*, *Mycoplasma*, *Chlamydophila*, *Coxiella*, or viral); or unknown. Revise within the first 48 hours as more data become available and pay attention to the processes of care, such as oxygenation, rapid identification, and appropriate treatment of complications. Ensure appropriate follow-up after discharge has occurred.[55,56]

NEED FOR FUTURE STUDIES TO RESOLVE OR ANSWER QUESTION

Several authors of the systematic reviews and observational studies reviewed previously indicate the best way to assess the need to treat for atypical pathogens for all CAP empirically is with well-designed, prospective trials. One suggestion is a randomized controlled trial of β-lactam monotherapy compared with β-lactam combined with a macrolide in patients with CAP with mortality as its primary outcome.[19] However, in light of the lower mortality rate of *Mycoplasma* and *Chlamydophila* and newer emphasis on earlier time points for assessment, it is recommended to use an early assessment time as at least a coprimary endpoint to assess for an earlier clinically relevant outcome. Such an outcome assessment may be better to identify differential effects of two treatments for infections with low mortality rates. The implementation of such trials, however, will be difficult to conduct in countries that have guidelines that recommend routine coverage of atypical pathogens, including the United States, Canada, the United Kingdom, Germany, and Japan. Controlled trials in countries in which atypical coverage is optional seem feasible.[5] Furthermore, in countries in which macrolide-resistant *Mycoplasma* has become common, the use of a macrolide is expected to have less benefit.

For future trials it is critical for researchers to explore more extensively the possibility of atypical infection by performing comprehensive microbiologic studies and by assessing the potential immunomodulating effect of the macrolides with measurements of various proinflammatory markers during the course of severe CAP. However, the emergence of rapid, diagnostic tests that have the potential for point-of-care diagnosis of atypical pathogens may preclude the use of empiric therapy with the possibility to provide specific pathogen-directed therapy.

SUMMARY

The present controversy regarding the need to cover atypical pathogens in the empiric therapy for CAP is related to several issues, including the relevance of terminology, imprecise diagnostic methods at present, and perceived contradictory results of published evidence. However, limitations of clinical trial methodology limit interpretation of the actual benefit of providing coverage because many atypical pneumonias are eventually self-limited. Studies evaluating the time to clinical recovery and the use of earlier endpoints for evaluation suggest that appropriate therapy provides a benefit if an atypical pathogen is a pathogen. Because recent surveillance studies suggest these pathogens are common and until there is the availability of accurate, cost-effective, and easily interpreted laboratory tests to provide the etiologic diagnosis at the time of point of care, the authors support empiric therapy for atypical pathogens.

REFERENCES

1. File TM Jr, Tan JS, Plouffe JF. The role of atypical pathogens in respiratory infection. Infect Dis Clin North Am 1998;12:569–92.
2. File TM Jr. Atypical pneumonia. In: Jong EC, Stevens DL, editors. Netter's infectious diseases. Philadelphia: Elsevier Saunders; 2011. p. 146–52.
3. Marrie TJ. Empiric treatment of community-acquired pneumonia: always include treatment for atypical agents. Infect Dis Clin North Am 2004;18:829–42.
4. Marrie TJ, Costain N, La Scola B, et al. The role of atypical pathogens in community-acquired pneumonia. Semin Respir Crit Care Med 2012;33:244–56.
5. Bartlett JG. Is activity against "atypical" pathogens necessary in the treamtnet protocols for community-acquired pneumonia? Issues with combination therapy. Clin Infect Dis 2008;47:S232–6.
6. te Witt R, van Leeuwen WB, van Belkum A. Specific diagnostic tests for atypical respiratory tract pathogens. Infect Dis Clin North Am 2010;24:229–48.
7. Hammerschlag MR, Kohlhoff SA. Treatment of chlamydial infections. Expert Opin Pharmacother 2012;13:545–52.
8. Marrie TJ, Poulin-Costello M, Beecroft MD, et al. Etiology of community-acquired pneumonia in an ambulatory setting. Respir Med 2005;99:60.
9. Ciloniz C, Ewig S, Polverins E, et al. Microbial aetiology of community-acquired pneumonia and its relation to severity. Thorax 2011;66:340.
10. Lui G, Ip M, Lee N, et al. Role of atypical pathogens among adult hospitalized patients with community-acquired pneumonia. Respirology 2009;14:1098–105.
11. Arnold FW, Summersgill JT, LaJoie AS, et al. A worldwide perspective of atypical pathogens in community-acquired pneumonia. Am J Respir Crit Care Med 2007; 175:1086–93.
12. File TM Jr. New diagnostic tests for pneumonia: what is their role in clinical practice? Clin Chest Med 2011;32:417–30.
13. File TM Jr, Garau J, Blasi F, et al. Guidelines for empiric antimicrobial prescribing in community-acquired pneumonia. Chest 2004;125:1888–901.
14. Niederman MS, Luna CM. Community-acquired pneumonia guidelines: a global perspective. Semin Respir Crit Care Med 2012;33:298–310.
15. Mandell LA, Wunderink RG, Anzueto A, et al. Infectious Diseases Society of America/American Thoracic Society Consensus Guidelines on the Management of community-acquired pneumonia in adults. Clin Infect Dis 2007;44(Suppl 2) S1–S46.
16. Lim WS, Baudouin SV, George RC, et al. BTS guidelines for the management of community acquired pneumonia in adults: update 2009. Thorax 2009; 64(Suppl 3):iii1.
17. Oosterheert JJ, Bonten MJ, Hak E, et al. How good is the evidence for the recommended empirical antimicrobial treatment of patients hospitalized because of community-acquired pneumonia? A systematic review. J Antimicrob Chemother 2003;52:555–63.

18. Mills GD, Oehley MR, Arrol B. Effectiveness of B lactam antibiotics compared with antibiotics active against atypical pathogens in nonsevere community acquired pneumonia: meta-analysis. BMJ 2005;330:456–60.

19. Shefet D, Robenshtock E, Paul M, et al. Empiric antibiotic coverage of atypical pathogens for community acquired pneumonia in hospitalized adults. Cochrane Database Syst Rev 2005;(2):CD004418. 37.

20. Maimon N, Nopmaneejumruslers C, Marras TK. Antibacterial class not obviously important in outpatient pneumonia: a meta-analysis. Eur Respir J 2008;31: 1068–76, 38.

21. Gleason PP, Meehan TP, Fine JM, et al. Associations between initial antimicrobial therapy and medical outcomes for hospitalized elderly patients with pneumonia. Arch Intern Med 1999;159:2562–72.

22. Stahl JE, Barza M, DesJardin J, et al. Effect of macrolides as part of initial empiric therapy on length of stay in patients hospitalized with community-acquired pneumonia. Arch Intern Med 1999;159:2576–80.

23. Dudas V, Hopefl A, Jacobs R, et al. Antimicrobial selection for hospitalized patients with presumed community-acquired pneumonia: a survey of nonteaching US community hospitals. Ann Pharmacother 2000;34:446–52.

24. Houck PM, MacLehose RF, Niederman MS, et al. Empiric antibiotic therapy and mortality among Medicare pneumonia inpatients in 10 western states: 1993, 1995, and 1997. Chest 2001;119:1420–6.

25. Waterer GW, Somes GW, Wunderink RG. Monotherapy may be suboptimal for severe bacteremic pneumococcal pneumonia. Arch Intern Med 2001;161:1837.

26. Martínez JA, Horcajada JP, Almela M, et al. Addition of a macrolide to a beta-lactam-based empirical antibiotic regimen is associated with lower in-hospital mortality for patients with bacteremic pneumococcal pneumonia. Clin Infect Dis 2003;36:389.

27. Baddour LM, Yu VL, Klugman KP, et al. Combination antibiotic therapy lowers mortality among severely ill patients with pneumococcal bacteremia. Am J Respir Crit Care Med 2004;170:440.

28. Metersky ML, Ma A, Houck PM, et al. Antibiotics for bacteremic pneumonia: improved outcomes with macrolides but not fluoroquinolones. Chest 2007;131:466.

29. Rodríguez A, Mendia A, Sirvent JM, et al. Combination antibiotic therapy improves survival in patients with community-acquired pneumonia and shock. Crit Care Med 2007;35:1493.

30. Dwyer R, Ortqvist A, Aufwerber E, et al. Addition of a macrolide to a ss-lactam in bacteremic pneumococcal pneumonia. Eur J Clin Microbiol Infect Dis 2006;25: 518.

31. Chokshi R, Restrepo MI, Weeratunge N, et al. Monotherapy versus combination antibiotic therapy for patients with bacteremic Streptococcus pneumoniae community-acquired pneumonia. Eur J Clin Microbiol Infect Dis 2007;26:447.

32. Marrie TJ, Michalyk D, Man P. A critical pathway for treating community-acquired pneumonia. The Canadian Journal of CME 2001;13(1):43–59.

33. Mandell LA, Marrie TJ, Grossman RF, et al. The Canadian Community-Acquired Pneumonia Working Group. Canadian guidelines for the initial management of community-acquired pneumonia: an evidence-based update by the Canadian Infectious Diseases Society and the Canadian Thoracic Society. Clin Infect Dis 2000;31:383–421.

34. Niederman MS, Mandell LA, Anzueto A, et al. Guidelines for the management of adults with community-acquired pneumonia: diagnosis, assessment of severity, antimicrobial therapy, and prevention. Am J Respir Crit Care Med 2001;163:1730–54.

35. Asadi L, Eurich DT, Gamble JM, et al. Impact of guideline concurrent antibiotics and macrolide beta lactam combinations in 3203 patients hospitalized with pneumonia. A prospective cohort study. Clin Microbiol Infect 2012. Jan 30. http://dx.doi.org/10.1111/j.1469-0691.2012.03783.x. [Epub ahead of print].
36. Asadi L, Eurich DT, Gamble JM, et al. Guideline adherence and macrolides reduced mortality in outpatients with pneumonia. Respir Med 2012;106:451–8.
37. Asadi L, Sligl WI, Eurich DT, et al. Macrolide-based regimens and mortality in hospitalized patients with community-acquired pneumonia: a systematic review and meta-analysis. Clin Infect Dis 2012;55(3):371–80.
38. Kingston JR, Chanock RM, Mufson MA, et al. Eaton agent pneumonia. JAMA 1961;176:118–23.
39. Rasch JR, Mogabgab WJ. Therapeutic effect of erythromycin on *Mycoplasma pneumoniae*. Antimicrob Agents Chemother (Bethesda) 1965;5:693–9.
40. Shames JM, George RB, Holliday WB, et al. Comparison of antibiotics in the treatment of mycoplasmal pneumonia. Arch Intern Med 1970;125:680–4.
41. Shah SS, Test M, Sheffler-Collins S, et al. Marolide therapy and outcomes in a multicenter cohort of children hospitalized with *Mycoplasma pneumoniae* pneumonia. J Hosp Med 2012;7:311–7.
42. Suzuki S, Yamazaki T, Narita M, et al. Clinical evaluation of macrolide-resistant *Mycoplasma pneumoniae*. Antimicrob Agents Chemother (Bethesda) 2006;50:709–12.
43. Kawai Y, Miyashita N, Yamguchi T, et al. Clinical efficacy of macrolide antibiotics against genetically determined macrolide-resistant *Mycoplasma pneumoniae* pneumonia in paediatric patients. Respirology 2012;17:354–62.
44. Tsai TF, Finn DR, Plikaytis BD, et al. Legionnaires' disease: clinical features of the epidemic in Philadelphia. Ann Intern Med 1979;90:509–17.
45. Rello J, Yu VL. Legionnaires' disease: a rational approach to therapy. J Antimicrob Chemother 2003;51:1119–29.
46. Heath CH, Grove DI, Looke DFM. Delay in appropriate therapy of *Legionella* pneumonia associated with increased mortality. Eur J Clin Microbiol Infect Dis 1996;15:286–90.
47. Teh B, Grayson ML, Jonhson PD, et al. Doxycycline vs. macrolides in combination therapy for treatment of community-acquired pneumonia. Clin Microbiol Infect 2012;18:E71–3.
48. File TM Jr, Low DE, Eckburg PB, et al. Integrated Analysis of FOCUS 1 and FOCUS 2: Randomized, doubled-blinded, multicenter phase 3 trials of the efficacy and safety of ceftaroline fosamil versus ceftriaxone in patients with community-acquired pneumonia. Clin Infect Dis 2010;51:1395–405.
49. File TM Jr, Low DE, Eckburg PB, et al, Focus 1 investigators. Randomized, doubled-blinded, multicenter phase 3 trials of the efficacy and safety of ceftaroline fosamil versus ceftriaxone in patients with community-acquired pneumonia. J Antimicrob Chemother 2011;66(Suppl 3):19–32.
50. Low DE, File TM Jr, Eckburg PB, et al. FOCUS 2: a randomized, double-blinded, multicentre, Phase III trial of the efficacy and safety of ceftaroloine fosamil versus cefrriaxone in community-acquired pneumonia. J Antimicrob Chemother 2011;66(Suppl 3):33–44.
51. File T Jr, Eckburg P, Low D, et al. Assessment of outcomes at an early time point may identify a differential effect of macrolide therapy on community-acquired pneumonia due to atypical pathogens. Presented at the 22nd European Congress of Clinical Microbiology and Infectious Diseases. London, March 31, 2012, P 721.

52. Talbot GH, Powers JH, Fleming TR, et al. Progress on developing endpoints for registrations clinical trials of community-acquired bacterial pneumonia and acute bacterial skin and skin structure infections: update from the Biomarkers Consortium of the Foundation for the National Institutes of Health. Clin Infect Dis 2012; 55(8):1114–21.
53. Kim JH, Gallis HA. Observations on spiraling empiricism: its causes, allure and perils with particular reference to antibiotic therapy. Am J Med 1989;87:201–6.
54. Ewig S, Torres A. Community-acquired pneumonia as an emergency: time for an aggressive intervention to lower mortality. Eur Respir J 2011;38:253–60.
55. Majumdar SR, Eurich DT, Gamble JM, et al. Oxygen saturations less than 92% are associated with major adverse outcomes in outpatients with pneumonia: a population-based cohort study. Clin Infect Dis 2011;52:325–31.
56. Johnstone J, Eurich DT, Majumdar SR, et al. Long-term morbidity and mortality after hospitalization with community-acquired pneumonia: a population-based study. Medicine 2008;87:329–34.

Does Empirical Therapy with a Fluoroquinolone or the Combination of a β-Lactam Plus a Macrolide Result in Better Outcomes for Patients Admitted to the General Ward?

Jörg Ruhe, MD, MPH*, Donna Mildvan, MD

KEYWORDS

- Community-acquired pneumonia • Fluoroquinolone • β-lactam • Macrolide
- Outcome

KEY POINTS

- Current guidelines recommend therapy with a fluoroquinolone or a β-lactam plus a macrolide for the treatment of hospitalized adults with community-acquired pneumonia who do not require admission to an intensive care unit.
- A review of the currently existing literature on this topic is presented.
- Both regimens should be considered equivalent unless specific patient circumstances warrant the preference of one regimen over the other.
- Further prospective randomized studies are needed to clarify currently existing controversies in the literature.

INTRODUCTION

Community-acquired pneumonia (CAP) is a frequent cause of morbidity and mortality in the United States and worldwide, in particular among older patients and those with significant comorbid conditions. In the United States, 5 to 6 million episodes of CAP occur each year, and about 20% of these require hospital admission.[1] Despite the availability of effective antibiotic therapy, CAP is still associated with mortality rates of 6% to 23% and a 30-day readmission rate as high as 20%.[2] *Streptococcus pneumoniae* is the most common causative agent of CAP, but other species such as

Division of Infectious Diseases, Beth Israel Medical Center, Albert Einstein College of Medicine, First Avenue at 16th Street, New York, NY 10003, USA
* Corresponding author.
E-mail address: jruhe@chpnet.org

Infect Dis Clin N Am 27 (2013) 115–132
http://dx.doi.org/10.1016/j.idc.2012.11.004
0891-5520/13/$ – see front matter © 2013 Elsevier Inc. All rights reserved.

Haemophilus influenzae and the so-called atypical bacteria (*Legionella* species, *Mycoplasma pneumoniae*, and *Chlamydophila pneumoniae*) are also frequently identified.[3] However, in clinical practice settings, a causative pathogen is often not identified; thus, the administration of effective empirical therapy is frequently warranted.

Therapy has been complicated by the emergence of antibiotic resistance over the last 4 decades, especially among *S pneumoniae*.[4] Among 1817 *S pneumoniae* isolates obtained from patients with respiratory infections in 45 US medical centers during the winter of 2002 to 2003, resistance rates to different agents were as follows: penicillin 34.2% (older, pre-2008 penicillin breakpoints were used in this study), ceftriaxone 6.9%, erythromycin 29.5%, tetracycline 16.2%, ciprofloxacin 2.3%, and moxifloxacin 0.5%.[5] 22.2% of isolates were multidrug resistant, defined as intermediate-level or high-level resistance to penicillin and at least 2 of 4 other drugs (erythromycin, trimethoprim/sulfamethoxazole, chloramphenicol, and tetracycline). Compared with data on isolates from 1994 to 1995, resistance rates to most drugs had plateaued or declined, with the exception of the fluoroquinolones; resistance, especially to ciprofloxacin, has become relatively more prevalent. Clinical Laboratory Standards Institute (CLSI) penicillin breakpoint minimum inhibitory concentrations (MICs) for nonmeningeal isolates were significantly increased in 2008.[6] Based on these new parameters, it is estimated that currently about 14% of pneumococcal strains in the United States are nonsusceptible (includes intermediate-level and high-level resistance) to penicillin and about 9% are nonsusceptible to ceftriaxone.[7] Risk factors for the presence of penicillin-resistant *S pneumoniae* have been identified and include previous β-lactam use, stay in a nursing home, long-term care facility, or homeless shelter, and previous respiratory infections.[8,9]

However, the effect of β-lactam resistance among *S pneumoniae* on the clinical outcome of patients treated with these agents has been the subject of intensive investigation and debate. To summarize, based on data from observational studies, penicillin or cephalosporin therapy does not seem to lead to adverse outcomes among most patients who are treated for nonmeningeal infections caused by strains with relatively low levels of nonsusceptibility.[10,11] This is likely because sufficiently high local tissue concentrations can be achieved through appropriate drug dosing even in the presence of decreased susceptibility. In contrast, *S pneumoniae* resistance to macrolides or fluoroquinolones has clearly been correlated with treatment failures among patients treated with these agents.[12,13]

Current and previous guidelines by the Infectious Diseases Society of America and the American Thoracic Society on the management of CAP in adults admitted to a non–intensive care hospital unit recommend the use of either a respiratory fluoroquinolone (such as moxifloxacin, gemifloxacin, or levofloxacin) or a β-lactam (preferred agents are cefotaxime, ceftriaxone, or ampicillin) plus a macrolide.[3] Both regimens provide adequate coverage for the most common causative agents mentioned earlier. Oral stepdown therapy is recommended once the patient's clinical status has improved and stabilized. The total treatment duration should be at least 5 days. These recommendations are mainly based on the results of several large cohort studies that have demonstrated a significant benefit of either regimen compared with cephalosporin monotherapy.[14–16] The effectiveness of either treatment option has been further substantiated by several clinical trials.[3] Consequently, these results also raise the question whether 1 of these regimens, fluoroquinolone monotherapy or β-lactam plus macrolide combination therapy, is superior to the other on a direct head-to-head comparison. Over the last decade, several studies including randomized clinical trials, observational cohort studies, and meta-analyses have addressed this question and revealed some interesting and controversial results. This article provides a brief summary and overview of these studies categorized by their main results (please also see **Table 1**) and summarizes the potential implications for future clinical practice and research.

Studies That Favor Fluoroquinolone Therapy

Finch and colleagues[17] conducted a multicenter clinical trial on 628 patients requiring hospitalization for CAP who were randomized to receive either moxifloxacin 400 mg intravenously (i.v.) daily or amoxicillin/clavulanate 1.2 g i.v. 3 times daily with or without clarithromycin 500 mg twice daily. Patients were treated for 7 to 14 days; therapy could be switched to oral forms of the same drugs after a minimum of 3 days. The study, which was designed as a noninferiority trial, showed significantly higher clinical cure rates in the moxifloxacin group at both 5 to 7 days posttherapy (93.4% vs 85.4%, respectively; $P = .004$) and at days 21 to 28 posttherapy (83.7% vs 74.3%). According to Finch and colleagues,[17] this outcome benefit in the fluoroquinolone group was seen to be independent of whether a macrolide was added to amoxicillin/clavulanate or not; however, the absolute number of patients who received a macrolide and the number of patients who had an atypical pathogen identified and were treated with a macrolide were not reported. Clinical cure rates were also higher for both nonsevere and severe disease. Furthermore, patients in the fluoroquinolone group were found to have a significantly faster return to apyrexia, hospital stay was 1 day shorter, and mortality was lower (3% vs 5.3%) than in patients in the comparator group. Causative organisms were isolated in 194 (31%) patients; S pneumoniae (55.4%) and H influenzae (19.6%) were the most commonly identified species. Atypical pathogens were seen in 14%. Among evaluable patients, bacteriologic success rates were also higher in the moxifloxacin group (93.7%) than the comparator group (81.7%). These findings could not be explained by higher rates of resistance to amoxicillin/clavulanate (the MIC90 was 0.25 mg/L). Drug-related adverse events were similar in both groups.

In a prospective, randomized, open-label study in 40 North American medical centers by File and colleagues,[18] 590 patients were randomized to receive either i.v. and/or oral levofloxacin or i.v. ceftriaxone and/or oral cefuroxime axetil; among 230 clinically evaluable patients in the β-lactam arm, 50 (22%) also received erythromycin or doxycycline, which could be added at the investigator's discretion. Most (53%) of the patients were treated on an outpatient basis. A higher clinical success rate at 5 to 7 days posttherapy was found in the levofloxacin group (96%) than in the comparator group (90%; 95% confidence interval −10.7 to −1.3). Bacterial eradication rates of typical respiratory pathogens (S pneumoniae and H influenzae) were also higher in the levofloxacin group (98% vs 85%, respectively). One hundred and fifty atypical pathogens were identified in the study cohort; 101 of these were C pneumoniae. However, among clinically evaluable patients with treatment failure, only 2 with atypical pneumonia received β-lactam monotherapy. None of the pathogens isolated on admission were resistant to levofloxacin, whereas 5 pathogens were resistant to ceftriaxone and 19 were resistant to cefuroxime axetil. It is possible that the lack of universal coverage with antiatypical agents, the use of older agents among those who did receive atypical coverage, and the higher resistance levels to the study drug in the comparator group contributed to the observed outcome differences.

Treatment success measured by mortality rates was also higher among fluoroquinolone-treated patients in a prospective, observational, cohort study done in a single medical center in Spain between 2000 and 2003.[19] Of 459 hospitalized patients, 250 received levofloxacin (54%) and 209 received (46%) ceftriaxone plus clarithromycin, both for a minimum of 7 days. The latter regimen was the preferred

Table 1
Overview of studies that compare the efficacy of fluoroquinolone versus β-lactam ± macrolide therapy for the treatment of patients with CAP

Study, Year of Publication	Study Location	Study Type	No. of Enrolled Patients	Fluoroquinolone (FQ) Arm	β-Lactam Arm	Main Outcome
A. Studies That Demonstrated Better Outcomes with Fluoroquinolone Therapy						
Finch et al,[17] 2002	Multicenter study from Europe, Israel, South Africa	Randomized, open-label trial	628	Moxifloxacin	Amoxicillin/clavulanate ± clarithromycin (optional)	Higher clinical success rate in FQ arm (93.4% vs 85.4%; P = .004) in per protocol analysis
File et al,[18] 1997	Multicenter study from North America	Randomized, open-label trial	590	Levofloxacin	Ceftriaxone (and/or cefuroxime axetil) ± erythromycin or doxycycline (optional)	Higher clinical success rate at 5–7 d in FQ arm (96%) than β-lactam arm (90%; 95% CI −10.7 to −1.3)
Querol-Ribelles et al,[19] 2005	Single center study in Spain	Prospective cohort study	459	Levofloxacin	Ceftriaxone plus clarithromycin	Higher mortality rate in β-lactam arm (12%) than in FQ arm (6%; P = .024)
Welte et al,[21] 2005	Multicenter study from 5 European countries	Randomized, open-label trial	397	Moxifloxacin	Ceftriaxone ± erythromycin	Faster clinical improvement including more rapid sustained defervescence in FQ group
Dresser et al,[22] 2001	Multicenter study from North America	Randomized, double-blind trial	283	Gatifloxacin	Ceftriaxone ± erythromycin	No statistically significant difference in clinical or microbiological cure rates. Geometric mean cost $1.053 less in FQ group

Source	Setting	Study design	No.	FQ regimen	Comparator regimen	Outcome
Vardakas et al,[23] 2008	—	Meta-analysis of randomized trials	23 trials included	Different regimens used among included studies	Different regimens used among included studies	Higher clinical success rates among patients treated with FQ. However, no difference in mortality
B. Studies That Demonstrated Better Outcomes with β-Lactam Plus Macrolide Therapy						
Lodise et al,[24] 2007	Single center study in the United States	Retrospective cohort study	515	Levofloxacin	Extended-spectrum cephalosporin (91%) or β-lactam/β-lactam inhibitor (9%) plus azithromycin	Lower mortality (18.4% vs 36.6%; $P = .05$) in the β-lactam group among patients with severe CAP
Zervos et al,[25] 2004	Multicenter study from North America and Europe	Randomized, open-label trial	212	Levofloxacin	Ceftriaxone plus azithromycin	Comparable clinical efficacy, but better bacteriologic eradication rates in β-lactam group (100%) than in FQ group (44%)
C. Studies That Demonstrated Comparable Efficacy of Both Regimens						
Portier et al,[1] 2005	80 French hospitals	Randomized, open-label trial	346	Moxifloxacin	Amoxicillin/clavulanate ± roxithromycin	Similar clinical and microbiological success rates of both regimens
Fogarty et al,[26] 2004	33 medical centers in the United States	Randomized, open-label trial	269	Levofloxacin	Ceftriaxone plus i.v. erythromycin followed by oral amoxicillin/clavulanate plus clarithromycin	No statistically significant difference in clinical success rates between both regimens

(continued on next page)

Table 1
(continued)

Study, Year of Publication	Study Location	Study Type	No. of Enrolled Patients	Fluoroquinolone (FQ) Arm	β-Lactam Arm	Main Outcome
Torres et al,[27] 2003	Multicenter study from Europe and South Africa	Randomized, double-blind trial	564	Moxifloxacin	Amoxicillin/ clavulanate plus clarithromycin	Similar clinical success rates of both regimens (93.5% and 93.9%, respectively) at 7–10 d posttherapy
Lode et al,[28] 2002	Multicenter study from 4 continents	Randomized, open-label trial	345	Gemifloxacin	Intravenous ceftriaxone/oral cefuroxime ± a macrolide	No statistically significant difference in clinical success rates between both regimens
Petermann et al,[29] 2001	Multicenter study from Europe, South Africa, and Australia	Randomized, open-label trial	527	Clinafloxacin	Ceftriaxone ± erythromycin	No statistically significant difference in clinical success rates between both regimens
Katz et al,[30] 2004	40 medical centers in the United States	Randomized, open-label trial	221	Moxifloxacin	Ceftriaxone ± azithromycin	Similar clinical cure rates (83.3% vs 79.6%, respectively)
Bratzler et al,[31] 2008	Centers for Medicare and Medicaid Services database	Retrospective cohort study	24,780	Fluoroquinolone	Cephalosporin (second or third generation) plus a macrolide	Both treatment modalities resulted in significantly better survival rates at days 14 and 30 compared with third-generation cephalosporin monotherapy

Gleason et al,[14] 1999	Medicare database	Retrospective cohort study	12,945	Ciprofloxacin or ofloxacin	Third-generation cephalosporin plus a macrolide	Both treatment modalities resulted in significantly better survival rates at day 30 compared with third-generation cephalosporin monotherapy
Erard et al,[32] 2004	Two Swiss medical centers	Randomized, open-label trial	129	Levofloxacin	Ceftriaxone ± clarithromycin	Similar rates of clinical resolution and length of stay
Frank et al,[33] 2002	Multicenter study from the United States	Randomized, open-label trial	236	Levofloxacin	Azithromycin plus ceftriaxone	Similar clinical success rates were observed in both treatment arms
Asadi et al,[34] 2012	—	Meta-analysis of randomized trials and observational studies	23 studies included	Different regimens used among included studies	Different regimens used among included studies	Similar mortality rates on comparison of respiratory fluoroquinolone (5.8%) and β-lactam/macrolide combination therapy (5.3%; $P = .22$)

treatment choice throughout the first 20 months; levofloxacin was primarily used during the following 26 months. Only 63% of patients in the levofloxacin group had a Pneumonia Severity Index (PSI) score of IV or V, compared with 73% in the ceftriaxone/macrolide group (P = .02).[20] The main result of this study was that significantly fewer patients died in the levofloxacin group (n = 15; 6%) than in the comparator group (n = 25; 12%) (P = .024). All deaths occurred among patients with either PSI class IV or V. Among 28 *S pneumoniae* strains isolated from blood cultures, all were susceptible to levofloxacin, but 7% and 39% were resistant to ceftriaxone and erythromycin, respectively. However, none of the isolates was resistant to both agents. Rates of a switch to different antibiotic regimens did not differ significantly between the 2 cohorts. The limitations in study design and the difference in pneumonia severity in the 2 treatment groups need to be taken into account when interpreting these results.

Similar clinical success rates, not a faster clinical improvement, measured by earlier sustained defervescence (median onset, 3 vs 4 days; $P<.019$), a more rapid decrease of pretreatment C-reactive protein levels, and faster resolution of specific patient-reported symptoms of pneumonia, were reported in a randomized, non-blinded, multicenter study from several European countries among patients who received moxifloxacin monotherapy, rather than the comparator ceftriaxone 2 g daily with or without i.v. erythromycin.[21] Both groups were similar with regard to a variety of underlying clinical characteristics including PSI scores. Mean duration of therapy was 10.1 days in the moxifloxacin group (a switch to the oral formulation occurred after a mean of 5.9 days on i.v. therapy) and 9.5 days in the cephalosporin group (no oral stepdown regimen was permitted). Only 59 (38%) of 156 patients in the ceftriaxone group were also treated with concomitant erythromycin (permitted if the clinician suspected the presence of an atypical organism). Results of clinical efficacy were not stratified by the presence of macrolide therapy.

In a study by Dresser and colleagues[22] (n = 233 evaluable patients), monotherapy with gatifloxacin was as clinically effective with regard to clinical cure and microbiological eradication rates as combination therapy with ceftriaxone with or without erythromycin, but was associated with potential cost savings in an independent cost analysis. Oral conversion was achieved in 98% of patients in each group.

Vardakas and colleagues[23] presented a meta-analysis on clinical trials published between 1980 and 2008 that compared the efficacy of fluoroquinolone monotherapy with either β-lactam and macrolide combination therapy or monotherapy with a macrolide, ketolide, or a β-lactam in patients with CAP. Twenty-three trials were included in the analysis; 8 of these were double blinded. The investigators found no difference in mortality between patients who received fluoroquinolones and patients who received comparator regimens. However, pneumonia was cured or improved according to predefined criteria in significantly more patients in the fluoroquinolone group than in the comparator group (odds ratio [OR] 1.17, 95% confidence interval [CI] 1.00–1.36). Comparator drug regimens in 6 (40%) of the 15 studies that were evaluated in this subanalysis consisted of only β-lactam or macrolide monotherapy. Furthermore, fluoroquinolones were reported to be more effective in studies that only used a β-lactam and macrolide combination therapy comparator (OR 1.39, 95% CI 1.02–1.90). Among the 9 studies included for the latter comparison, patients in 4 studies did not routinely receive a macrolide, only at the discretion of the treating physician. When the outcomes of patients with severe pneumonia from 7 studies were analyzed, fluoroquinolones were again found to be significantly more effective. However, the addition of a macrolide was required in only 1 of these 7 studies, and it was optional in 5 other studies. There was no difference in the effectiveness between fluoroquinolone and comparator regimens if only trials of high quality according to predefined criteria were included in the analysis.

Studies That Show Similar or Superior Efficacy of β-Lactam and Macrolide Combination Therapy

One cohort study, but no randomized clinical trial, has to our knowledge demonstrated clinical superiority of β-lactam/macrolide combination therapy over fluoroquinolone monotherapy.

A retrospective cohort study by Lodise and colleagues[24] showed clinical superiority of β-lactam/macrolide combination therapy. They analyzed data from the Upstate New York Veterans Affairs (VA) network generated between October 1999 and May 2003. Five hundred and fifteen patients hospitalized with CAP received either combination therapy consisting of a β-lactam and a macrolide (n = 261) or levofloxacin monotherapy (n = 254). Combination therapy consisted of azithromycin combined with ceftriaxone (91%) or a β-lactam/β-lactamase inhibitor (9%). The 2 groups were similar with regard to age, comorbid diseases, previous antibiotic use, mean PSI scores, and APACHE-II scores. This also applied to the subgroup of patients who presented with the most severe pneumonia (PSI category V). The main outcome measures of the study were 14-day and 30-day mortality. No mortality difference between the 2 treatment arms was found among patients with lower PSI scores I to IV. Mortality was significantly lower by day 14 (8.2% vs 26.8%; $P = .02$) and by day 30 (18.4% vs 36.6%; $P = .05$) among patients with severe pneumonia (PSI category V) in the β-lactam/macrolide combination group compared with those in the levofloxacin group. The overall length of stay was longer in the combination group (6.0 days vs 5.0 days; $P = .01$); after subanalysis of length of stay within the 5 PSI classes, only patients on combination therapy in class IV had a significantly longer hospital stay (5 vs 4 days). It may be difficult to generalize the findings of this study to other patient populations as patients admitted to the VA health care system have unique underlying demographic and clinical characteristics. Furthermore, clinicians choosing the most appropriate treatment regimen for patients with a PSI V score, especially if these require admission to an intensive care unit, would likely prefer the combination of a third-generation cephalosporin plus a macrolide or a fluoroquinolone or even broader-spectrum coverage than fluoroquinolone monotherapy based on current treatment guidelines.[3]

An open-label multicenter trial randomized patients (n = 212) to either combination therapy with i.v. ceftriaxone and azithromycin or to monotherapy with daily i.v. levofloxacin at a dose of 500 mg.[25] Patients who improved clinically could switch to oral therapy, which consisted of oral azithromycin in the combination arm (the addition of oral cefuroxime axetil was permitted if a macrolide-resistant S pneumoniae strain was isolated) or to oral levofloxacin. The investigators found similar rates of clinical success at the end of study visit (89.2% vs 85.1%, respectively). In contrast, bacteriologic cure rates were higher among patient with documented S pneumoniae infections: Only 44% of the isolates were eradicated in the fluoroquinolone group compared with 100% in the combination group. The investigators concluded that combination therapy was at least as effective as levofloxacin monotherapy.

In addition, a significant body of literature consisting of several randomized clinical trials and large prospective cohort studies has been published that demonstrates equal clinical efficacy of the 2 therapeutic regimens among patients admitted for CAP to a non–intensive care unit. A brief review of the most important of these studies follows.

In an open-label trial performed in 80 French hospitals, 346 hospitalized patients were randomized to receive a 10-day course of either oral moxifloxacin 400 mg daily or oral amoxicillin/clavulanate 1000/125 mg 3 times daily plus roxithromycin (an erythromycin derivate licensed in Europe) 150 mg twice daily, all for 10 days.[1] No specific information on the severity of pneumonia was provided, but the fact that all patients received oral therapy throughout their hospital stay suggests a relatively stable, less seriously ill patient population. In their intent-to-treat analysis, clinical success at the test-of-cure visit 5 to 7 days after the end of therapy was not significantly different between the 2 groups (83% and 77.7%, respectively). Bacteriologic success (a causative pathogen was identified in 19% of patients) was also similar in both groups; however, no specific data on antibiotic resistance among identified isolates were provided. Rates of adverse events also did not differ between the 2 groups.

In another open-label study performed in 33 medical centers in the United States, 269 seriously ill patients were randomized to therapy with levofloxacin 500 mg i.v. daily followed by oral administration of the same regimen, or to therapy with ceftriaxone 1 to 2 g daily and i.v. erythromycin followed by administration of oral amoxicillin/clavulanate 875 mg twice daily and clarithromycin 500 mg twice daily.[26] The average APACHE II score was ~ 16 and the median duration of therapy was 13 and 11 days in each group, respectively. Levofloxacin was considered as efficacious as the comparator regimen with regard to clinical success in the intent-to-treat population (72.7% vs 64.2%, respectively). Both regimens were well tolerated. Among patients requiring vasopressor therapy, clinical success was achieved in 11 (69%) of 16 patients treated with levofloxacin and 7 (50%) of 14 patients treated with the β-lactam/macrolide combination. In this study, 101 (39%) of 256 identified organisms were atypical organisms (Chlamydophila pneumoniae n = 47, Legionella pneumophila n = 25, Mycoplasma pneumoniae n = 29). These results further emphasize the need for empirical coverage of these organisms.

A multicenter study from several European countries and South Africa on 564 patients with CAP treated in inpatient and outpatient settings showed similar efficacy of oral moxifloxacin monotherapy (n = 233) and oral amoxicillin/clarithromycin combination therapy (n = 143) at days 7 to 10 after the end of therapy (93.6% and 93.7%, respectively) and at days 28 to 35 after the end of therapy (both 94.2%).[27] Patients with class IV and V PSI scores comprised only 18% of the study population. Rates of resolution of clinical symptoms during therapy did not differ significantly between the 2 treatment groups.

Lode and colleagues[28] performed a multicenter open-label trial that investigated the efficacy of oral gemifloxacin compared with ceftriaxone (and oral stepdown therapy with cefuroxime) with or without macrolide therapy in 69 medical centers in 15 countries. One hundred and seventy-two patients were randomized to fluoroquinolone monotherapy, and 173 patients were enrolled in the cephalosporin arm; among the latter, 38% of clinically evaluable patients also had a macrolide administered. Mean duration of therapy was 10.3 days in both arms. Clinical and microbiological success rates were equivalent in both groups. Among patients with a PSI score of IV or V (total n = 47), clinical success rates were 87% and 83.3%, respectively (not significant). In this study, a causative bacterial agent was identified in 170 patients; 89 (52.4%) of these were atypical pathogens. Further analysis based on whether a macrolide was added or not did not reveal any difference in patient outcome. Both treatment arms were generally well tolerated.

Another similar multicenter, open-label, randomized study from Europe, South Africa, and Australia showed equal clinical and microbiological efficacy of clinafloxacin monotherapy compared with ceftriaxone with or without erythromycin.[29]

A randomized, open-label, multicenter study compared i.v. and oral moxifloxacin monotherapy with i.v. ceftriaxone (followed by oral cefuroxime) with or without azithromycin.[30] Similar clinical cure rates were found in the moxifloxacin group (n = 108) and the comparator group (n = 113) (83.3% and 79.6%, respectively); among the latter, 70% of patients were treated with ceftriaxone and azithromycin combination therapy. Ten patients also received metronidazole.

Using a large data set from the Centers for Medicare and Medicaid Services, Bratzler and colleagues[31] compared mortality data among 24,780 patients admitted with CAP to non–intensive care wards from July to March in 1998 to 1999 and 2000 to 2001. Compared with monotherapy with a third-generation cephalosporin as the reference, both therapies with fluoroquinolone monotherapy and with cephalosporin plus macrolide combination therapy were associated with a statistically significantly lower 14-day mortality (adjusted OR 0.7 [0.5–0.8] and 0.7 [0.6–0.9], respectively) and 30-day mortality (adjusted OR 0.7 [0.6–0.9] and 0.7 [0.6–0.9], respectively). On further subgroup analysis of 30-day mortality based on PSI score, these outcome differences were only found among patients with high PSI scores IV and V, but not in patients with lower risk classes II and III. However, it was surprising that macrolide monotherapy was also associated with a significantly better outcome among PSI class IV and V patients compared with third-generation cephalosporin monotherapy. This result raises the concern that unidentified confounding variables may even compromise the validity of such large cohort studies on CAP treatment outcomes. Other therapies including macrolide monotherapy, second-generation monotherapy, and cephalosporin plus fluoroquinolone combination therapy did not perform statistically differently when compared with third-generation monotherapy.

A previous study of similar design by Gleason and colleagues[14] on 12,945 Medicare inpatients treated between October 1994 and September 1995 came to similar conclusions: Both fluoroquinolone monotherapy and combination therapy with a nonpseudomonal third-generation cephalosporin plus a macrolide were associated with significantly better 30-day mortality rates than third-generation cephalosporin monotherapy. It should be taken into account that older fluoroquinolones (ciprofloxacin and ofloxacin) with less in vitro activity against *S pneumoniae* compared with the newer respiratory fluoroquinolones were used in this study.

Other studies not discussed in detail have also described equal clinical efficacy of β-lactam/macrolide combination therapy and fluoroquinolone monotherapy.[32,33]

A systematic review and meta-analysis on the effect of macrolide-based regimens on the mortality of patients hospitalized with CAP has recently been published.[34] A total of 23 studies, including 5 randomized clinical trials, were analyzed. Overall, a 22% reduction in mortality among patients who received macrolide-based regimens compared with patients treated with nonmacrolides was detected. Of specific importance for this discussion, 2 predefined subgroup analyses on studies that compared β-lactam/macrolide combinations with fluoroquinolones were performed. These consisted of (1) all 5 randomized trials (no study heterogeneity was observed) and (2) 4 of the 5 randomized trials together with 12 observational studies and a total of 12,624 patients (moderate study homogeneity was observed). Both subanalyses revealed no difference in mortality between the 2 treatment options.

INTERPRETATION OF THE EVIDENCE

Given the large number of people affected by CAP worldwide each year, providing the most effective and best tolerated therapy for patients with CAP is of high importance as even a small true difference in efficacy between different therapies would have a significant effect on global health. Ideally, narrow-spectrum pathogen-directed therapy could be used to effectively treat the causative organisms and preserve the patient's commensal microflora as much as possible. However, currently available, routine, diagnostic tests such as Gram stain and culture from respiratory specimens have limited sensitivity and applying their results has not led to better outcomes compared with empirical therapy in at least 1 study.[35,36] Thus, empirical broad-spectrum therapy with either 1 of the regimens discussed is recommended by current CAP guidelines unless other specific pathogens (eg, methicillin-resistant *Staphylococcus aureus*) are suspected.

As outlined earlier, a significant number of studies with different strengths and weaknesses have addressed the efficacy and safety of these first-line CAP treatment strategies: fluoroquinolone monotherapy or β-lactam plus macrolide combination therapy. Most found similar results. However, several investigations suggested or demonstrated superiority of either 1 of the regimens; most of these studies, including 3 randomized clinical trials, found a more rapid clinical response within the first days of therapy, higher clinical cure rates, and/or improved mortality (the latter was only found in 1 cohort study) among patients treated with fluoroquinolone. This section presents additional considerations that are relevant for the interpretation of these results, especially with regard to the suggested superiority of fluoroquinolones in the treatment of patients hospitalized with CAP.

First, lending support to the potential advantage of fluoroquinolones for treatment of CAP is the high oral bioavailability of agents in this class, allowing for early and convenient once-daily oral stepdown therapy. This therapy may translate into a shorter length of hospital stay compared with combination therapy, as has been observed in some studies, and could be associated with significant cost savings.[22] Moreover, as observed in multiple clinical trials, fluoroquinolones were well tolerated and associated with few serious side effects, similar to the comparator arms.[17,18]

On the other hand, it is also fair to note that fluoroquinolones may have seemed to outperform comparator arms in several of the studies reviewed because of important study design issues.

One such concern relates to the implications of empirical therapy assignments in the face of increasingly widespread antibiotic resistance to the most important pathogen, *S pneumoniae*. Although it is possible that higher pneumococcal resistance rates to the β-lactams and macrolides compared with the fluoroquinolones overall are responsible for the observed poorer outcomes of the former treatment regimen, it also possible that the stepdown switch to oral cefuroxime in some trials may have conferred a disadvantage to the β-lactam/macrolide arm. In one of the largest studies on the effect of penicillin resistance, Yu and colleagues[10] published a prospective, international, cohort study on 844 patients hospitalized with *S pneumoniae* bacteremia in 2003. Among a total of 360 patients who received monotherapy, receipt of discordant therapy (ie, administration of an antibiotic agent to which the organism was found to be nonsusceptible) with penicillin, cefotaxime, or ceftriaxone was not related to an increased mortality risk compared with receipt of concordant therapy. However, patients treated with cefuroxime for bacteremic infections caused by a cefuroxime-resistant *S pneumoniae* isolate had a significantly higher risk of death than patients on concordant cefuroxime therapy (4 [36.4%] of 11 patients vs 4 [5.8%] of 53 patients; $P = .02$). Cefuroxime was given in many of the studies reviewed once the patient was stable for conversion to oral therapy. In a recent study on 891 *S pneumoniae* isolates from 22 centers in the United States, only 70% were cefuroxime susceptible.[7] High-dose amoxicillin or amoxicillin/clavulanate is considered to be the preferred oral treatment option, especially if a causative organism has not been identified and/or the patient resides in an area where β-lactam resistance is prevalent.[37]

Because fluoroquinolones provide excellent coverage for atypical organisms, another consideration in interpreting the body of evidence concerns whether or not the comparator regimens included empirical coverage for atypicals. In 3 clinical trials that showed improved outcomes among patients who received fluoroquinolones, the addition of a macrolide in the β-lactam treatment arm was optional and was, to the extent reported, given in only 22% to 38% of patients. Thus, an unknown number of patients with CAP caused by an atypical organism may not have received effective therapy. Studies aimed at determining the cause of CAP indicate that about 20% to 30% of CAP is caused by *Legionella* species, *Mycoplasma pneumoniae*, or *Chlamydophila pneumonia*.[38] Although the necessity of providing antibiotic therapy against these organisms has been debated, a more recent meta-analysis described higher treatment failures among patients who received β-lactam monotherapy and whose pneumonia was caused by *Legionella pneumophila*, but not by other atypical pathogens.[39]

Macrolides also seem to produce significant immunomodulatory effects that include the suppression of specific transcription factors with resultant decreased production of proinflammatory cytokines such as tumor necrosis factor alpha, interleukin (IL)-1, IL-6, IL-8, and transforming growth factor-β, decreased neutrophil chemotaxis to the airways, and increased production of antiinflammatory cytokines such as IL-10.[40] Thus, macrolides could provide an additional therapeutic benefit independent of their antimicrobial activity, and their omission could bias trials in favor of the quinolone comparator. This interpretation may be supported by several observational studies that have shown a positive effect on length of stay and mortality among patients who were treated with a macrolide-containing regimen versus treatment with other monotherapies or combination therapies that did not contain a macrolide.[16,41,42] Not all comparators in these studies, however, provided other forms of atypical coverage. Furthermore, a few studies suggest that the addition of a macrolide to β-lactam therapy is associated with lower mortality rates among patients with documented bacteremic, β-lactam–susceptible *S pneumoniae* pneumonia when compared with β-lactam monotherapy.[43–45] In vitro studies detected no synergistic effect between the 2 drug classes.[46] Interpretation of the latter studies is complicated, however, by their retrospective and observational design, the possible presence of unidentified atypical copathogens, and the potentially incomplete adjustment for other confounders such as severity of disease.

Many additional and relevant open questions remain, including the potential for either of the first-line drug regimens to cause collateral damage (ie, to promote subsequent downstream colonization or infection with drug-resistant organisms). The worldwide emergence of antibiotic resistance among many important pathogens has been declared a major health threat by the World Health Organization and antibiotic resistance has been clearly linked to previous exposure to antibiotics.[47] To examine the contribution of the 2 first-line empirical CAP regimens to development of resistance, the authors performed a retrospective cohort study on 175 patients treated with either moxifloxacin monotherapy (n = 41) or ceftriaxone/azithromycin combination therapy (n = 134) for CAP and recorded the rates of subsequent colonization or infection with multidrug-resistant organisms (methicillin-resistant *Staphylococcus aureus*, vancomycin-resistant enterococci, multidrug-resistant gram-negative organisms, and *Clostridium difficile*) among these patients within the next 6 months.[48] Both cohorts were similar with regard to several characteristics including age, CURB-65 score, and underlying comorbidities. On logistic regression analyses, moxifloxacin therapy remained an independent predictor of subsequent isolation of multidrug-resistant organisms (adjusted OR 6.5, 95% CI 1.8–23.1; $P = .004$). Rates of isolation of drug-susceptible organisms did not differ between the 2 groups. Other studies demonstrated high rates of fluoroquinolone resistance to *Mycobacterium tuberculosis* among patients who had erroneously been diagnosed with CAP (rather than pulmonary tuberculosis) and were treated with a respiratory fluoroquinolone.[49]

The important question regarding a therapeutic advantage of either empirical regimen for patients with more serious disease remains unanswered, especially among patients with a PSI score of IV or V. Many studies were underpowered to derive an interpretable conclusion about this patient population, although 1 study by Lodise found a statistically significantly higher mortality difference of 18.6% at day 14 and 18.2% at day 30 in favor of β-lactam plus macrolide combination therapy (compared with levofloxacin monotherapy) among 90 seriously ill patients with a PSI score of V.[24]

In summary, many studies have examined and compared the clinical efficacy and tolerability of fluoroquinolone monotherapy versus β-lactam plus macrolide combination therapy. These studies differ significantly with regard to multiple criteria including study design, antibiotic agents used, number of patients enrolled, severity of disease, local prevalence of antibiotic resistance, geographic location, and sources of financial support for the study. Although most studies reported similar clinical efficacy of both treatment regimens, only a few described a statistically significant clinical benefit of 1 regimen more than the other.

However, after reviewing the existing literature, the authors conclude that neither of the 2 first-line regimens has been proved to have clear-cut clinical superiority. This view is strongly supported by a recently published meta-analysis that found no significant difference in mortality with either treatment option on evaluation of relevant clinical trials with or without the inclusion of additional observational studies.[34] Thus, clinicians should choose either 1 of the preferred first-line therapies for patients who present with CAP. Therapeutic decision making should be individualized taking into account additional patient information such as the presence of drug allergies, local resistance patterns, patient comorbidities, and risk factors for the presence of a β-lactam–resistant *S pneumoniae* isolate such as recent use of antibiotics with activity against respiratory pathogens (for these patients, current guidelines recommend considering the prescription of an alternative regimen).[3]

NEED FOR FUTURE STUDIES

Ideally, a large, randomized, single-blind, or preferably double-blind, multicenter trial to answer the question on the best empirical treatment modality for CAP would include the following: (1) a newer respiratory fluoroquinolone compared with a third-generation cephalosporin with the mandatory addition of a macrolide; (2) a second-generation macrolide such as azithromycin with a greater antimicrobial spectrum of activity, better oral absorption, and higher tolerability than erythromycin; (3) oral step-down therapy in the β-lactam/macrolide arm consisting of high-dose amoxicillin or amoxicillin/clavulanate; (4) adequately powered sample size to detect a small but clinically relevant difference in outcome; (5) an adequate number of patients with serious disease (but who do not require admission to an intensive care unit) to allow meaningful subanalysis of the outcome of these patients and data analysis that can be stratified by severity of disease; (6) analysis of the effect of treatment regimens on early clinical improvement after 3 to 5 days of therapy, patient length of stay, 30-day readmission rates, and cost of therapy; (7) a thorough search for causative pathogens and data on rates of microbiological failure; and (8) assessment of the effect of treatment regimen on the subsequent colonization or infection with drug-resistant organisms and *C difficile*.

The authors recognize that such a study may not be conducted in the near future as it would require major industry/government/academic collaborations, a generous funding source, and enrollment of large numbers of patients from multiple medical centers. A different but potentially even more promising approach to optimize CAP therapy while minimizing collateral damage was recently outlined in the literature.[35] This strategy would consist of the routine use of diagnostic modalities, such as *S pneumoniae* and *Legionella pneumophila* urinary antigens, on patient arrival in the emergency department, and optimally, with the future addition of molecular method-ologies that test for the presence of important bacterial and viral pathogens in respi-ratory specimens. This strategy would allow physicians to prescribe effective and narrower-spectrum therapy and, in many instances, reduce the need for broad-spectrum empirical coverage with either of the currently recommended first-line regimens.

SUMMARY

Until such time as an adequately powered study resolves the outstanding questions regarding the potential superiority of either of the first-line empirical treatment regi-mens for CAP, our literature review supports currently existing guidelines that recom-mend the use of either monotherapy with a respiratory fluoroquinolone or combination therapy with both a β-lactam such as ceftriaxone and a macrolide for the treatment of adult patients hospitalized with CAP to a non–intensive care unit. Although limited existing data point to the possible superiority of the fluoroquinolones, many important unresolved issues do not permit endorsement of one regimen over the other, but argue for individualized choices between the first-line regimens in the clinical setting. The future of CAP treatment may also be changing, with promising new diagnostic modal-ities likely to promote the shift from empirical to rational pathogen-directed therapy for CAP.

REFERENCES

1. Portier H, Brambilla C, Garre M, et al. Moxifloxacin monotherapy compared to amoxicillin-clavulanate plus roxithromycin for nonsevere community-acquired pneumonia in adults with risk factors. Eur J Clin Microbiol Infect Dis 2005; 24(6):367–76.
2. File TM Jr, Marrie TJ. Burden of community-acquired pneumonia in North Amer-ican adults. Postgrad Med 2010;122(2):130–41.
3. Mandell LA, Wunderink RG, Anzueto A, et al. Infectious Diseases Society of America/American Thoracic Society consensus guidelines on the management of community-acquired pneumonia in adults. Clin Infect Dis 2007;44(Suppl 2): S27–72.
4. Whitney CG, Farley MM, Hadler J, et al. Increasing prevalence of multidrug-resistant *Streptococcus pneumoniae* in the United States. N Engl J Med 2000; 343(26):1917–24.
5. Doern GV, Richter SS, Miller A, et al. Antimicrobial resistance among *Strepto-coccus pneumoniae* in the United States: have we begun to turn the corner on resistance to certain antimicrobial classes? Clin Infect Dis 2005;41(2):139–48.
6. Weinstein MP, Klugman KP, Jones RN. Rationale for revised penicillin suscepti-bility breakpoints versus *Streptococcus pneumoniae*: coping with antimicrobial susceptibility in an era of resistance. Clin Infect Dis 2009;48(11):1596–600.

7. Jacobs MR, Good CE, Windau AR, et al. Activity of ceftaroline against recent emerging serotypes of Streptococcus pneumoniae in the United States. Antimicrob Agents Chemother 2010;54(6):2716–9.

8. Ruhe JJ, Myers L, Mushatt D, et al. High-level penicillin-nonsusceptible Streptococcus pneumoniae bacteremia: identification of a low-risk subgroup. Clin Infect Dis 2004;38(4):508–14.

9. Moreno F, Crisp C, Jorgensen JH, et al. The clinical and molecular epidemiology of bacteremias at a university hospital caused by pneumococci not susceptible to penicillin. J Infect Dis 1995;172(2):427–32.

10. Yu VL, Chiou CC, Feldman C, et al. An international prospective study of pneumococcal bacteremia: correlation with in vitro resistance, antibiotics administered, and clinical outcome. Clin Infect Dis 2003;37(2):230–7.

11. Turett GS, Blum S, Fazal BA, et al. Penicillin resistance and other predictors of mortality in pneumococcal bacteremia in a population with high human immunodeficiency virus seroprevalence. Clin Infect Dis 1999;29(2):321–7.

12. Daneman N, McGeer A, Green K, et al. Macrolide resistance in bacteremic pneumococcal disease: implications for patient management. Clin Infect Dis 2006; 43(4):432–8.

13. Davidson R, Cavalcanti R, Brunton JL, et al. Resistance to levofloxacin and failure of treatment of pneumococcal pneumonia. N Engl J Med 2002;346(10):747–50.

14. Gleason PP, Meehan TP, Fine JM, et al. Associations between initial antimicrobial therapy and medical outcomes for hospitalized elderly patients with pneumonia. Arch Intern Med 1999;159(21):2562–72.

15. Houck PM, MacLehose RF, Niederman MS, et al. Empiric antibiotic therapy and mortality among Medicare pneumonia inpatients in 10 western states: 1993, 1995, and 1997. Chest 2001;119(5):1420–6.

16. Brown RB, Iannini P, Gross P, et al. Impact of initial antibiotic choice on clinical outcomes in community-acquired pneumonia: analysis of a hospital claims-made database. Chest 2003;123(5):1503–11.

17. Finch R, Schürmann D, Collins O, et al. Randomized controlled trial of sequential intravenous (i.v.) and oral moxifloxacin compared with sequential i.v. and oral co-amoxiclav with or without clarithromycin in patients with community-acquired pneumonia requiring initial parenteral treatment. Antimicrob Agents Chemother 2002;46(6):1746–54.

18. File TM Jr, Segreti J, Dunbar L, et al. A multicenter, randomized study comparing the efficacy and safety of intravenous and/or oral levofloxacin versus ceftriaxone and/or cefuroxime axetil in treatment of adults with community-acquired pneumonia. Antimicrob Agents Chemother 1997;41(9):1965–72.

19. Querol-Ribelles JM, Tenías JM, Querol-Borras JM, et al. Levofloxacin versus ceftriaxone plus clarithromycin in the treatment of adults with community-acquired pneumonia requiring hospitalization. Int J Antimicrob Agents 2005;25(1):75–83.

20. Fine MJ, Auble TE, Yealy DM, et al. A prediction rule to identify low-risk patients with community-acquired pneumonia. N Engl J Med 1997;336(4):243–50.

21. Welte T, Petermann W, Schürmann D, et al. Treatment with sequential intravenous or oral moxifloxacin was associated with faster clinical improvement than was standard therapy for hospitalized patients with community-acquired pneumonia who received initial parenteral therapy. Clin Infect Dis 2005;41(12): 1697–705.

22. Dresser LD, Niederman MS, Paladino JA. Cost-effectiveness of gatifloxacin vs ceftriaxone with a macrolide for the treatment of community-acquired pneumonia. Chest 2001;119(5):1439–48.

23. Vardakas KZ, Siempos II, Grammatikos A, et al. Respiratory fluoroquinolones for the treatment of community-acquired pneumonia: a meta-analysis of randomized controlled trials. CMAJ 2008;179(12):1269–77.
24. Lodise TP, Kwa A, Cosler L, et al. Comparison of beta-lactam and macrolide combination therapy versus fluoroquinolone monotherapy in hospitalized Veterans Affairs patients with community-acquired pneumonia. Antimicrob Agents Chemother 2007;51(11):3977–82.
25. Zervos M, Mandell LA, Vrooman PS, et al. Comparative efficacies and tolerabilities of intravenous azithromycin plus ceftriaxone and intravenous levofloxacin with step-down oral therapy for hospitalized patients with moderate to severe community-acquired pneumonia. Treat Respir Med 2004;3(5):329–36.
26. Fogarty C, Siami G, Kohler R, et al. Multicenter, open-label, randomized study to compare the safety and efficacy of levofloxacin versus ceftriaxone sodium and erythromycin followed by clarithromycin and amoxicillin-clavulanate in the treatment of serious community-acquired pneumonia in adults. Clin Infect Dis 2004; 38(Suppl 1):S16–23.
27. Torres A, Muir JF, Corris P, et al. Effectiveness of oral moxifloxacin in standard first-line therapy in community-acquired pneumonia. Eur Respir J 2003;21(1): 135–43.
28. Lode H, File TM Jr, Mandell L, et al. Oral gemifloxacin versus sequential therapy with intravenous ceftriaxone/oral cefuroxime with or without a macrolide in the treatment of patients hospitalized with community-acquired pneumonia: a randomized, open-label, multicenter study of clinical efficacy and tolerability. Clin Ther 2002;24(11):1915–36.
29. Petermann W, Alegre-Martin J, Odenholt I, et al. A prospective, randomized, multicenter comparative study of clinafloxacin versus a ceftriaxone-based regimen in the treatment of hospitalized patients with community-acquired pneumonia. Scand J Infect Dis 2001;33(11):832–7.
30. Katz E, Larsen LS, Fogarty CM, et al. Safety and efficacy of sequential i.v. to p.o. moxifloxacin versus conventional combination therapies for the treatment of community-acquired pneumonia in patients requiring initial i.v. therapy. J Emerg Med 2004;27(4):395–405.
31. Bratzler DW, Ma A, Nsa W. Initial antibiotic selection and patient outcomes: observations from the National Pneumonia Project. Clin Infect Dis 2008;47(Suppl 3): S193–201.
32. Erard V, Lamy O, Bochud PY, et al. Full-course oral levofloxacin for treatment of hospitalized patients with community-acquired pneumonia. Eur J Clin Microbiol Infect Dis 2004;23(2):82–8.
33. Frank E, Liu J, Kinasewitz G, et al. A multicenter, open-label, randomized comparison of levofloxacin and azithromycin plus ceftriaxone in hospitalized adults with moderate to severe community-acquired pneumonia. Clin Ther 2002;24(8): 1292–308.
34. Asadi L, Sligl WI, Eurich DT, et al. Macrolide-based regimens and mortality in hospitalized patients with community-acquired pneumonia: a systematic review and meta-analysis. Clin Infect Dis 2012;55(3):371–80.
35. Bartlett JG. Diagnostic tests for agents of community-acquired pneumonia. Clin Infect Dis 2011;52(Suppl 4):S296–304.
36. Van der Eerden MM, Vlaspolder F, de Graaff CS, et al. Comparison between pathogen directed antibiotic treatment and empirical broad spectrum antibiotic treatment in patients with community acquired pneumonia: a prospective randomised study. Thorax 2005;60(8):672–8.

37. File TM Jr, Lode H, Kurz H, et al. Double-blind, randomized study of the efficacy and safety of oral pharmacokinetically enhanced amoxicillin-clavulanate (2,000/125 milligrams) versus those of amoxicillin-clavulanate (875/125 milligrams), both given twice daily for 7 days, in treatment of bacterial community-acquired pneumonia in adults. Antimicrob Agents Chemother 2004;48(9):3323–31.

38. Bartlett JG. Is activity against "atypical" pathogens necessary in the treatment protocols for community-acquired pneumonia? Issues with combination therapy. Clin Infect Dis 2008;47(Suppl 3):S232–6.

39. Mills GD, Oehley MR, Arrol B. Effectiveness of beta lactam antibiotics compared with antibiotics active against atypical pathogens in non-severe community acquired pneumonia: meta-analysis. BMJ 2005;330(7489):456.

40. Healy DP. Macrolide immunomodulation of chronic respiratory diseases. Curr Infect Dis Rep 2007;9(1):7–13.

41. Metersky ML, Ma A, Houck PM, et al. Antibiotics for bacteremic pneumonia: improved outcomes with macrolides but not fluoroquinolones. Chest 2007;131(2):466–73.

42. Stahl JE, Barza M, DesJardin J, et al. Effect of macrolides as part of initial empiric therapy on length of stay in patients hospitalized with community-acquired pneumonia. Arch Intern Med 1999;159(21):2576–80.

43. Martínez JA, Horcajada JP, Almela M, et al. Addition of a macrolide to a beta-lactam-based empirical antibiotic regimen is associated with lower in-hospital mortality for patients with bacteremic pneumococcal pneumonia. Clin Infect Dis 2003;36(4):389–95.

44. Baddour LM, Yu VL, Klugman KP, et al. Combination antibiotic therapy lowers mortality among severely ill patients with pneumococcal bacteremia. Am J Respir Crit Care Med 2004;170(4):440–4.

45. Waterer GW, Somes GW, Wunderink RG. Monotherapy may be suboptimal for severe bacteremic pneumococcal pneumonia. Arch Intern Med 2001;161(15):1837–42.

46. Lin E, Stanek RJ, Mufson MA. Lack of synergy of erythromycin combined with penicillin or cefotaxime against Streptococcus pneumoniae in vitro. Antimicrob Agents Chemother 2003;47(3):1151–3.

47. Piddock LJ. The crisis of no new antibiotics–what is the way forward? Lancet Infect Dis 2012;12(3):249–53.

48. Goldstein RC, Lalite S, Mildvan D, et al. Fluoroquinolone- and ceftriaxone-based therapy of community-acquired pneumonia (CAP) in hospitalized patients (pts) and the risk of subsequent colonization and infection with multidrug-resistant (MDR) organisms. Abstract 205. Infectious Diseases Society of America. Boston, October 20–23, 2011.

49. Ginsburg AS, Hooper N, Parrish N, et al. Fluoroquinolone resistance in patients with newly diagnosed tuberculosis. Clin Infect Dis 2003;37(11):1448–52.

What is the Best Antimicrobial Treatment for Severe Community-Acquired Pneumonia (Including the Role of Steroids and Statins and Other Immunomodulatory Agents)

Oriol Sibila, MD[a,b], Marcos I. Restrepo, MD, MSc[a,c,d],
Antonio Anzueto, MD[a,c],*

KEYWORDS

- Community-acquired infections • Pneumonia • Therapeutics • Intensive care unit

KEY POINTS

- Patients with severe community-acquired pneumonia (CAP) refers to the sickest patients with CAP, who require hospitalization, usually in the intensive care unit, and who need intensive therapies including mechanical ventilation and vasopressor support.
- Several risk factors present in patients with severe CAP are associated with different pathogens including *Pseudomonas aeruginosa*, community-associated methicillin-resistant *Staphylococcus aureus* (CA-MRSA), which suggest appropriate specific empirical antimicrobial coverage.
- A combination of antimicrobials with antipneumococcal agents is highly recommended for patients with severe CAP involving atypical pathogens (especially *Legionella* spp) and gram-positive and gram-negative respiratory pathogens according to multiple clinical practice guidelines.
- The use of immunomodulatory agents is a matter of significant interest in patients with severe CAP, and includes the use of a macrolide agent as part of the combination of antimicrobial therapy. In addition, the use of adjunctive therapies such as corticosteroids, statins, and so forth. remain a matter of debate and of clinical interest in selected patients.

Financial Support: Dr Sibila is supported by Instituto de Salud Carlos III (BAE11/00102), Sociedad Espanola de Neumologia y Cirugia Toracica (SEPAR), Societat Catalana de Pneumologia (SOCAP) and Fundacio Catalana de Pneumologia (FUCAP). Dr Restrepo's time is partially protected by Award Number K23HL096054 from the National Heart, Lung, and Blood Institute. The content is solely the responsibility of the authors and does not necessarily represent the official views of the National Heart, Lung, and Blood Institute or the National Institutes of Health. The funding agencies had no role in the preparation, review, or approval of the article. The views expressed in this article are those of the author and do not necessarily represent the views of the Department of Veterans Affairs. Conflicts of Interest: Dr Marcos I. Restrepo participated as a consultant in the data safety monitoring board for clinical trials run by Theravance, Trius, and Pfizer (Wyeth). Dr Antonio Anzueto has served in the speaker's bureaus of Pfizer, Boehringer Ingelheim, GlaxoSmithKline, Astra-Zeneca; and in the advisory board of Glaxo SmithKline, Boehringer Ingelheim, Bayer-Healthcare, and Pfizer.
^a University of Texas Health Science Center at San Antonio, San Antonio, TX, USA; ^b Servei de Pneumologia, Hospital de la Santa Creu i Sant Pau, Barcelona, Spain; ^c South Texas Veterans Health Care System, San Antonio, TX, USA; ^d Veterans Evidence Based Research Dissemination and Implementation Center (VERDICT)
* Corresponding author. South Texas Veterans Health Care System, Audie L. Murphy Division at San Antonio, 7400 Merton Minter Boulevard (11C6), San Antonio, TX 78229.
E-mail address: anzueto@uthscsa.edu

Infect Dis Clin N Am 27 (2013) 133–147
http://dx.doi.org/10.1016/j.idc.2012.11.014
0891-5520/13/$ – see front matter © 2013 Elsevier Inc. All rights reserved.

id.theclinics.com

INTRODUCTION

Community-acquired pneumonia (CAP) and influenza are the leading causes of death from infectious diseases in the United States.[1,2] The sickest patients with CAP are those who require hospitalization and are usually admitted to the intensive care unit (ICU). The term severe CAP identifies a group of patients with severe disease, who are prone to complications and poor outcomes and require a higher level of care. Increased mortality in patients with severe CAP who do not receive adequate empirical antibiotics that cover the infection pathogen(s) is well documented.[3–6] Several risk factors associated with different pathogens have been recognized and should be considered so that appropriate antibiotics are selected. In addition, there is evidence that outcomes are considerably better in patients with severe CAP when a combination of antibiotics is used rather than a single agent.[7] The use of macrolides is still a matter of debate, although the weight of observational data supports macrolide use in severe CAP.[7–11] Despite potent antibiotics effective against most pathogens, different adjunctive therapies have been tested in severe CAP.[12] These treatments are directed to the host response rather than the pathogen. Potential immunomodulatory therapies with antiinflammatory agents (eg, corticosteroids), anticoagulants (eg, activated protein C) or statins, and angiotensin-converting enzyme (ACE) inhibitor have been tested in severe CAP in recent years. The most recent and relevant data regarding different antimicrobial and adjunctive therapies in patients with severe CAP are reviewed in this article.

SEVERE CAP

The definition of severe is still matter of controversy. Previous reports have suggested that patients with severe CAP are those who require therapeutic interventions that can only be provided in a higher acuity level of care such as an ICU and have a higher risk of dying. Several tools have been developed to predict mortality, safe management in the outpatient setting, and hospitalization or ICU admission of patients with CAP.[13–18] The pneumonia severity index (PSI) score and the CURB-65 are the most studied and validated scores. They are currently recommended by multiple clinical practice guidelines for patients with CAP who do not require ICU admission[19–23] and therefore are at a lower risk of dying. Several other scores have been evaluated to better predict the need for ICU admission, need for mechanical ventilation/vasopressor support, and risk of death of patients with CAP. Such tools include the Infectious Diseases Society of America/American Thoracic Society (IDSA/ATS) guidelines,[19] PS-CURXO80,[24] SMART-COP,[16] and the SCAP scores.[17] However, due the lack of sufficient sensitivity to identify criteria, it is recommended that these criteria do not replace physicians' clinical judgment when deciding severity of CAP.[25] Need for mechanical ventilation, vasopressor support, and ICU admission are still considered fundamental components to define severe CAP.[26]

Treatment of severe CAP remains a controversial issue. Until better diagnostic test are available in the clinical setting, initial treatment is usually empirical. Different studies have shown increased mortality in patients with severe CAP who do not receive empirical antibiotics that cover the infecting pathogen.[3–6] Current guidelines emphasize the importance of appropriate, aggressive, and early management of patients with CAP who are cared for in the ICU.[19,27] Traditionally, antimicrobial agents have been considered the cornerstone of therapy against severe CAP. However, with the aim of understanding severe CAP as a systemic disease, there are other nonantimicrobial therapies that should also be considered in this group of patients.

ANTIMICROBIAL TREATMENT

Appropriate antimicrobial empirical coverage of the most likely pathogens is crucial in the management of patients with severe CAP. Observational data suggested that delay in treatment, even with appropriate antibiotics, is associated with poor outcomes in all cases of sepsis and CAP specifically.[28] Severe CAP has a distinct microbial cause compared with other cases of CAP, with higher representation of gram-negative bacteria and *Staphylococcus aureus*.[29–31] Extensive interest has focused on severe CAP caused by *Pseudomonas aeruginosa* and community-associated methicillin-resistant *Staphylococcus aureus* (CA-MRSA). *P aeruginosa* has been reported in patients with severe CAP with specific risk factors, such as chronic or prolonged use of broad-spectrum antibiotic therapy, bronchiectasis, malnutrition, human immunodeficiency virus, and other forms of immunosuppression.[32–35] CA-MRSA has been linked as a secondary infection in patients with influenza infection, and has been associated with skin infections.[36] **Table 1** shows the most common pathogens associated with severe CAP and their associated comorbid conditions. All patients with severe CAP should be stratified according to the risk factor of different potentially causative microorganisms.

If a patient has no risk factors for *Pseudomonas aeruginosa* or MRSA infection, the initial antibiotic treatment should always include 2 antibiotics. The combination therapy should include one antibiotic (β-lactam) to cover *Pneumococcus* (including drug-resistant isolates) and other likely respiratory pathogens, and therapy against atypical pathogens especially *Legionella* spp, such as a macrolide (azithromycin or clarithromycin) or a respiratory fluoroquinolone (levofloxacin at the highest dose of 750 mg/d or moxifloxacin).[19,20,27,37,38]

Table 1
Risk factors associated with most important pathogens in severe CAP

Pathogen	Risk Factor
Pseudomonas aeruginosa	Structural lung diseases, bronchiectasis, COPD, corticosteroid treatment, previous antibiotic treatment, enteral tube feeding
Gram-negative *Bacilli*	Diabetes mellitus, decreased functional status, comorbidities (cardiopulmonary, renal, central nervous system or hepatic, neoplasia), chronic aspiration
Staphylococcus aureus	Decreased functional status, CVD, intravenous drug use, diabetes mellitus, renal failure, influenza
CA-MRSA	Previous influenza infection, skin infections
Streptococcus pneumoniae	Smoking, COPD, low socioeconomic status, sulfur dioxide air pollution, alcoholism, dementia, seizures, congestive heart failure, CVD, HIV infection
DRSP	Alcoholism, β-lactams within 3 months, presence of more than 1 coexisting disease, immunosuppressive
Legionella pneumophila	Chronic steroid use, hematologic malignancy, humid weather, male sex, smoking, diabetes mellitus, cancer, ESRD, HIV infection
Anaerobes	High dental plaque index or periodontal disease, aspiration

Abbreviations: CA-MRSA, community-associated methicillin-resistant *S aureus*; COPD, chronic obstructive pulmonary disease; CVD, cerebrovascular disease; DRSP, drug-resistant *S pneumoniae*; ESRD, end-stage renal disease; HIV, human immunodeficiency virus.

Several studies in the last decade have shown that outcomes are considerably better in patients with severe CAP when a combination of antibiotics is used rather than a single agent.[7–11,39,40] The odds ratio (OR) for death among patients receiving monotherapy after adjusting for severity of disease of illness across these studies ranged from 1.5 to 6 times greater than that for patients receiving combination therapy.[41] In addition, the mortality benefit is seen in those with the most severe disease.[8,10,11,39,42] However, data are limited to a few randomized control trials, and most of the results come from observational studies that have evaluated the benefit of using combination therapy versus monotherapy in patients with severe CAP admitted to the ICU.[43,44] Recent concerns of the arrhythmogenic properties of macrolides suggest careful selection of appropriate patients.

Risk of Pseudomonas aeruginosa

In patients at risk of severe CAP caused by P aeruginosa, the treatment should include at least 3 antibacterial medications, an initial empirical combination of appropriate antipseudomonal coverage (with a β-lactam antipseudomonal therapy) plus an antipseudomonal fluoroquinolone (levofloxacin 750 mg/d or ciprofloxacin 400 mg 3 times a day) or an antipseudomonal aminoglycoside.[19] The downside of a combination with an aminoglycoside is that atypicals, particularly Legionella sp are not covered by this approach. In addition, the guidelines recommend including an antimicrobial agent with activity against atypical pathogens (eg, Legionella pneumophila) using a regime that includes a fluoroquinolone, or if fluoroquinolone is not present, the association of a macrolide. Patients at risk for adverse events caused by macrolides or fluoroquinolones should receive doxycycline. Failure to identify a pathogen has not been associated with a worse outcome particularly in the severely ill, but the empirical regimen should cover S pneumoniae and atypical pathogens.[5,45]

Risk of MRSA

Centers of Disease Control and Prevention (CDC) recommended empirically covering for MRSA in community-dwelling hosts that present with influenza infection.[46] Vancomycin or linezolid has been recommended as first-line therapy.[47] Optimal management of these patients remains uncertain, and is extrapolated from anecdotal experiences with small case series,[36,48] studies of hospital-acquired pneumonia,[49,50] and laboratory investigations using in vitro experiments and animal models of MRSA pneumonia.[51,52]

Newer antimicrobials such as ceftaroline, a fifth-generation cephalosporin, may have clinical value for patients with MRSA infection, but further data are required.[53,54] However, clinical efficacy against severe CAP MRSA infections has not yet been reported.

Macrolides

Of all the combinations recommended by the guidelines, the one that has acquired a critical role is the use of macrolides in association with other antimicrobials. Initially, Waterer and colleagues[8] found that single effective drug therapy for severe bacteremic pneumococcal pneumonia was associated with a greater risk of death than dual effective therapy. Several other studies suggested a benefit of having a macrolide added to β-lactam therapy in patients with bacteremic pneumococcal pneumonia[4,7,9,39,55] and ventilator-associated pneumonia.[56] In severe CAP, Rodriguez and colleagues[10] found that in the subset of ICU patients with CAP and shock, combination antibiotic therapy improved survival rates (OR = 1.69; 95% confidence interval [CI], 1.09–2.60; $P = .01$), suggesting that combination therapy may be beneficial in more severe cases. Restrepo and colleagues[11] reported that macrolide therapy decreased mortality in a retrospective cohort study of 237 patients with severe sepsis due to pneumonia (hazard ratio 0.3; 95% CI 0.2–0.7). In addition, Martin-Loeches and colleagues,[57] in a prospective observational study of 208 patients with severe CAP admitted to the ICU, showed that combination therapy with macrolides improves survival in intubated patients.

This effect is presumed to be secondary to the immunomodulatory effect rather than the antimicrobial effects,[58] particularly associated with the host inflammatory response.[59,60] Macrolides are known to possess a myriad of immunomodulatory effects, including alterations in leukocyte function, cytokine expression, apoptosis, and mucus production.[61,62] Another possible explanation for the observed benefit of macrolides is that atypical bacterial pathogens, which are covered with macrolide treatment, are frequently coinfections in patients with CAP.[63,64]

Despite the large number of publications, obligatory use of a macrolide in severe CAP has so far not been included in guidelines because of the observational, and usually retrospective, nature of all studies that showed a clear benefit. Unfortunately, prospective, randomized, double-blind pharmaceutical industry trials that could have provided key data either failed to enroll patients with severe CAP or did not include a macrolide in at least 1 arm of therapy.[41]

In conclusion, current recommendations regarding antimicrobial treatment in severe CAP include the use of empirical combination therapy with 2 or more antimicrobial agents according to the risk of *Pseudomonas* or MRSA infection and constant atypical coverage, mainly for infection with *Legionella* sp.

ADJUNCTIVE THERAPIES

Mortality due to severe pneumonia has not varied in recent years, suggesting that other factors than microorganisms are crucial in the evolution of the disease.[65] Different adjunctive therapeutic measures directed to the host response rather than the pathogen have been evaluated (**Box 1**).

One of the key factors determining the evolution of pneumonia is the host inflammatory response. It is well known that the presence of pathogens in the distal airway and alveolar space creates a complex inflammatory response with the interaction of several defense mechanisms and the production of inflammatory mediators and acute phase proteins. These inflammatory molecules promote migration of defensive cells such as neutrophils, lymphocytes, and platelets through the circulatory system to

---

Box 1
Potential adjunctive therapies in severe CAP

- Corticosteroids
- Statins
- Angiotensin-converting enzyme inhibitors
- Anticoagulant agents
  - Human activated protein C
  - Tissue factor pathway inhibitor
- Surfactant
- Immunoglobulin
- Interferon γ

inflammatory sites.[66] This process will be beneficial as long as it is limited to the control of local infection. If this reaction is over proportioned, several systemic consequences have a negative influence on the clinical evolution of the infection.[67]

Studies on severe pneumonia have shown that, even though the inflammatory response is initially compartmentalized,[68] an increase of inflammatory cytokines in serum is also detected and related to poor prognosis.[69–72] Recent studies showed that an excessive inflammatory response was associated with treatment failure,[73] ICU admission,[74] and mortality[75] in patients with CAP.

Corticosteroids

Corticosteroids inhibit the expression and action of many molecules involved in the acute inflammatory response associated with severe pneumonia as a result of their molecular mechanisms of action[76,77] and increase gene transcription of different anti-inflammatory molecules (eg, lipocortin 1, β-2 receptors) in a mechanism called transactivation. In addition, corticosteroids decrease gene transcription of several inflammatory molecules, such as cytokines, chemokines, or adhesion molecules, in a mechanism called transrepression.[77] Different experimental studies have shown that acute administration of corticosteroids reduces inflammatory cytokines in severe CAP.[78,79]

Few studies have evaluated the impact of corticosteroid treatment on severe CAP in clinical practice. A pilot study by Monton and colleagues[80] on patients with pneumonia requiring mechanical ventilation detected the possible immunosuppressive effect of corticosteroids in severe pneumonia. In this study, a decrease in proinflammatory cytokines, such as interleukin (IL)-6 and tumor necrosis factor (TNF)-α, was observed in serum and in bronchoalveolar lavage of patients who received corticosteroids as coadjuvant treatment to the antibiotic treatment. Furthermore, in the group of patients receiving corticosteroids, a trend to lower mortality was also observed. However, the study was limited by the small sample size (n = 20). A retrospective study with 308 patients with severe CAP (defined as PSI score class IV and V) showed that mortality decreased in patients who received simultaneous administration of systemic corticosteroids with antibiotic treatment (OR 0.28, 95% CI 0.113–0.732).[81]

Several randomized controlled trials have evaluated the effect of corticosteroids on CAP. Confalonieri and colleagues[82] assessed the efficacy and safety of continuous infusion of hydrocortisone in 46 patients with CAP requiring ICU admission. Twenty-three patients received an intravenous bolus of 200 mg of hydrocortisone followed by an infusion of 10 mg/h for 7 days. These investigators demonstrated a reduction in mortality in the group treated with hydrocortisone, better modulation of systemic inflammatory response (determined by serum C-reactive protein), and significant improvement in clinical end points, such as chest radiographs, multiple organ dysfunction syndrome severity scale, Pao_2/Fio_2 ratio, and ICU and hospital stay. However, the small sample size and differences among groups at admission (placebo group had lower Pao_2/Fio_2 ratio and lower levels of C-reactive protein) limited the generalizability of the results.

Other randomized controlled trials on patients with less severe CAP who required hospitalization have conflicting results. Snijeder and colleagues[83] studied the impact of 40 mg of prednisolone once daily for 7 days compared with placebo among 213 patients hospitalized with CAP. The investigators found no differences regarding the rate of 30-day mortality, time to clinical stability, or length of hospital stay. However, patients treated with corticosteroids had faster decline in serum C-reactive protein levels compared with placebo. By contrast, late clinical failure (>72 hours from admission) was more common in the corticosteroid group. The investigators performed a subanalyses on patients with severe CAP, and found no differences among groups. Meijvis and colleagues[84] evaluated the effect of intravenous dexamethasone (5 mg once a day) versus placebo in the first 4 days after admission for CAP. The investigators found no differences in the main outcomes, including in-hospital mortality, ICU admission, and severe adverse events. However, patients treated with corticosteroids had a shorter length of hospital stay compared with the placebo group. In this study, only about 20% of the patients included in the study had severe CAP, but no statistical significant differences were observed in the subgroup analysis.

In conclusion, scientific evidence is still limited to suggest the clinical use of systemic corticosteroids in patients with severe CAP despite their antiinflammatory properties.[85]

Statins

Statins, or 3-hydroxy 3-methylglutaryl coenzyme A (HMG-CoA) reductase inhibitors, are extensively used in medical practice as cholesterol-lowering agents. Statin therapy has been shown to decrease coronary and cerebrovascular events, and decrease mortality from coronary artery disease and stroke.[86,87] For that reason, they are 1 of the most prescribed drugs in the United States and worldwide.[88] Statins have also been shown to have other multiple properties with potential applications. They are able to decrease the production of proinflammatory cytokines such as TNF-α, IL-1, and IL-6.[89] Some data suggest that statins interfere with the recognition of different microbial products and depress the associated inflammatory cascade.[90] In addition, the multiple properties of statins include antioxidant, antiapoptotic, and antithrombotic activity, which may play a crucial role in the management of infections.[86]

Observational studies have suggested that patients who were taking statins at the time of development of pneumonia or other infection were less likely to develop sepsis, death from sepsis, or complications leading to ICU admission.[91–96] A retrospective study on a cohort of 787 patients with a discharge diagnosis of pneumonia showed that use of statins at presentation was associated with decreased 30-day mortality (OR 0.36, 95%CI 0.14–0.92).[97] Another retrospective analysis of all CAP admissions in Denmark showed a significant decreased mortality with statin use at admission (adjusted mortality ratio 0.69, 95% CI 0.58–0.82).[98] Chalmers and colleagues,[99] in a prospective observational study, showed that patients with CAP on prescribed statins at admission had lower 30-day mortality (adjusted OR 0.46, 95% CI 0.25–0.85) and less development of complicated pneumonia (adjusted OR 0.44, 95% CI 0.25–0.79). These investigators showed that, although patients on prescribed statins had higher severity of illness scores at admission, C-reactive protein levels were significantly lower in patients compared with those who were not taking statin.[99] However, a large, prospective, observational, cohort study found no benefit with statin use on mortality or need for ICU admission when adjusted for potential confounders.[100] Yende and colleagues,[101] in a recent prospective cohort multicenter study of 1895 patients hospitalized with CAP, did not find any differences in the risk of developing severe sepsis and 90-day mortality among statin users compared with those who were not taking statins.

These studies have focused on the use of statins before the development of CAP, and it is possible that they are affected by healthy user bias. No study has examined the addition of statins as an adjunctive therapy once pneumonia has developed. Kruger and colleagues[102] performed a prospective, randomized, double-blind, placebo-controlled trial of atorvastatin (20 mg) versus a matched placebo control group. The investigators found that statin therapy was not associated with improved sepsis and inflammatory parameters. Further randomized clinical trials are needed to determine the impact of statins at admission for pneumonia, particularly among patients without risk for coronary artery disease or other indications for statins use.

Other Adjunctive Therapies

Similar to statins, previous use of ACE inhibitors has been associated with better clinical outcomes in patients with CAP, especially in Japanese cohorts.[103,104] These studies found that patients under treatment with ACE inhibitors experienced a decreased risk of developing pneumonia and decreased risk of mortality in CAP. Other studies performed on large cohorts of predominantly white patients with CAP have found mixed results in the association of ACE inhibitors and clinical outcomes.[97,105] Part of the discrepancy may be caused by the different classes of ACE inhibitors used. The risk of developing CAP may be greater for lipophilic ACE inhibitors compared with hydrophilic ACE inhibitors.[106,107] Given the conflicting data, it is unclear whether ACE inhibitors have a protective role in CAP. Once again, current studies do not justify initiation of treatment with ACE inhibitors after the development of CAP, and prospective randomized controlled trials are needed.

Activated protein C, an anticoagulant, has been evaluated as an adjunctive treatment in severe CAP. The PROWESS trial,[108] a randomized, double-blinded, placebo-controlled trial evaluating the effect of drotecogin α or activated protein C in patients with severe sepsis, showed an absolute risk reduction in 28-day mortality in patients on the treatment arm. Furthermore, most the benefit of the drug was seen in the CAP subgroup,[109] with the greatest reduction in mortality seen in *Streptococcus pneumoniae* infection (relative risk = 0.56, 95% CI 0.35–0.88). However, a recent randomized controlled trial on 1697 patients with septic shock did not find differences in mortality at 28 and 90 days between patients treated with drotecogin α versus placebo.[110] This motivated the company to remove the medication from the market.

Other potentially immunomodulatory therapies such as tissue factor pathway inhibitor, surfactant, immunoglobulin, or interferon γ have been evaluated,[12] although information regarding their effect is scarce and further studies are needed before they can be considered as a therapeutic option in severe CAP.

SUMMARY

Severe CAP is a complex condition with significant mortality that has not varied in the last recent years. Several antibiotic approaches and adjunctive therapies have been tested. Appropriate antibiotic therapy with early initiation of combination therapy is an important component in the management of severe CAP in the ICU. Increased antibiotic coverage for *P aeruginosa* and CA-MRSA when specific risk factors are present is required. The immunomodulatory effects of macrolide antibiotics may play a significant role in survival after severe CAP, although further randomized prospective trials are needed. Adjunctive therapies directed at the host response rather than the pathogens are attractive to improve outcomes. Corticosteroids, statins, ACE inhibitors, and anticoagulants have been used with some encouraging results, although data are still scarce. Future research is needed in these areas to decrease mortality due to severe CAP.

REFERENCES

1. Anonymous. Pneumonia and influenza death rates–United States, 1979–1994. MMWR Morb Mortal Wkly Rep 1995;44(28):535–7.

2. Marston BJ, Plouffe JF, File TM Jr, et al. Incidence of community-acquired pneumonia requiring hospitalization. Results of a population-based active surveillance Study in Ohio. The Community-Based Pneumonia Incidence Study Group. Arch Intern Med 1997;157(15):1709–18.
3. Garcia-Vidal C, Fernandez-Sabe N, Carratala J, et al. Early mortality in patients with community-acquired pneumonia: causes and risk factors. Eur Respir J 2008;32:733–9.
4. Lujan M, Gallego M, Fontanals D, et al. Prospective observational study of bacteremic pneumococcal pneumonia: effect of discordant therapy on mortality. Crit Care Med 2004;32:625–31.
5. Leroy O, Santre C, Beuscart C, et al. A five-year study of severe community-acquired pneumonia with emphasis on prognosis in patients admitted to an intensive care unit. Intensive Care Med 1995;21:24–31.
6. Torres A, Serra-Batlles J, Ferrer A, et al. Severe community-acquired pneumonia: epidemiology and prognostic factors. Am Rev Respir Dis 1991;144: 312–8.
7. Metersky ML, Ma A, Houck PM, et al. Antibiotics for bacteremic pneumonia: improved outcomes with macrolides but not fluoroquinolones. Chest 2007; 131(2):466–73.
8. Waterer GW, Somes GW, Wunderink RG. Monotherapy may be suboptimal for severe bacteremic pneumococcal pneumonia. Arch Intern Med 2001;161(15): 1837–42.
9. Martínez JA, Horcajada JP, Almela M, et al. Addition of a macrolide to a beta-lactam-based empirical antibiotic regimen is associated with lower in-hospital mortality for patients with bacteremic pneumococcal pneumonia. Clin Infect Dis 2003;36(4):389–95.
10. Rodríguez A, Mendia A, Sirvent JM, et al, CAPUCI Study Group. Combination antibiotic therapy improves survival in patients with community-acquired pneumonia and shock. Crit Care Med 2007;35(6):1493–8.
11. Restrepo MI, Mortensen EM, Waterer GW, et al. Impact of macrolide therapy on mortality for patients with severe sepsis due to pneumonia. Eur Respir J 2009; 33(1):153–9.
12. Wunderink RG, Mandell L. Adjunctive therapy in community acquired pneumonia. Semin Respir Crit Care Med 2012;33:311–8.
13. Fine MJ, Auble TE, Yealy DM, et al. A prediction rule to identify low-risk patients with community-acquired pneumonia. N Engl J Med 1997;336(4):243–50.
14. Lim WS, van der Eerden MM, Laing R, et al. Defining community acquired pneumonia severity on presentation to hospital: an international derivation and validation study. Thorax 2003;58(5):377–82.
15. Chalmers JD, Mandal P, Singanayagam A, et al. Severity assessment tools to guide ICU admission in community-acquired pneumonia: systematic review and meta-analysis. Intensive Care Med 2011;37(9):1409–20.
16. Charles PG, Wolfe R, Whitby M, et al. SMART-COP: a tool for predicting the need for intensive respiratory or vasopressor support in community-acquired pneumonia. Clin Infect Dis 2008;47(3):375–84.
17. Espana PP, Capelastegui A, Gorordo I, et al. Development and validation of a clinical prediction rule for severe community-acquired pneumonia. Am J Respir Crit Care Med 2006;174(11):1249–56.
18. Chalmers JD, Taylor JK, Mandal P, et al. Validation of the Infectious Diseases Society of America/American Thoracic Society minor criteria for intensive care unit admission in community-acquired pneumonia patients without major criteria

or contraindications to intensive care unit care. Clin Infect Dis 2011;53(6): 503–11.

19. Mandell LA, Wunderink RG, Anzueto A, et al. Infectious Diseases Society of America/American Thoracic Society consensus guidelines on the management of community-acquired pneumonia in adults. Clin Infect Dis 2007;44(Suppl 2): S27–72.

20. Niederman MS, Mandell LA, Anzueto A, et al. Guidelines for the management of adults with community-acquired pneumonia. Diagnosis, assessment of severity, antimicrobial therapy, and prevention. Am J Respir Crit Care Med 2001;163(7): 1730–54.

21. Chalmers JD, Akram AR, Hill AT. Increasing outpatient treatment of mild community-acquired pneumonia: systematic review and meta-analysis. Eur Respir J 2011;37(4):858–64.

22. Chalmers JD, Singanayagam A, Akram AR, et al. Safety and efficacy of CURB65-guided antibiotic therapy in community-acquired pneumonia. J Antimicrob Chemother 2011;66(2):416–23.

23. British Thoracic Society, Myint PK, Kamath AV, Vowler SL, et al. Severity assessment criteria recommended by the British Thoracic Society (BTS) for community-acquired pneumonia (CAP) and older patients. Should SOAR (systolic blood pressure, oxygenation, age and respiratory rate) criteria be used in older people? A compilation study of two prospective cohorts. Age Ageing 2006;35(3):286–91.

24. Rello J, Rodriguez A, Lisboa T, et al. PIRO score for community-acquired pneumonia: a new prediction rule for assessment of severity in intensive care unit patients with community-acquired pneumonia. Crit Care Med 2009;37(2):456–62.

25. Ewig S, Woodhead M, Torres A. Towards a sensible comprehension of severe community-acquired pneumonia. Intensive Care Med 2011;37(2):214–23.

26. Restrepo MI, Anzueto A. Severe community-acquired pneumonia. Infect Dis Clin North Am 2009;23(3):503–20.

27. Woodhead M, Blasi F, Ewing S, et al. Guidelines for the management of adult lower respiratory tract infections. Eur Respir J 2005;26(6):1138–80.

28. Ibrahim EH, Sherman G, Ward S, et al. The influence of inadequate antimicrobial treatment of bloodstream infections on patient outcomes in the ICU setting. Chest 2000;118:146–55.

29. Restrepo MI, Jorgensen JH, Mortensen EM, et al. Severe community-acquired pneumonia: current outcomes, epidemiology, etiology, and therapy. Curr Opin Infect Dis 2001;14:703–9.

30. Ruiz M, Ewig S, Torres A, et al. Severe community-acquired pneumonia. Risk factors and follow-up epidemiology. Am J Respir Crit Care Med 1999;160: 923–9.

31. Paganin F, Lilienthal F, Bourdin A, et al. Severe community acquired pneumonia: assessment of microbial aetiology as mortality factor. Eur Respir J 2004;24: 779–85.

32. Arancibia F, Bauer TT, Ewig S, et al. Community-acquired pneumonia due to gram-negative bacteria and *Pseudomonas aeruginosa*: incidence, risk, and prognosis. Arch Intern Med 2002;162(16):1849–58.

33. Hatchette TF, Gupta R, Marrie TJ. *Pseudomonas aeruginosa* community-acquired pneumonia in previously healthy adults: case report and review of the literature. Clin Infect Dis 2000;31(6):1349–56.

34. Cordero E, Pachon J, Rivero A, et al. Community-acquired bacterial pneumonia in human immunodeficiency virus-infected patients: validation of severity

criteria. The Grupo Andaluz para el Estudio de las Enfermedades Infecciosas. Am J Respir Crit Care Med 2000;162(6):2063–8.

35. Luna CM, Famiglietti A, Absi R, et al. Community-acquired pneumonia: etiology, epidemiology, and outcome at a teaching hospital in Argentina. Chest 2000; 118(5):1344–54.

36. Francis JS, Doherty MC, Lopatin U, et al. Severe community-onset pneumonia in healthy adults caused by methicillin-resistant *Staphylococcus aureus* carrying the Panton-Valentine leukocidin genes. Clin Infect Dis 2005;40(1):100–7.

37. Mandell LA, Bartlett JG, Dowell SF, et al. Update of practice guidelines for the management of community-acquired pneumonia in immunocompetent adults. Clin Infect Dis 2003;37(11):1405–33.

38. Shefet D, Robenshtok E, Paul M, et al. Empirical atypical coverage for inpatients with community-acquired pneumonia: systematic review of randomized controlled trials. Arch Intern Med 2005;165(17):1992–2000.

39. Baddour LM, Yu VL, Klugman KP, et al, International Pneumococcal Study Group. Combination antibiotic therapy lowers mortality among severely ill patients with pneumococcal bacteremia. Am J Respir Crit Care Med 2004; 170(4):440–4.

40. García Vázquez E, Mensa J, Martínez JA, et al. Lower mortality among patients with community-acquired pneumonia treated with a macrolide plus a beta-lactam agent versus a beta-lactam agent alone. Eur J Clin Microbiol Infect Dis 2005;24(3):190–5.

41. Waterer GW, Rello J, Wunderink RG. Management of community-acquired pneumonia in adults. Am J Respir Crit Care Med 2011;183:157–64.

42. Tessmer A, Welte T, Martus P, et al. Impact of intravenous {beta}-lactam/macro-lide versus {beta}-lactam monotherapy on mortality in hospitalized patients with community acquired pneumonia. J Antimicrob Chemother 2009;63: 1025–33.

43. Moine P, Vercken JB, Chevret S, et al. Severe community-acquired pneumonia. Etiology, epidemiology, and prognosis factors. French Study Group for Community-Acquired Pneumonia in the Intensive Care Unit. Chest 1994; 105(5):1487–95.

44. Fogarty C, Siami G, Kholer R, et al. Multicenter, open label, randomized study to compare the safety and efficacy of levofloxacin versus ceftriaxone sodium and erythromycin followed by clarithromycin and amoxicillin-clavulanate in the treatment of serious community-acquired pneumonia in adults. Clin Infect Dis 2004; 38(S1):S16–23.

45. Leroy O, Saux P, Bedos JP, et al. Comparison of levofloxacin and cefotaxime combined with ofloxacin for ICU patients with community-acquired pneumonia who do not require vasopressors. Chest 2005;128(1):172–83.

46. Hageman JC, Uyeki TM, Francis JS, et al. Severe community-acquired pneu-monia due to *Staphylococcus aureus*, 2003–04 influenza season. Emerg Infect Dis 2006;12(6):894–9.

47. Kwong JC, Chua K, Charles PG. Managing severe community-acquired pneu-monia due to community methicillin-resistant *Staphylococcus aureus* (MRSA). Curr Infect Dis Rep 2012;14(3):330–8.

48. Geng W, Yang Y, Wu D, et al. Community-acquired, methicillin-resistant *Staph-ylococcus aureus* isolated from children with community-onset pneumonia in China. Pediatr Pulmonol 2010;45(4):387–94.

49. Bodi M, Ardanuy C, Rello J. Impact of Gram-positive resistance on outcome of nosocomial pneumonia. Crit Care Med 2001;29(Suppl 4):N82–6.

50. Welte T, Pletz MW. Antimicrobial treatment of nosocomial methicillin-resistant *Staphylococcus aureus* (MRSA) pneumonia: current and future options. Int J Antimicrob Agents 2010;36(5):391–400.

51. Stevens DL, Ma Y, Salmi DB, et al. Impact of antibiotics on expression of virulence-associated exotoxin genes in methicillin-sensitive and methicillin-resistant *Staphylococcus aureus*. J Infect Dis 2007;195(2):202–11.

52. Martinez-Olondris P, Rigol M, Soy D, et al. Efficacy of linezolid compared to vancomycin in an experimental model of pneumonia induced by methicillin-resistant *Staphylococcus aureus* in ventilated pigs. Crit Care Med 2012;40(1):162–8.

53. Jorgenson MR, Depestel DD, Carver PL. Ceftaroline fosamil: a novel broad-spectrum cephalosporin with activity against methicillin-resistant *Staphylococcus aureus*. Ann Pharmacother 2011;45(11):1384–98.

54. Germel C, Haag A, Soderquist B. In vitro activity of beta-lactam antibiotics to community-associated methicillin-resistant *Staphylococcus aureus* (CA-MRSA). Eur J Clin Microbiol Infect Dis 2012;31:475–80.

55. Mufson MA, Stanek RJ. Bacteremic pneumococcal pneumonia in one American city: a 20-year longitudinal stay, 1978–1997. Am J Med 1999;107(1A):34S–43S.

56. Giamarellos-Bourboulis EJ, Pechere JC, Routsi C, et al. Effect of clarithromycin in patients with sepsis and ventilator-associated pneumonia. Clin Infect Dis 2008;46(8):1157–64.

57. Martin-Loeches I, Lisboa T, Rodriguez A, et al. Combination antibiotic therapy with macrolides improves survival in intubated patients with community-acquired pneumonia. Intensive Care Med 2010;36(4):612–20.

58. Giamarellos-Bourboulis EJ, Baziaka F, Antonopoulou A, et al. Clarithromycin co-administered with amikacin attenuates systemic inflammation in experimental sepsis with *Escherichia coli*. Int J Antimicrob Agents 2005;25(2):168–72.

59. Giamarellos-Bourboulis EJ. Immunomodulatory therapies for sepsis: unexpected effects with macrolides. Int J Antimicrob Agents 2008;32(Suppl 1):S39–43.

60. Cazzola M, Matera MG, Pezzuto G. Inflammation–a new therapeutic target in pneumonia. Respiration 2005;72(2):117.

61. Giamarellos-Bourboulis EJ. Macrolides beyond the conventional antimicrobials: a class of potent immunomodulators. Int J Antimicrob Agents 2008;31(1):12–20.

62. Amsden GW. Anti-inflammatory effects of macrolides—an underappreciated benefit in the treatment of community-acquired respiratory tract infections and chronic inflammatory pulmonary conditions? J Antimicrob Chemother 2005; 55(1):10–21.

63. Lieberman D, Schlaeffer F, Boldur I, et al. Multiple pathogens in adult patients admitted with community acquired pneumonia: a one year prospective study of 346 consecutive patients. Thorax 1996;51:179–84.

64. Jokinen C, Heiskanen L, Juvonen H, et al. Microbial etiology of community-acquired pneumonia in the adult population of 4 municipalities in eastern Finland. Clin Infect Dis 2001;32:1141–54.

65. Alvarez-Lerma F, Torres A. Severe community-acquired pneumonia. Curr Opin Crit Care 2004;10(5):369–74.

66. Sibille Y, Reynolds HY. Macrophages and polymorphonuclear neutrophils in lung defense and injury. Am Rev Respir Dis 1990;141:471–501.

67. Martin C, Sauzx P, Mege JL, et al. Prognostic value of serum cytokines in septic shock. Intensive Care Med 1994;20:272–7.

68. Dehoux MS, Boutten A, Ostinelli J, et al. Compartmentalized cytokine production within the human lung in unilateral pneumonia. Am J Respir Crit Care Med 1994;150:710–6.

69. Sibila O, Agusti C, Torres A, et al. Experimental *Pseudomonas aeruginosa* pneumonia; evaluation of the associated inflammatory response. Eur Respir J 2007;30: 1167–72.
70. Puren AJ, Feldeman C, Savage N, et al. Patterns of cytokine expression in community-acquired pneumonia. Chest 1995;107:1342–9.
71. Monton C, Torres A, el-Ebiary M, et al. Cytokine expression in severe pneumonia: a bronchoalveolar study. Crit Care Med 1999;27:1745–53.
72. Fernandez-Serrano S, Dorca J, Coromines M, et al. Molecular inflammatory response measured in blood of patients with severe community-acquired pneumonia. Clin Diagn Lab Immunol 2003;10:813–20.
73. Menendez R, Cavalcanti M, Reyes S, et al. Markers of treatment failure in hospitalized community-acquired pneumonia. Thorax 2008;63:447–52.
74. Ramirez P, Ferrer M, Marti V, et al. Inflammatory biomarkers and prediction for intensive care unit admission in severe community-acquired pneumonia. Crit Care 2011;39(10):2211–7.
75. Menendez R, Martinez R, Reyes S, et al. Biomarkers improve mortality prediction by prognostic scales in community-acquired pneumonia. Thorax 2009;64:587–91.
76. De Bosscher K, Vanden Berghe W, Haegeman G. The interplay between the glucocorticoid receptor and nuclear factor-kappa beta or activator protein-1: molecular mechanisms for gene repression. Endocr Rev 2003;24:488–522.
77. Rhen T, Cidlowsky JA. Antiinflammatory action of glucocorticoids – new mechanisms for old drugs. N Engl J Med 2005;353:1711–23.
78. Sibila O, Luna CM, Agusti C, et al. Effects of glucocorticoids in ventilated piglets with severe pneumonia. Eur Respir J 2008;32:1037–46.
79. Li Y, Cui X, Li X, et al. Risk of death does not alter the efficacy of hydrocortisone therapy in a mouse *E. coli* pneumonia model: risk and corticosteroids in sepsis. Intensive Care Med 2008;34:568–77.
80. Montón C, Ewig S, Torres A, et al. Role of glucocorticoids on inflammatory response in nonimmunosuppressed patients with pneumonia: a pilot study. Eur Respir J 1999;14:218–20.
81. Garcia-Vidal C, Calbo E, Pascual V, et al. Effects of systemic steroids in patients with severe community-acquired pneumonia. Eur Respir J 2007;30:951–6.
82. Confalonieri R, Rubino G, Carbone A, et al. Hydrocortisone infusion for severe community-acquired pneumonia; a preliminary randomised study. Am J Respir Crit Care Med 2005;171:242–8.
83. Snijders D, Daniels JMA, De Graaff C, et al. Efficacy of corticosteroids in community-acquired pneumonia. A randomised double-blinded clinical trial. Am J Respir Crit Care Med 2010;181:975–82.
84. Meijvis S, Hardeman H, Remmelts H, et al. Dexamethasone and length of hospital stay in patients with community-acquired pneumonia: a randomized, double-blind, placebo-controlled trial. Lancet 2011;377:2023–30.
85. Sibila O, Agusti C, Torres A. Corticosteroids in severe pneumonia. Eur Respir J 2008;32:259–64.
86. Merx MW, Weber C. Statins in the intensive care unit. Curr Opin Crit Care 2006; 12:309–14.
87. LaRosa JC, He J, Vupputuri S. Effect of statins on risk of coronary disease. A meta-analysis of randomized controlled trials. JAMA 1999;282:2340–6.
88. Ross R. Atherosclerosis - an inflammatory disease. N Engl J Med 1999;340(2):115–26.
89. Zhang J, Cheng X, Liao YH, et al. Simvastatin regulates myocardial cytokine expression and improves ventricular remodeling in rats after acute myocardial infarction. Cardiovasc Drugs Ther 2005;19:13–21.

90. Weitz-Schmidt G, Welzenbach K, Brinkmann V, et al. Statins selectively inhibit leukocyte function antigen-1 by binding to a novel regulatory integrin site. Nat Med 2001;7:687–92.
91. Almog Y, Shefer A, Novack V, et al. Prior statin therapy is associated with a decreased rate of severe sepsis. Circulation 2004;110:880–5.
92. Thomsen RW, Hundborg HH, Johnsen SP, et al. Statin use and mortality within 180 days after bacteremia: a population-based cohort study. Crit Care Med 2006;34:1080–6.
93. Kruger P, Fitzsimmons K, Cook D, et al. Statin therapy is associated with fewer deaths in patients with bacteraemia. Intensive Care Med 2006;32:75–9.
94. Fernandez R, De Pedro VJ, Artigas A. Statin therapy prior to ICU admission: protection against infection or a severity marker? Intensive Care Med 2006;32: 160–4.
95. Hackam DG, Mamdani M, Li P, et al. Statins and sepsis in patients with cardiovascular disease: a population-based cohort analysis. Lancet 2006;367:413–8.
96. Liappis AP, Kan VL, Rochester CG, et al. The effect of statins on mortality in patients with bacteremia. Clin Infect Dis 2001;33:1352–7.
97. Mortensen EM, Restrepo MI, Anzueto A, et al. The impact of prior outpatient ACE inhibitor use on 30-day mortality for patients hospitalized with community-acquired pneumonia. BMC Pulm Med 2005;5:12.
98. Thomsen RW, Riis A, Kornum JB, et al. Preadmission use of statins and outcomes after hospitalization with pneumonia: population-based cohort study of 29,900 patients. Arch Intern Med 2008;168:2081–7.
99. Chalmers JD, Singanayagam A, Murray MP, et al. Prior statin use is associated with improved outcomes in community-acquired pneumonia. Am J Med 2008; 121(11):1002–7.
100. Majumdar SR, McAlister FA, Eurich DT, et al. Statins and outcomes in patients admitted to hospital with community acquired pneumonia: population based prospective cohort study. BMJ 2006;333:999.
101. Yende S, Milbrandt EB, Kellum JA, et al. Understanding the potential role of statins in pneumonia and sepsis. Crit Care Med 2011;39(8):1871–8.
102. Kruger PS, Harward ML, Jones MA, et al. Continuation of statin therapy in patients with presumed infection: a randomized controlled trial. Am J Respir Crit Care Med 2011;183(6):774–81.
103. Okaishi K, Morimoto S, Fukuo K, et al. Reduction of risk of pneumonia associated with use of angiotensin I converting enzyme inhibitors in elderly inpatients. Am J Hypertens 1999;12(8 Pt 1):778–83.
104. Takahashi T, Morimoto S, Okaishi K, et al. Reduction of pneumonia risk by an angiotensin I-converting enzyme inhibitor in elderly Japanese inpatients according to insertion/deletion polymorphism of the angiotensin I-converting enzyme gene. Am J Hypertens 2005;18(10):1353–9.
105. van de Garde EM, Souverein PC, Hak E, et al. Angiotensin-converting enzyme inhibitor use and protection against pneumonia in patients with diabetes. J Hypertens 2007;25(1):235–9.
106. Mukamal KJ, Ghimire S, Pandey R, et al. Antihypertensive medications and risk of community-acquired pneumonia. J Hypertens 2010;28(2):401–5.
107. Mortensen EM, Restrepo MI, Copeland LA, et al. Association of hydrophilic versus lipophilic angiotensin-converting enzyme inhibitor use on pneumonia-related mortality. Am J Med Sci 2008;336(6):462–6.
108. Bernard GR, Vincent JL, Laterre PF, et al. Efficacy and safety of recombinant human activated protein C for severe sepsis. N Engl J Med 2001;344:699–709.

109. Laterre PF, Garber G, Levy H, et al. Severe community-acquired pneumonia as a cause of severe sepsis: data from the PROWESS study. Crit Care Med 2005; 33:952–61.
110. Ranieri VM, Thompson BT, Barie PS, et al. Drotrecogin alfa (activated) in adults with septic shock. N Engl J Med 2012;366:2055–64.

How Important Are Anaerobic Bacteria in Aspiration Pneumonia

When Should They Be Treated and What Is Optimal Therapy

John G. Bartlett, MD

KEYWORDS

- Anaerobes • Aspiration • Lung abscess • Clindamycin
- Beta lactam/beta lactamase inhitor

KEY POINTS

- Anaerobic bacteria are infrequent pulmonary pathogens, but may cause serious disease.
- Clues for anaerobic pneumonia include aspiration risks, putrid discharge, indolent course, and necrotizing pneumonia.
- Treatment includes drainage of pleural collections and antimicrobials, including clindamycin or a β-lactamase/β-lactamase inhibitor.

HISTORICAL PERSPECTIVE

Anaerobic bacteria have been implicated in aspiration pneumonia and its sequelae, including lung abscess, necrotizing pneumonia, and empyema, since the early 1900s. The initial report was by Veillon in 1893.[1] There were multiple reports in the preantibiotic era; the classic studies of Smith with the animal model of aspiration pneumonia were reported in 1927,[2] and a plethora of reports came with the introduction of clindamycin and the "anaerobic bandwagon" of the 1970 to 1985 era. This development was facilitated by the use of diagnostic methods that yielded specimens valid for meaningful anaerobic culture combined with major laboratory advances with taxonomy and culture of anaerobes. Since 1985 there has been a dearth of new data and neglect of the prior work, reflecting a palpable disinterest in detecting pathogens in most pulmonary infections[3] and general reliance on antibiotic decisions based on empiricism.

The Animal Model

The classic studies of Smith[2] defined an important role for anaerobes in the pathophysiology of aspiration pneumonia leading to lung abscess. This investigator

Johns Hopkins University School of Medicine, 1830 East Monument Street, Room 447, Baltimore, MD 21205, USA
E-mail address: jb@jhmi.edu

Infect Dis Clin N Am 27 (2013) 149–155
http://dx.doi.org/10.1016/j.idc.2012.11.016
0891-5520/13/$ – see front matter © 2013 Elsevier Inc. All rights reserved.

performed a series of methodical studies in the 1920s. First he noted that the bacteria in the walls of lung abscess in patients who died with lung abscess resembled the morphology of the bacteria in the gingival crevice. Because lung abscesses were clinically associated with gingival crevice disease, he postulated that aspiration of these inocula was the pathophysiologic mechanism. To test this thesis, he examined gingival crevice material and generated inocula with the 4 dominant bacteria, a spirochete (anaerobic, but not clearly identified), a gram-positive coccus (presumed to be Peptostreptococcus based on gram-stain features or, less likely, Peptococcus), and a small, fragile anaerobic gram-negative vacillus (presumed *Bacteroides melaninogenicus*). He used a mouse model and tested these agents with intratracheal inoculation alone and in various combinations in an attempt to simulate aspiration pneumonia leading to lung abscess. He found all 4 agents were generally needed, thus establishing an early model of bacterial synergy with inocula of 4 anaerobes leading to lung abscess.

Clindamycin

Lincomycin was introduced in 1997 and was soon replaced by its successor, clindamycin. The drug had 3 important target pathogens, *Staphylococcus aureus*, nonenterococcal streptococci, and nearly all clinically important anaerobic bacteria. This agent, combined with gentamicin or other aminoglycosides, quickly became favored for intra-abdominal and pelvic infections because most involved a mixed flora of coliforms sensitive to aminoglycosides and anaerobes sensitive to clindamycin. These relative roles in the pathophysiology were well illustrated with rodent models of intra-abdominal sepsis, showing coliforms caused bacteremia, sepsis, and death; by contrast, anaerobes caused abscesses.[4–7] In fact, simply the capsular polysaccharide of *Bacteroides fragilis*, which is similar to that of *B melaninogenicus*, induced abscesses.[7] This point is emphasized because it contributes to the totality of data, indicating pathogenic potential of selected anaerobic bacteria.

With regard to lung abscess, clindamycin was compared with penicillin, which was considered the standard drug in the early 1980s.[8] The trial (**Table 1**) was discontinued prematurely due to clear evidence that clindamycin was superior. Then a sequel study comparing intravenous penicillin versus clindamycin by Gudiol and colleagues[9] in Spain showed nearly identical results. These studies established clindamycin as a favored agent for treating lung abscess and possibly as a precursor in aspiration pneumonia in the 1980s. The record of this drug was subsequently tarnished by its role in pseudomembraneous colitis. Conclusions were also limited due to its spectrum that included most streptococci. It should be acknowledged that metronidazole is a drug that is active versus virtually all clinically important anaerobes, but does not work well in anaerobic lung infections.[10,11] The presumed reason is that metronidazole

Table 1 Comparative trial of penicillin versus clindamycin for primary lung abscess		
	Clindamycin n = 19	Penicillin n = 20
Duration of fever (mean)	4.4 d	7.6 d[a]
Duration fetid sputum (mean)	4.2 d	8.2 d[a]
Failure at 20 d	0	2
Cure/completed follow-up	13/13	8/15

[a] $P = <.05$.

Data from Levison ME, Mangura CT, Lorber B, et al. Clindamycin compared with penicillin for the treatment of anaerobic lung abscess. Ann Intern Med 1983;98:466–71.

has minimal activity versus most microaerophilic and aerobic streptococci that are found in many or most lung infections involving anaerobic bacteria. These streptococci are resistant to metronidazole and sensitive to clindamycin.

Cultures

A great challenge with "selling" anaerobes is that they are rarely cultured in microbiology laboratories. The reason is that anaerobes are fragile, fastidious, slow growing require specialized culture systems (anaerobic jars or anaerobic chambers) and specimens that are uncontaminated by normal flora, and then take a long time to identify. In many cases the completed cultures return from the laboratory long after the patient is discharged. It is likely that most physicians in contemporary practice have seen many patients with lung infections involving anaerobes but never saw a microbiology report to verify this; the exception might be on empyema. The laboratory demands for retrieving and identifying anaerobics are especially great with lung infections because the need for uncontaminated specimens requires specialized methods including transthoracic needle aspiration (rarely performed), transtracheal aspiration (as developed in the 1970s and now rarely performed),[12] or fiber optic bronchoscopy with quantitation as developed in the 1980s[13] (and also rarely performed now). The combined impact is great neglect for achieving a microbial diagnosis in patients with pneumonia. The need for an invasive procedure to obtain a specimen valid for anaerobic culture and the challenge of specialized microbiology needed to cultivate and to identify the microbes has dissuaded attempts to recognize anaerobes. The methods of the 1980s were expensive, tedious, and invasive but resulted in data that now permit prediction of anaerobes and empiric use of antibiotics that is likely to be effective. The data from most of these studies are now dated, but presumably still relevant (**Table 2**).[14–32]

Note that the use of transtracheal aspiration (TTA) for the collection of uncontaminated pulmonary secretions that were uncontaminated by upper airway flora was validated by obtaining sterile TTA specimens in healthy medical students and the bronchoscopy technique using a double-lumen catheter with a distal occluding plug was validated with in vitro tests and then bronchoscopy on volunteers, including the investigators.[33] Also note that the data from Wang and colleagues[19] for lung abscess are skewed because they were performed in Taiwan, where the K1 strain of *Klebsiella pneumoniae* is a poorly understood pathogen that predominates in lung and liver abscesses.[34]

With regard to specific anaerobes, the dominant isolates in the larger series[33,35] show a dominance of *B melaninogenicus*, *Fusobacterium nucleatum*, and Peptostreptococcus, organisms that seem to be the same as those reported by Smith, as noted previously (**Table 3**).[33,35]

WHAT HAPPENED AFTER 1985?

There have been virtually no large series reporting bacteriology results in pulmonary infections that include specimens and microbiology appropriate for detecting anaerobes in the past 25 years except for a few from Asia and Bulgaria,[18–20,31] which use molecular techniques of uncertain significance for anaerobes.[36] This dearth of interest in microbiology was fostered by the contemporary era of empiricism in the management of lung infections fostered in the United States by (1) Clinical Laboratory Improvement Amendments 1988, that essentially eliminated housestaff laboratories; (2) the Medicare requirement of the 6-hour "door to needle time"; and (3) guidelines for empiric "standard" antibiotic selection that worked well. In the United States, the

Table 2
Frequency of recovering anaerobic bacteria using transtracheal aspiration, transthoracic needle aspiration, or pleural fluid specimens

Condition (Citation)	Frequency Anaerobes/Total
Lung abscess	
Beerens and Tahon,[14] 1965	22/26 (85%)
Brook and Finegold,[15] 1979	9/10 (90%)
Guidiol et al,[9] 1990	37/41 (90%)
Bartlett,[16] 1987	53/57 (93%)
Mori et al,[17] 1993	24/55 (45%)
De et al,[18] 2002	13/13 (100%)
Wang et al,[19] 2005	18/46 (39%)
Takayangi et al,[20] 2010	32/122 (26%)
Aspiration pneumonia	
Lorber and Swenson,[21] 1974	29/47 (62%)
Gonzalez and Calia,[22] 1975	17/17 (100%)
Bartlett,[23] 1979	61/70 (87%)
Brook and Frazier,[24] 1993	69/74 (93%)
Empyema	
Berens and Tahon-Castel,[14] 1965	23/45 (51%)
Sullivan et al,[25] 1973	42/482 (9%)
Bartlett,[26] 1977	63/83 (76%)
Varkey et al,[27] 1981	28/72 (39%)
Mavroudis et al,[28] 1981	25/100 (25%)
Grant and Finley,[29] 1985	26/90 (29%)
Lammer et al,[30] 1985	20/70 (29%)
Brook and Frazier,[24] 1993	70/197 (36%)
Boyanova et al,[31] 2004	147/198 (74%)

Table 3
Anaerobic bacteriology of lung infections involving these agents

Anaerobes	Bartlett,[34] 1993	Feingold et al,[33] 1985
Period reviewed	1968–75	1975–85
Cases	193	196
Total anaerobes	461	656
Dominant agents		
B melaninogenicus	76	45
Bacteroides (other)	75	258
F nucleatum	56	58
Peptostreptococcus	87	66

Data from Finegold SM, George WL, Mulligan ME. Anaerobic infections. Part I. Dis Mon 1985;31:1–77, and Bartlett JG. Anaerobic bacterial infections of the lung and pleural space. Clin Infect Dis 1993;16(Suppl 4):S248–55.

Medicare data for more than 34,000 patients hospitalized with pulmonary infections show a possible pathogen is reported in 7.6% of cases.[3] Nevertheless, a recent report from Sweden showed that the use of multiple diagnostic methods, including semi-quantitative polymerase chain reaction, to detect selected (aerobic) bacteria identified a likely pathogen in 89% of cases.[36] This report did not include any method to detect anaerobes, but it makes the point that anaerobes are uncommon in most cases of Community-acquired pneumonia (CAP) and the author's study with transtracheal aspiration in patients with nosocomial pneumonia showing anaerobes were relatively common in transtracheal aspirates but probably not important.[37]

WHAT IS THE CASE FOR ANAEROBES?

1. Anaerobic bacteria are the dominant agents in the normal oral flora and dominant pathogens in sophisticated studies of selected dental infections, such as pyorrhea, gingivitis, and oral abscesses. Thus, their role as potential pathogens and the dominant inoculum with aspiration seem well established.
2. Anaerobic bacteria play a relatively well-confirmed role in selected types of pulmonary infections that are uncommon but distinctive, with common clinical features that include indolent course, putrid discharge, and response to antibiotics directed at anaerobes, including clindamycin or β-lactam-β-lactamase inhibitors that are now favored for most cases of lung abscess.
3. Putrid discharge as sometimes found with lung abscess or empyema cases is often considered diagnostic of anaerobic infection because these agents, as all microbiologists know well, are the only microbes that produce the short-chain volatile fatty acids responsible for this distinctive odor.
4. The experimental studies by Smith as reviewed earlier[2] are an elegant demonstration of pathogenic potential and synergy. More recent studies show specific virulence factors, such as the capsular polysaccharide that promotes abscess formation.[4–7]
5. Why do currently recommended antibiotics work if anaerobes are important? Most cases of pneumonia probably do not involve anaerobic bacteria; it is the select categories noted earlier. In addition, the antimicrobials that are commonly used for CAP and other common lung infections (β-lactams, macrolides, and fluoroquinolones) probably have sufficient activity versus upper airway anaerobes to explain a response.

Interpretation Based on Evidence

The evidence summarized here makes a strong case for a role for selected anaerobes because pulmonary pathogens are selected types of pulmonary infections. However, most pulmonary infections do not involve anaerobes. The clues to the subset that do involve anaerobes are well characterized clinically and bacteriologically: The clues include the following:

- Probable aspiration as evidenced by dysphagia (inability to drink water rapidly) or reduced consciousness plus infection in a dependent pulmonary segment, usually a posterior segment of a lower lobe or superior segment with aspiration in the recumbent position or basilar segments with aspiration in the upright position.
- Putrid discharge (sputum, breath, empyema fluid), diagnostic of anaerobes
- Indolent course (nonspecific)
- Necrosis of tissue with necrotizing pneumonia, lung abscess, or empyema with a bronchopleural fistula.

Recommendations

Anaerobic bacteria are infrequent pulmonary pathogens but may cause serious disease that often defies traditional microbiological evaluations. The specific clues are noted earlier, but the following 2 points are emphasized:

- *Microbiology*: It is difficult to acquire appropriate microbiology because most specimen sources are contaminated by normal oral flora, and many laboratories do not perform adequate anaerobic microbiology. The specimen source is a big problem. Transtracheal aspiration is no longer performed. Transthorasic aspiration is rare and bronchoscopy with a protected brush is sometimes performed, but standard methods do not include anaerobic cultures in most laboratories. Pleural fluid should be obtained when available, and these specimens need Gram stain and cultures for anaerobes should be routine because of the high yield in prior reports (see **Table 2**).
- *Treatment*: Drain large pleural collections and use the antibiotics that are standard for anaerobic lung infections: Either clindamycin or a β-lactam/β-lactamase inhibitor. If metronidazole is used, it must be combined with β-lactam for concurrent aerobic and microaerophilic streptococci.

REFERENCES

1. Veillon A. Sur un Microcoque anaerobe trouvé dans suppurations fetides. CR Soc Biol 1893;5:897.
2. Smith DT. Experimental aspiratory abscess. Arch Surg 1927;14:231.
3. Bartlett JG. Diagnostic tests for agents of community-acquired pneumonia. Clin Infect Dis 2011;52(Suppl 4):S296–304.
4. Bartlett JG, Louie TJ, Gorbach SL, et al. Therapeutic efficacy of 29 antimicrobial regimens in experimental intra-abdominal sepsis. Rev Infect Dis 1981;3:535–42.
5. Kasper DL, Onderdonk AB, Crabb J, et al. Protective efficacy of immunization with capsular antigen against experimental infection with Bacteroides fragilis. J Infect Dis 1979;140:724–31.
6. Wang Y, Kalka-Moll WM, Roehrl MH, et al. Structural basis of the abscess-modulating polysaccharide A2 from Bacteroides fragilis. Proc Natl Acad Sci U S A 2000;97:13478–83.
7. Bartlett JG, Onderdonk AB, Louie T, et al. A review. Lessons from an animal model of intra-abdominal sepsis. Arch Surg 1978;13:853–7.
8. Levison ME, Mangura CT, Lorber B, et al. Clindamycin compared with penicillin for the treatment of anaerobic lung abscess. Ann Intern Med 1983;98:466–71.
9. Gudiol F, Manresa F, Pallares R, et al. Clindamycin vs. penicillin for anaerobic lung infections. High rate of penicillin failures associated with penicillin-resistant Bacteroides melaninogenicus. Arch Intern Med 1990;150:2525–9.
10. Sanders CV, Hanna BJ, Lewis AC. Metronidazole in the treatment of anaerobic infections. Am Rev Respir Dis 1979;120:337–43.
11. Perlino CA. Metronidazole vs. clindamycin treatment of anaerobic pulmonary infection. Failure of metronidazole therapy. Arch Intern Med 1981;141:1424–7.
12. Bartlett JG, Rosenblatt JE, Finegold SM. Percutaneous transtracheal aspiration in the diagnosis of anaerobic pulmonary infection. Ann Intern Med 1973;79:535–40.
13. Wimberley N, Faling LJ, Bartlett JG. A fiberoptic bronchoscopy technique to obtain uncontaminated lower airways secretions for bacterial culture. Am Rev Respir Dis 1979;119:337–43.

14. Beerens H, Tahon-Castel M. Infections humaines à bactéries anaerobes non toxigénes. Brussels (Belgium): Presses Acadèmiques Européenes; 1965. p. 91–114.
15. Brook I, Finegold SM. Bacterioloogy and thereapy of lung abscess in children. J Pediatr 1979;94:10–2.
16. Bartlett JG. Anaerobic bacterial infections of the lung. Chest 1987;91:901–9.
17. Mori T, Ebe T, Takahashi M, et al. Lung abscess: analysis of 66 cases from 1979 to 1991. Intern Med 1993;32:278–84.
18. De A, Varaiua A, Mathur M. Anaerobes in pleuropulmonary infections. Indian J Med Microbiol 2002;20:150–2.
19. Wang JL, Chen KY, Fang CT, et al. Changing bacteriology of adult community-acquired lung abscess in Taiwan: Klebsiella pneumoniae versus anaerobes. Clin Infect Dis 2005;40:915–22.
20. Takayanagi N, Kagiyama N, Ishiguro T, et al. Etiology and outcome of community-acquired lung abcess. Respiration 2010;80:98–105.
21. Lorber B, Swenson RM. Bacteriology of aspiration pneumonia: a prospective study of community-and hospital-acquired cases. Ann Intern Med 1974;81:329–31.
22. Gonzalez-C CL, Calia FM. Bacteriologic flora of aspiration-induced pulmonary infections. Arch Intern Med 1975;135:711–4.
23. Bartlett JG. Anaerobic bacterial pneumonitis. Am Rev Respir Dis 1979;119(1):19–23.
24. Brook I, Frazier EH. Aerobic and anaerobic microbiology of empyema. A retrospective review in two military hospitals. Chest 1993;103:1502–7.
25. Sullivan KM, O'Toole RD, Fisher RH, et al. Anaerobic empyema thoracis. Arch Intern Med 1973;131:521–7.
26. Bartlett JG. Diagnostic accuracy of transtracheal aspiration bacteriologic studies. Am Rev Respir Dis 1977;115:772–82.
27. Varkey B, Rose D, Kutty CPK, et al. Empyema thoracis during a ten-year period: analysis of 72 cases and comparison to a previous study (1952 to 1967). Arch Intern Med 1981;141:1771–6.
28. Mavroudis C, Symmonds JB, Minagi H, et al. Improved survival in management of empyema thoracis. J Thorac Cardiovasc Surg 1981;82:49–57.
29. Grant DR, Finley RJ. Empyema: analysis of treatment techniques. Can J Surg 1985;28:449–51.
30. Lemmer J, Botham MJ, Orringer MB. Modern management of adult thoracic empyema. J Thorac Cardiovasc Surg 1985;90:849–55.
31. Boyanova L, Djambazov F, Gergova G, et al. Anaerobic microbiology in 198 cases of pleural empyema: a Bulgarian study. Anaerobe 2004;10:261–7.
32. Hunter JV, Chadwick M, Hutchinson G, et al. Use of gas liquid chromatograph in the clinical diagnosis of anaerobic pleuropulmonary infection. Br J Dis Chest 1985;79:1–8.
33. Finegold SM, George WL, Mulligan ME. Anaerobic infections. Part I. Dis Mon 1985;31:1–77.
34. Wimberly NW, Bass JB Jr, Boyd BW, et al. Use of a bronchoscopic protected catheter brush for the diagnosis of pulmonary infections. Chest 1982;81:556–62.
35. Bartlett JG. Anaerobic bacterial infections of the lung and pleural space. Clin Infect Dis 1993;16(Suppl 4):S248–55.
36. Johansson N, Kalin M, Tiveljung-Lindell A, et al. Etiology of community-acquired pneumonia: increased microbiological yield with new diagnostic methods. Clin Infect Dis 2010;50:202–9.
37. Bartlett JG, O'Keefe P, Tally FP, et al. Bacteriology of hospital-acquired pneumonia. Arch Intern Med 1986;146:868–71.

What is the Role of Respiratory Viruses in Community-Acquired Pneumonia?

What is the Best Therapy for Influenza and Other Viral Causes of Community-Acquired Pneumonia?

Andrew T. Pavia, MD

KEYWORDS

- Respiratory viruses • Respiratory viral infections • Influenza • Antiviral agents
- Viral pneumonia

KEY POINTS

- Respiratory viruses, particularly influenza and RSV, are a common cause of CAP.
- Respiratory viruses are detected in 45% to 75% of children and 15% to 54% of adults hospitalized with CAP.
- Coinfection with viruses and bacteria is common: 22% to 33% of children and 4% to 30% of adults hospitalized with CAP.
- The role of *Streptococcus pneumonia* relative to viral causes of CAP may have decreased because of widespread use of pneumococcal conjugate vaccines in children.
- Neuraminidase inhibitors reduce ICU admission and mortality among patients hospitalized with influenza, including those with pneumonia, and should be started when influenza is suspected.
- Differentiating viral CAP from mixed infection and bacterial CAP remains challenging, but better approaches could reduce antibiotic overuse.

Respiratory viruses including influenza have long been appreciated as a cause of community-acquired pneumonia (CAP), particularly among children, people with serious medical comorbidities, and military recruits. Recent advances in molecular virology have led to the discovery of previously unrecognized respiratory viruses, including human metapneumovirus (hMPV), parainfluenza virus (PIV) 4, human coronaviruses (HCoV) HKU1 and NL-63, and human bocavirus. Polymerase chain reaction (PCR)–based testing has allowed detection of newer agents and improved the ability to detect old viral infections, such as influenza virus and rhinovirus (**Table 1**).

Division of Pediatric Infectious Diseases, Department of Pediatrics, University of Utah, 295 Chipeta Way, Salt Lake City, UT 84108, USA
E-mail address: andy.pavia@hsc.utah.edu

Infect Dis Clin N Am 27 (2013) 157–175
http://dx.doi.org/10.1016/j.idc.2012.11.007

Table 1 Viruses associated with pneumonia	
Common	**Less Common or Predominantly in Specific Hosts or Settings**
Respiratory syncytial virus	Measles
Influenza virus A and B	Cytomegalovirus
Human metapneumovirus[a]	Varicella zoster virus
Adenovirus	Herpes simplex virus
Parainfluenza virus 1, 2, 3, and 4[a]	Epstein-Barr virus
Human coronavirus types 229e, OC43, HKU1,[a] and NL-63[a]	Hantavirus
Rhinovirus[a]	Enterovirus
Bocavirus[a]	Parechovirus[a]
	Severe acute respiratory syndrome coronavirus

[a] Those recently discovered or recently appreciated as associated with pneumonia. The role of all bocavirus and parechovirus has not been clearly established.

Widespread use of newer vaccines against *Streptococcus pneumoniae* and *Haemophilus influenzae* has changed the epidemiology of childhood and adult pneumonia. These changes have led to recognition of the greater and more widespread role of respiratory viruses in CAP in all age groups. Although not addressed in this article, respiratory viruses are a very important cause of severe pneumonia and respiratory failure in patients who are immunocompromised, particularly recipients of hematopoietic stem cell transplant.[1,2]

One challenge is that respiratory viruses in patients with CAP can be the sole cause of a viral pneumonia (often referred to as primary viral pneumonia); can be present as a coinfection (virus- bacteria or virus-virus); and can act as a predisposing factor to facilitate or worsen bacterial pneumonia. Moreover, detection of some viruses in the upper respiratory tract of asymptomatic patients is relatively common and therefore may indicate convalescent shedding or asymptomatic infection.[3]

There are several critical questions that are not fully answered. What is the role of individual viruses in pneumonia? What is the prevalence of specific viruses among patients of CAP? Which patients are most likely to have viral pneumonia? What does the detection of a respiratory virus from a patient with CAP tell about the cause? How should viral detection effect clinical management and when can antibiotics be avoided or stopped?

SPECIFIC VIRUSES
Respiratory Syncytial Virus

Respiratory syncytial virus (RSV) is a paramyxovirus that causes upper respiratory tract infection (URI) and bronchiolitis in children but is also associated with a substantial proportion of CAP among children. RSV has been detected in 3% to 31% of children hospitalized with CAP. The incidence and severity varies with age; younger children are generally more likely to have RSV-associated pneumonia and are the most severely affected. Important studies in the mid-1990s demonstrated that RSV was an important cause of CAP in adults.[4,5] Dowell and coworkers[5] studied noninstitutionalized adults admitted to two Ohio hospitals and found that 53 (4.4%) of 1195 adults admitted during the RSV seasons and 4 (1%) of 390 in the off-season had serologic evidence of RSV infection. RSV has been identified in 4% to 7% of adults with CAP.[6–9]

RSV-associated CAP seems to be more common and severe among older adults.[10] Using viral surveillance, hospitalization, and mortality data, Zhou and colleagues[11] from the Centers for Disease Control and Prevention (CDC) estimated that the rate of hospitalization for RSV for persons older than 65 was 86 per 100,000 persons per year, compared with a hospitalization rate for influenza of 309 per 100,000 in that age group. RSV was listed in the discharge codes in fewer than 2% of the hospitalizations for RSV among older persons, suggesting marked underrecognition. RSV causes substantial mortality. Thompson and colleagues[12] estimated that during the 1990s, RSV was associated with an average of more than 11,000 deaths each year in the United States. Most of these deaths were in persons older than 65.

In studies comparing adults with RSV and pneumonia with those with influenza or other causes, wheezing is more common,[5] but clinical characteristics cannot reliably differentiate those with RSV.[13]

Influenza Virus

Pneumonia was recognized as a complication of influenza during the pandemic of 1918 to 1919, long before the virus was identified. During the "Asian influenza" pandemic of 1957 to 1958, Louria and coworkers[14] and others codified the concept that influenza could cause a primary viral pneumonia or lead to bacterial pneumonia with each having distinct pathologic appearance. Animal studies are beginning to yield insights into the nature of the complex and synergistic interaction in the lung between influenza and *S pneumoniae* and *Staphylococcus aureus*,[15,16] which is thought to be responsible for much of the mortality during pandemics.[17]

Among patients hospitalized with influenza, radiographic pneumonia has been reported in 16% to 55%, with lower rates in studies among children.[18–21] Patients admitted with influenza who have pneumonia are more likely to be admitted to the intensive care unit or die.[19,22] Differentiating viral pneumonia caused by influenza from bacterial coinfection or superinfection is not always clear. The classical presentation of superinfection is biphasic, with typical influenza-like illness that begins to resolve over several days followed by acute deterioration with the development of chest pain and new infiltrates, and bacteriologic evidence of infection, but this represents a minority.

Human Metapneumovirus

Dutch researchers first described hMPV in 2001 in children with bronchiolitis.[23] Subsequent studies identified it as an important cause of acute respiratory infections in children and adults, with a worldwide distribution.[24,25] hMPV is a paramyxovirus in the subfamily pneumovirineae that includes RSV, but hMPV is most closely related to avian pneumovirus. In temporal climates, infection occurs predominantly in the winter months, and there is significant year-to-year variation. Clinical manifestations of hMPV infection include asymptomatic infections, colds, febrile seizures, bronchiolitis, asthma exacerbations, chronic obstructive pulmonary disease (COPD) exacerbations, pneumonia, and respiratory failure. Symptomatic infection occurs in all age groups,[24–30] but pneumonia is most commonly seen among younger children, older adults, and those with underlying medical conditions.[23,31] In prospective studies of adults hospitalized in Rochester, New York, and Nashville, Tennessee, with acute respiratory illness, the prevalence of hMPV infection and clinical characteristics of patients were similar to patients with influenza and RSV.[29,30] Using prospective surveillance in central Tennessee, Widmer and coworkers[30] estimated the incidence of hospitalization for hMPV among persons older than 65 years was 220 per 100,000 compared with 254 per 100,000 and 123 per 100,000 for RSV and influenza virus, respectively.

Adenovirus

Shortly after the discovery of adenovirus in 1953, it was recovered from military personnel with acute respiratory disease, thus making it one of the first viruses clearly linked with pneumonia.[32] Adenoviruses are lytic nonenveloped DNA viruses, which contrasts with most respiratory viruses that are RNA viruses. More than 50 serotypes have been described. Adenoviruses cause a wide variety of infections, including conjunctivitis, epidemic keratoconjunctivitis, pharyngitis, URI, pneumonia, meningitis, hepatitis, and gastroenteritis. Conjunctivitis, pharyngitis, or rash may be present with pneumonia and provide a clue to the cause, but this is uncommon. Serotypes differ in tissue tropism and their tendency to cause severe respiratory disease, although the mechanisms for this are poorly understood. Severe respiratory disease is associated with adenovirus serotypes 5, 7, 14, and 21. Historically, adenovirus pneumonia has been primarily documented among children; immunocompromised adults[33]; and outbreaks in hospitalized patients[34,35] and healthy adults in closed settings, such as military recruits.[36-38] However, severe disease can occur in immunocompetent adults.[39] The genetic diversity of adenoviruses has limited the sensitivity of culture and PCR-based diagnostics, so the true rate of adenoviral pneumonia may be underestimated.

Adenovirus vaccine was used in the US military for more than two decades, resulting in a marked decrease in adenoviral pneumonia among recruits. When the sole manufacturer ceased production there was a marked resurgence in adenoviral disease.[36,40] Beginning in 2005, a new variant of serotype 14 emerged as a cause of severe lower respiratory tract disease in immunocompetent adults in the community[41] and in the military.[42]

Parainfluenza Virus

PIVs are paramyxovirus that are antigenically divided in to four serotypes (PIV1–4).[43] They are common causes of acute respiratory infections including URI, croup, bronchiolitis, and pneumonia.[44,45] Seasonal outbreaks occur in the fall and spring. Most infections are mild, but in a prospective surveillance study of children in three regions, Weinberg and coworkers[45] found that PIVs were associated with an average annual rate of 100 hospitalizations per 100,000 persons younger than 5 years or roughly 23,000 hospitalizations per year. Similar population-based estimates for adults are not available. In one study, Marx and coworkers[46] used serology to detect PIV1 from 2.5% of 721 and PIV3 from 3.1% of 705 adults hospitalized with lower respiratory tract infection. However, they predominantly tested patients hospitalized during "the parainfluenza season."

Most pneumonia associated with PIVs occurs in infants, young children, and immunocompromised hosts. However, PIV has been detected in 0% to 8% of adults with CAP.[6-9,47,48] PIV3 is more commonly associated with pneumonia than other types, although fewer studies have systematically sought PIV4.

Non–Severe Acute Respiratory Syndrome Coronaviruses

HCoV 229E and OC43 have been long recognized as causes of viral URI and were linked to pneumonia in children and immunocompromised adults.[49] Two novel HCoV, NL63[50] and HKU1,[51] were identified in the past decade. All four HCoV show distinct winter seasonality. They are associated with upper and lower respiratory tract infections in all age groups.[52-54] In a prospective study from Scotland that included a control group of patients with no respiratory symptoms, HCoV HKU1, HCoV NL63, and HCoV OC43 were isolated significantly more often from patients with lower respiratory tract infections than from control subjects, supporting the etiologic role of these viruses.[52] In a prospective study of hospitalized patients with pneumonia in Thailand, coronaviruses were detected by PCR in 5.9% of 734 patients in the first year of the study. However, in the second year when a control group was included, coronaviruses were detected in only 1.8% of 1156 patients and were detected in 2.1% of control subjects.[55] Thus, this study did not demonstrate an epidemiologic association of coronaviruses with pneumonia, but it is unclear if this was caused by variation in intensity of the season. In a prospective study of patients with severe pneumonia undergoing bronchoalveolar lavage about half of whom were transplant recipients, coronaviruses were detected in 5.8%, mostly as the sole pathogen.[56] Thus, the role of coronaviruses in pneumonia has not been completely clarified but it seems clear that they cause some cases of CAP in normal hosts and cause severe pneumonia in transplant patients.

Rhinovirus

Rhinoviruses are among the most common cause of respiratory infections in people of all ages. However, elucidating their role in pneumonia has proved complex.[57] The use of PCR and sequencing has greatly enhanced detection of rhinoviruses in severely ill patients and led to the recognition of a third rhinovirus species, genogroup C.[58] Many rhinovirus PCR assays also detect other picornaviruses, particularly enterovirus, which complicates the literature. Rhinoviruses were long known to cause common colds, otitis media, asthma exacerbations, and exacerbations of COPD, but lower respiratory tract infections were thought to be rare, perhaps because of the belief that rhinoviruses grow poorly at 37°C. Recent data clearly demonstrate that rhinoviruses can replicate at body temperature[59] and infect cells of the lower respiratory tract.[60] Rhinovirus infection of respiratory endothelium induces potent inflammatory responses, but in contrast in several other respiratory viruses does not induce cell lysis.[61]

Studies using PCR consistently identify rhinoviruses in nasopharyngeal or pharyngeal specimens from children and adults with lower respiratory tract infections.[62–65] Rhinovirus has also been detected in 4% to 45% of children[66–70] and 2% to 17% of adults with CAP (**Tables 2** and **3**).[6–9,47,48] Determining whether rhinovirus has a causal role in any single case of CAP is particularly problematic because of the high rate of codetection of rhinovirus with other viruses and bacteria, and because of the detection of rhinovirus in asymptomatic patients, representing convalescent shedding or asymptomatic infection. Shedding generally does not persist beyond 2 to 3 weeks, but few studies have done careful molecular subtyping, making it difficult to separate shedding from reinfection. The rates of rhinovirus detection in asymptomatic patients are generally substantially lower than among patients with lower respiratory tract infection or pneumonia. In a review of published studies of viral detection in asymptomatic subjects, Jartti and coworkers[3] found a mean rate of rhinovirus/enterovirus detection by PCR of 15%, with higher rates among children and very low rates (2%) among the elderly. In preliminary results from the CDC Etiology of Pnemonia in the Community (EPIC) Study, rhinovirus was detected in 31% of 1320 children hospitalized with CAP and 22% of 442 control children who were undergoing elective surgery.

It seems likely that rhinovirus is a cause of CAP, but questions remain. Are some rhinovirus strains more likely to cause CAP? Are higher viral loads in the nasopharynx better predictors of lower respiratory tract infection and rhinovirus pneumonia? Does coinfection with rhinovirus facilitate infection with a second viral or bacterial pathogen and does rhinovirus coinfection increase the severity?

Table 2
Cause of community-acquired pneumonia in hospitalized children and role of viruses in six recent studies

	Juven et al,[68] 2000 (N = 254)	Michelow et al,[69] 2004 (N = 154)	Cevey-Macherel et al,[66] 2009 (N = 99)	Tsolia et al,[70] 2004 (N = 75)	Garcia-Garcia[78] (N = 884)	Jain et al,[67] 2011 (N = 1320[a])
Age	1 mo–17 y	2 mo–17 y	2 mo–5 y	5–14 y	<14 y	1 mo–17 y
Any pathogen	85%	79%	86%	77%	Not stated	82%
Any bacteria	53%	60%	52%	40%	2.2%	10%
Any virus	62%	45%	66%	65%	73%[b]	77%
Coinfection	30%	23%	33%	28%	22%	23%
RSV	29%	13%	13%	3%	31%	25%
Influenza virus	4%	22%	14%	7%	5%	4%
hMPV	NS	NS	13%	1%	5%	1%
Adenovirus	7%	7%	7%	12%	13%	1%
Parainfluenza virus	10%	13%	13%	8%	5%	1%
Rhinovirus/enterovirus[c]	24%	4%	33%	45%	19%	31%
Coronavirus	3%	NS	7%	NS	1%	<1%

Abbreviation: NS, not sought.

[a] Preliminary results from an ongoing study.
[b] Includes detection of bocavirus in 13%.
[c] Most assays identify both rhinovirus and enterovirus.

Table 3
Cause of community-acquired pneumonia in hospitalized adults and role of viruses in six recent studies

	Charles et al,[47] 2008 (N = 885)	Johansson et al,[7] 2010 (N = 184)	Johnstone et al,[8] 2008 (N = 193)	Lieberman et al,[9] 2010 (N = 183)	Jennings et al,[6] 2008 (N = 225)[a]	Templeton et al,[48] 2005 (N = 105)
Age	Not stated	Mean 63	Median 71	Mean 60	Median 70	Median 60
Any pathogen	46%	67%	39%	Not stated	58%	76%
Any bacteria	38%	58%[b]	20%	Not stated	48%	46%
Any virus	15%	29%	15%	32%	34%	54%
Coinfection	9%	23%	4%	Not stated	30%	27%
RSV	2%	4%	3%	7%	4%	3%
Influenza virus	8%	8%	4%	4%	12%	10%
hMPV	NS	2%	4%	1%	0%	0%
Adenovirus	<1%	2%	1%	2%	4%	4%
Parainfluenza virus	<1%	4%	2%	0%	1%	8%
Rhinovirus/ enterovirus[c]	5%	7%	2%	5%	13%	17%
Coronavirus	NS	2%	2%	13%	2%	13%

Abbreviation: NS, not sought.
[a] Includes those with complete viral testing.
[b] PCR assays were used for bacterial pathogens including *Streptococcus pneumoniae, Haemophilus influenza, Moraxella, Legionella* sp, *Mycoplasma pneumoniae,* and *Chlamydophila pneumoniae.*
[c] Most assays identify both rhinovirus and enterovirus.

Other Viruses

Table 1 shows the range of viruses associated with CAP. Human bocavirus is a recently described parvovirus that has been frequently detected in respiratory secretions of children with respiratory tract infection.[71,72] The role of bocavirus in CAP remains unclear. Interpretation of human bocavirus detection has been complicated by relatively common detection in asymptomatic children and prolonged detection after infection. However, in a study of Thai patients hospitalized with pneumonia, Fry and colleagues[73] found that compared with control patients, detection of human bocavirus was associated with hospitalization for pneumonia. Four patients with human bocavirus and pneumonia were older than 65. However, 83% of pneumonia patients with human bocavirus had coinfection with another pathogen. Brieu and coworkers[72] detected human bocavirus in 10.8% of 508 children hospitalized with respiratory illness and none of 68 control subjects. Pneumonia was diagnosed in four of the children with human bocavirus. Most bocavirus-infected children had a coinfection, but viral loads were higher in the mono-infected children. Christensen and coworkers[74] detected bocavirus in 10% of 1154 children with respiratory tract infection and a similar proportion of control subjects. Of those with bocavirus, a second virus was detected in 75%. Bocavirus viral load greater than 10^6 copies/mL was not associated with respiratory infection; higher viral load was however associated with LRTI. Thus, the exact role of bocavirus in pneumonia remains unclear.

Varicella zoster virus, herpes simplex virus, cytomegalovirus, and measles virus can cause severe pneumonia in immunocompromised hosts, but can cause pneumonia in otherwise normal hosts. Parechoviruses are rapidly emerging as important causes of sepsis and meningitis in infants. Parechoviruses have been occasionally isolated from children with pneumonia.[75,76] The systematic investigation of parechovirus infections is just beginning and their true role in CAP is unknown.

RESPIRATORY VIRUSES IN CAP IN CHILDREN

Viral infections are the most common cause of CAP in children in recent studies where sensitive molecular methods were used.[66–70,77,78] It is challenging to compare individual studies because of differences in populations studied (age, severity of illness); seasons; samples obtained; agents sought; and the technologies used (eg, viral culture, viral or bacterial PCR, viral or bacterial serology). Moreover, the introduction of conjugate vaccines for *H influenza* and *S pneumonia* has decreased the incidence of these important pathogens compared with older studies.[79,80] Several recent studies of hospitalized children with CAP that use PCR to enhance viral detection are summarized in **Table 2**. A virus was detected in 45% to 77% of children and a potential bacterial cause in 2% to 60%. The frequency of coinfection ranged from 22% to 33%. Mixed bacterial viral infections were found in 28% to 33% and viral-viral infections in 8% to 14%.[66,69,70] In general, viral infections are more predominant among infants and children younger than 5 years old compared with older children.

RSV (3%–30%), influenza virus (4%–22%), and rhinovirus (4%–45%) were the viruses most commonly detected. The highly variable rates of detection of hMPV (1%–13%) and PIV (1%–13%) may reflect differences in the populations studied or year-to-year variation in the epidemiology of these infections. The ongoing CDC EPIC study[67] when finished will encompass approximately 2400 children over 2.5 years and include population-based data from three cities. This will provide more detailed and stable estimates of the role of viruses in CAP among children.

It is remarkable that no pathogen can be identified in 14% to 23% of pediatric CAP in recent studies, suggesting the need for improved diagnostics and the possibility of unrecognized pathogens.

RESPIRATORY VIRUSES IN CAP IN ADULTS

It is likely that the epidemiology of CAP in adults has also changed in recent years because of the indirect impact of pneumococcal conjugate vaccine in children and the increasing age of the population. In four recent studies of adult patients hospitalized with CAP that used at a minimum blood and sputum culture plus urinary antigen detection, *S pneumoniae* was detected in 7% to 38%.[6–8,47] The highest proportion of *S pneumoniae* (38%) was in the study of Johansson and coworkers,[7] which included the use of PCR to detect *S pneumoniae* in sputum. The apparently lower proportion of *S pneumoniae* has led to speculation that viruses now cause an increasing proportion of CAP in adults. It is hard to determine if this is true or reflects recent advances in viral diagnosis, the difficulty of establishing the cause of pneumonia, and the prevalence of dual infections.

Table 3 summarizes six prospective studies that included viral PCR to determine the cause of CAP in 1762 hospitalized adults (a small number of outpatients are included in the study by Templeton and coworkers[48]). At least one virus was detected in 15% to 54%. In the five studies that reported bacterial causes, bacterial pathogens were detected in 20% to 58% and coinfection was detected in 4% to 30%. Viral infections are generally a more prominent cause of CAP among older adults.[81] Johnstone and coworkers[8] reported that patients with viral infections were significantly older than those without viral infections (median age, 76 vs 64 years), and were more likely to have underlying cardiac disease (66% vs 32%) and to be frail. Influenza virus was among the most commonly detected viruses in adults hospitalized with CAP, detected in 4% to 12%. RSV was detected in 2% to 7% of adults. Influenza and RSV detection were highly seasonal. Detection of rhinovirus/enterovirus varied from 2% to 17%, but these viruses were often detected as a coinfection. Parainfluenza and coronaviruses were detected at variable rates (0%–8% and 2%–13%, respectively). HMPV and adenovirus were somewhat less commonly detected (0%–4% and <1%–4%, respectively). A putative pathogen could not be detected in 24% to 61% of patients in these studies despite the use of multiple methods including PCR for detection of viruses. This proportion is considerably higher than in studies of CAP in children, but the reasons are unclear. Possible explanations include a greater role of bacterial infection for which current diagnostics remain inadequate, the greater role of viral infection and coinfection in children, greater incidental detection of viral shedding in children, or lower viral copy number in the nasopharynx of adults with viral infections of the lower respiratory tract, making detection more difficult.

QUESTIONS
What is the Role of Mixed Infections in CAP?

When sophisticated diagnostic tests are applied, more than one pathogen can be identified in 23% to 33% of children and 4% to 30% of adults in prospective studies of CAP (see **Tables 2** and **3**). This raises several important questions. What proportion of patients in whom a virus is detected by PCR truly has a bacterial coinfection? Does viral-bacterial coinfection influence the course of illness?

The clinical interaction between influenza and *S pneumoniae* and *S aureus* has long been appreciated, and is a major contributor to influenza mortality.[16,17,82] Several pathologic mechanisms have been proposed including epithelial damage, changes in airway function, upregulation of receptors, and changes in the innate immune reponse.[16] It is becoming clear that similar interactions may occur with other respiratory viruses, including RSV, hMPV, and possibly rhinovirus and PIV.[83,84]

Clinical evidence from prospective studies on the role of coinfection on severity is somewhat conflicting. There is a suggestion that viral-bacterial coinfection is associated with more severe disease among adults. Johansson and coworkers[7,85] found that compared with those with only bacterial infections, adults with coinfection were much more likely to have pneumonia severity index (PSI) scores of IV or V (62% vs 26%; odds ratio, 4.6; *P*<.001) and had longer length of stay (7 vs 4 days; *P* = .002). Templeton and coworkers[48] reported that age older than 60, rhinovirus in mixed infection, and mixed infection were all associated with PSI score classes IV and V. Similarly, Jennings and coworkers[6] reported that rhinovirus infection with pneumococcal infection was independently associated with more severe disease by either PSI or CURBAge criteria. In contrast, Charles and coworkers[47] reported similar 30-day mortality among those with coinfection and single infection (8% vs 5.4%).

What Findings Differentiate Viral Pneumonia from Mixed or Bacterial Pneumonia?

Differentiating viral pneumonia from infection with bacteria alone or mixed viral-bacterial infection could significantly decrease antibiotic use with the associated risk of adverse reactions and the selective pressure for the development of resistance. However, developing clinical and laboratory tools to differentiate has been challenging.

Viral pneumonia is more likely during fall, winter, and early spring when outbreaks of respiratory viruses are occurring.[6,8,86] Age less than 2 years[87] or older age among adults[8] is associated with an increased likelihood of viral pneumonia. Wheezing in children[78] and adults[5] has been significantly associated in some studies with viral pneumonia compared with mixed or bacterial infection. High temperature,[69] rigors,[6] and chest pain[8] are significantly more common on presentation in patients with bacterial or mixed infection. Significant overlap limits the use of these findings.

There has been significant interest in the ability of inflammatory markers to discriminate between viral and bacterial cause in CAP.[88] In children, procalcitonin and C-reactive protein are consistently higher among children with bacterial infection,[69,89,90] but it is unclear if specific cutoffs can be identified. Toikka and coworkers[90] found that procalcitonin (median, 2.09 vs 0.56 ng/mL; $P = .019$) and C-reactive protein concentrations (96 vs 54 mg/L; $P = .008$) were significantly higher in children with bacterial CAP than those with sole viral cause, but there was substantial overlap. Nascimento-Carvalho and coworkers,[89] however, reported that a cutoff of procalcitonin less than 2 ng/mL had a negative predictive value of 95% for excluding bacterial infection. In adults, procalcitonin levels are also higher in bacterial pneumonia.[91] However, procalcitonin values are not static; they increase rapidly during bacterial infection and fall during appropriate therapy. To get around the limitations of a single cutoff value, treatment algorithms using sequential procalcitonin levels have been studied in several randomized trials as a way to guide therapy.[88,92,93] For a complete discussion see the article by Niederman elsewhere in this issue.

Chest radiographs are only moderately useful in discriminating viral from bacterial CAP.[86,87,94,95] Interstitial infiltrates with a patchy distribution are typical of viral pneumonia, whereas alveolar infiltrates, particularly with a lobar pattern, are suggestive of bacterial infection. However, there is marked overlap. In one study, 72% of 134 children with bacterial infection had alveolar infiltrates, as did 49% of 81 children with only viral infection ($P = .001$). Exclusively interstitial infiltrates were present in 28% of children with bacterial infection and 49% of those with viral infection.[87] The presence of pleural effusions was predictive of bacterial infection in several studies.[69,78]

It is tempting to hypothesize that the use of sensitive PCR assays in conjunction with biomarkers, such as procalcitonin, could lead to diagnostic algorithms with adequate predictive value to improve the use antibiotics in CAP, but this has not been adequately studied.

What is the Best Treatment of Influenza Virus in CAP?

Effective antiviral therapy may prevent the development of CAP, and treatment of patients with influenza-associated pneumonia may improve outcomes. However, the evidence base is not optimal. Two classes of drugs are available for the treatment of influenza virus infection: the adamantanes (amantadine and rimantidine) and neuraminidase inhibitors (oseltamivir [Tamiflu] and zanamivir [Relenza]). Widespread and stable resistance to the adamantanes has rendered this class of limited use.[96] Oseltamivir and zanamivir were initially studied in randomized controlled trials among adults and children with uncomplicated influenza.[97] These studies demonstrated reductions in the time to the primary endpoint of resolution of all symptoms of approximately 1.25 days when neuraminidase inhibitors were begun within 48 hours of symptom onset; larger benefits were seen for return to functional status. Few patients with risk factors for complications were enrolled in these studies and with low rate of events the individual studies did not demonstrate reductions in hospitalizations or pneumonia. Kaiser and coworkers[98] performed a pooled analysis of oseltamivir clinical trials including 1340 patients, and reported statistically significant reductions in the development of lower respiratory tract infections resulting in antibiotic use and in hospitalizations and a nonsignificant reduction in pneumonia. Although statistically significant, the absolute risk reductions in generally healthy patients were relatively modest.

A critical question is whether treatment is beneficial among patients at high risk of complications, those with more severe disease requiring hospitalization, or with lower respiratory tract infections caused by influenza (with or without bacterial coinfection). A large body of carefully conducted but observational studies in seasonal[99–101] and pandemic 2009 H1N1 influenza[19,22,102–109] demonstrated improved outcomes among hospitalized patients treated with neuraminidase inhibitors including decreased intensive care unit admission and mortality. Benefits were independently demonstrated among children,[108] pregnant women,[104] and critically ill patients.[109] A formal meta-analysis by Hsu and colleagues[110] concluded that among high-risk patients, oral oseltamivir may reduce mortality, hospitalization, and duration of symptoms, but the quality of the evidence was deemed low. Earlier initiation of therapy is associated with the greatest benefit, but among hospitalized patients, benefits were observed when oseltamivir was started as late as 5 days after symptom onset compared with no therapy.

Bacterial coinfection is an important cause of severe pneumonia and mortality in patients with influenza and pneumonia. In studies among critically ill children[111] and adults[82] with pandemic 2009 H1N1 influenza, bacterial infection, particularly with methicillin-resistant S aureus, was associated with mortality. It is not possible from existing data to conclusively demonstrate that oseltamivir in addition to appropriate antibiotic therapy improves outcomes in patients with documented bacterial coinfection, but animal data[15,16] and limited observational data suggest an independent benefit of antiviral therapy.

Thus, antiviral therapy with neuraminidase inhibitors should be started empirically in all hospitalized patients in whom influenza is suspected without waiting for laboratory confirmation, including those with CAP.[96,112] Influenza testing and empiric antiviral therapy in addition to antibiotic therapy is appropriate for patients at increased risk of influenza complications who present with signs of CAP during outbreaks of seasonal influenza. It is important to remember that current rapid antigen-based influenza tests have relatively low sensitivity and a negative test does not rule out influenza.[113,114]

Resistance to oseltamivir became widespread among seasonal strains of H1N1 influenza in 2008 in the H275Y mutation in the neuraminidase gene,[115,116] and sporadic resistance to oseltamivir has emerged on therapy and been transmitted in other strains, including pandemic 2009 H1N1 influenza.[117–119] These strains remain sensitive to zanamivir, but it is only available as a dry powder for inhalation, which is not appropriate for treatment of children younger than 5 years old and is not recommended for those with asthma or COPD because of the risk of bronchospasm. Continued spread of oseltamivir resistance would greatly reduce the ability to treat influenza-associated CAP.

What is the Best Treatment for Other Respiratory Viruses in CAP

Although effective therapy exists for influenza-related CAP in children and adults, options for the treatment of other viruses are extremely limited. Ribavirin has broad antiviral activity in vitro that includes RSV, hMPV, PIV, and influenza, but there are scarce data to demonstrate clinical use. Observational studies of inhaled ribavirin for RSV demonstrated limited benefits among severely immunocompromised patients[120] but the single randomized trial was underpowered.[121] Among other populations, the benefits are questionable and the costs and risks limit the use of inhaled ribabirin.[122] Palivizumab, a monoclonal antibody directed against the fusion glycoprotein of RSV, is recommended for the prevention of RSV hospitalization in specific subgroups of premature infants and infants with some types of congenital heart disease or chronic lung disease. Unfortunately, it has not demonstrated any value in the treatment of RSV disease.

Based on anecdotal experience, intravenous ribavirin may have a potential role for overwhelming viral pneumonia in severely immunocompromised patients caused by RSV, hMPV, or PIV.[123] Cidofovir has potent activity against adenovirus and case reports suggest clinical benefit in immunocompromised patients with adenovirus infection.[124,125] Cidofovir should be considered for patients with overwhelming adenovirus pneumonia including adenovirus type 14.[126] Because of the toxicity and difficulty with administration, cidofovir is not appropriate for CAP in immunocompetent hosts. An orally available prodrug of cidofovir, CMX001, is in advanced development and may prove useful for a wider array of patients with adenovirus pneumonia.[127] Pleconaril, a drug with activity against picornaviruses including rhinovirus, inhibits viral uncoating. A clinical trial showed reduction in the duration of symptoms for naturally occurring colds.[128] Pleconaril is no longer in development but this class of agents could be useful in lower respiratory tract disease caused by picornaviruses.

Because of the ubiquity of respiratory viruses, most pools of intravenous immunoglobulin have significant titers of antibody, including neutralizing antibody against common respiratory viruses. Intravenous immunoglobulin should be considered for hypogammaglobulinemic and severely immunocompromised patients with viral pneumonia.

UNANSWERED QUESTIONS AND FUTURE DIRECTIONS

Much remains to be learned about viral infections in CAP and how to translate the knowledge into improved patient care. How can it be determined if the detection of a virus in the upper airway in a patient with CAP indicates a causal role? This problem is common to interpreting prospective studies and tests in individual patients. The problem is more difficult for rhinovirus and coronaviruses that have been detected in 2% to 45% and 0% to 6% of asymptomatic subjects, respectively, by PCR than for influenza and hMPV, which are rarely detected in the absence of symptoms.[3] Some studies have shown higher viral loads in patients with pneumonia, suggesting that quantitative assays might increase the specificity.[74,129–132]

Which patients with CAP should be tested for viral infections and how should it alter clinical care? Detection of influenza infection can clearly lead to use of antivirals and in most cases limit the use of antibiotics. The use of sensitive and specific influenza tests is appropriate for children and adults with CAP during influenza season, and is recommended in recent guidelines.[133,134] In younger children with moderate to severe CAP and immunocompromised patients viral pneumonia is common and testing for an array of viral causes of pneumonia can direct therapy and improve infection control. However, additional studies are needed to determine the impact of viral testing in other groups. The combined use of biologic markers and viral testing holds the promise of correctly identifying patients for whom antibiotic exposure can be safely limited. This would be facilitated by tests that can accurately detect multiple viruses with rapid turnaround time and that can be deployed in a variety of settings.

There is a critical need for influenza antivirals that are effective for viruses resistant to oseltamivir. Moreover, effective treatments, including antiviral agents, immunomodulatory agents, or siRNA, are needed for respiratory viruses other than influenza. RSV and hMPV are particularly attractive targets, because an effective drug could decrease morbidity, hospitalization, and mortality in many young children, older adults, and immunocompromised patients. Targets have been identified, but clinical development has been slow.[135,136] Effective vaccines against respiratory viruses could have a substantial impact on CAP by preventing primary viral pneumonia and preventing secondary bacterial infections.

REFERENCES

1. Ison MG, Michaels MG. RNA respiratory viral infections in solid organ transplant recipients. Am J Transplant 2009;9(Suppl 4):S166–72.
2. Kim YJ, Boeckh M, Englund JA. Community respiratory virus infections in immunocompromised patients: hematopoietic stem cell and solid organ transplant recipients, and individuals with human immunodeficiency virus infection. Semin Respir Crit Care Med 2007;28:222–42.
3. Jartti T, Jartti L, Peltola V, et al. Identification of respiratory viruses in asymptomatic subjects: asymptomatic respiratory viral infections. Pediatr Infect Dis J 2008;27:1103–7.
4. Falsey AR, Cunningham CK, Barker WH, et al. Respiratory syncytial virus and influenza A infections in the hospitalized elderly. J Infect Dis 1995;172:389–94.
5. Dowell SF, Anderson LJ, Gary HE Jr, et al. Respiratory syncytial virus is an important cause of community-acquired lower respiratory infection among hospitalized adults. J Infect Dis 1996;174:456–62.
6. Jennings LC, Anderson TP, Beynon KA, et al. Incidence and characteristics of viral community-acquired pneumonia in adults. Thorax 2008;63:42–8.
7. Johansson N, Kalin M, Tiveljung-Lindell A, et al. Etiology of community-acquired pneumonia: increased microbiological yield with new diagnostic methods. Clin Infect Dis 2010;50:202–9.
8. Johnstone J, Majumdar SR, Fox JD, et al. Viral infection in adults hospitalized with community-acquired pneumonia: prevalence, pathogens, and presentation. Chest 2008;134:1141–8.
9. Lieberman D, Shimoni A, Shemer-Avni Y, et al. Respiratory viruses in adults with community-acquired pneumonia. Chest 2010;138:811–6.
10. Falsey AR, Hennessey PA, Formica MA, et al. Respiratory syncytial virus infection in elderly and high-risk adults. N Engl J Med 2005;352:1749–59.
11. Zhou H, Thompson WW, Viboud CG, et al. Hospitalizations associated with influenza and respiratory syncytial virus in the United States, 1993–2008. Clin Infect Dis 2012;54:1427–36.
12. Thompson WW, Shay DK, Weintraub E, et al. Mortality associated with influenza and respiratory syncytial virus in the United States. JAMA 2003;289:179–86.
13. Walsh EE, Peterson DR, Falsey AR. Is clinical recognition of respiratory syncytial virus infection in hospitalized elderly and high-risk adults possible? J Infect Dis 2007;195:1046–51.
14. Louria D, Blumenfeld H, Ellis J, et al. Studies on influenza in the pandemic of 1957–58. II. Pulmonary complications of Influenza. J Clin Invest 1959;38:213–65.
15. Iverson AR, Boyd KL, McAuley JL, et al. Influenza virus primes mice for pneumonia from Staphylococcus aureus. J Infect Dis 2011;203:880–8.
16. McCullers JA. Insights into the interaction between influenza virus and pneumococcus. Clin Microbiol Rev 2006;19:571–82.
17. Morens DM, Taubenberger JK, Fauci AS. Predominant role of bacterial pneumonia as a cause of death in pandemic influenza: implications for pandemic influenza preparedness. J Infect Dis 2008;198:962–70.
18. Ampofo K, Gesteland PH, Bender J, et al. Epidemiology, complications, and cost of hospitalization in children with laboratory-confirmed influenza infection. Pediatrics 2006;118:2409–17.

19. Jain S, Benoit SR, Skarbinski J, et al. Influenza-associated pneumonia among hospitalized patients with 2009 pandemic influenza A (H1N1) virus—United States, 2009. Clin Infect Dis 2012;54:1221–9.

20. Lee N, Chan PK, Lui GC, et al. Complications and outcomes of pandemic 2009 influenza A (H1N1) virus infection in hospitalized adults: how do they differ from those in seasonal influenza? J Infect Dis 2011;203:1739–47.

21. Murata Y, Walsh EE, Falsey AR. Pulmonary complications of interpandemic influenza A in hospitalized adults. J Infect Dis 2007;195:1029–37.

22. Louie JK, Acosta M, Winter K, et al. Factors associated with death or hospitalization due to pandemic 2009 influenza A(H1N1) infection in California. JAMA 2009;302:1896–902.

23. Schildgen V, van den Hoogen B, Fouchier R, et al. Human metapneumovirus: lessons learned over the first decade. Clin Microbiol Rev 2011;24:734–54.

24. Falsey AR, Erdman D, Anderson LJ, et al. Human metapneumovirus infections in young and elderly adults. J Infect Dis 2003;187:785–90.

25. Williams JV, Harris PA, Tollefson SJ, et al. Human metapneumovirus and lower respiratory tract disease in otherwise healthy infants and children. N Engl J Med 2004;350:443–50.

26. Foulongne V, Guyon G, Rodiere M, et al. Human metapneumovirus infection in young children hospitalized with respiratory tract disease. Pediatr Infect Dis J 2006;25:354–9.

27. Caracciolo S, Minini C, Colombrita D, et al. Human metapneumovirus infection in young children hospitalized with acute respiratory tract disease: virologic and clinical features. Pediatr Infect Dis J 2008;27:406–12.

28. Falsey AR. Human metapneumovirus infection in adults. Pediatr Infect Dis J 2008;27:S80–3.

29. Walsh EE, Peterson DR, Falsey AR. Human metapneumovirus infections in adults: another piece of the puzzle. Arch Intern Med 2008;168:2489–96.

30. Widmer K, Zhu Y, Williams JV, et al. Rates of hospitalizations for respiratory syncytial virus, human metapneumovirus, and influenza virus in older adults. J Infect Dis 2012;206:56–62.

31. Hamelin ME, Cote S, Laforge J, et al. Human metapneumovirus infection in adults with community-acquired pneumonia and exacerbation of chronic obstructive pulmonary disease. Cin Infect Dis 2005;41:498–502.

32. Hilleman MR, Werner JH. Recovery of new agent from patients with acute respiratory illness. Proc Soc Exp Biol Med 1954;85:183–8.

33. Ison MG. Adenovirus infections in transplant recipients. Clin Infect Dis 2006;43:331–9.

34. Gerber SI, Erdman DD, Pur SL, et al. Outbreak of adenovirus genome type 7d2 infection in a pediatric chronic-care facility and tertiary-care hospital. Clin Infect Dis 2001;32:694–700.

35. Sanchez MP, Erdman DD, Torok TJ, et al. Outbreak of adenovirus 35 pneumonia among adult residents and staff of a chronic care psychiatric facility. J Infect Dis 1997;176:760–3.

36. Gray GC, Goswami PR, Malasig MD, et al. Adult adenovirus infections: loss of orphaned vaccines precipitates military respiratory disease epidemics. For the Adenovirus Surveillance Group. Clin Infect Dis 2000;31:663–70.

37. Dudding BA, Top FH Jr, Winter PE, et al. Acute respiratory disease in military trainees: the adenovirus surveillance program, 1966-1971. Am J Epidemiol 1973;97:187–98.

38. van der Veen J, Oei KG, Abarbanel MF. Patterns of infections with adenovirus types 4, 7 and 21 in military recruits during a 9-year survey. J Hyg (Lond) 1969;67:255–68.

39. Hakim FA, Tleyjeh IM. Severe adenovirus pneumonia in immunocompetent adults: a case report and review of the literature. Eur J Clin Microbiol Infect Dis 2008;27:153–8.
40. Potter RN, Cantrell JA, Mallak CT, et al. Adenovirus-associated deaths in US military during postvaccination period, 1999-2010. Emerg Infect Dis 2012;18: 507–9.
41. Lewis PF, Schmidt MA, Lu X, et al. A community-based outbreak of severe respiratory illness caused by human adenovirus serotype 14. J Infect Dis 2009;199: 1427–34.
42. Metzgar D, Osuna M, Kajon AE, et al. Abrupt emergence of diverse species B adenoviruses at US military recruit training centers. J Infect Dis 2007;196: 1465–73.
43. Henrickson KJ. Parainfluenza viruses. Clin Microbiol Rev 2003;16:242–64.
44. Iwane MK, Edwards KM, Szilagyi PG, et al. Population-based surveillance for hospitalizations associated with respiratory syncytial virus, influenza virus, and parainfluenza viruses among young children. Pediatrics 2004;113:1758–64.
45. Weinberg GA, Hall CB, Iwane MK, et al. Parainfluenza virus infection of young children: estimates of the population-based burden of hospitalization. J Pediatr 2009;154:694–9.
46. Marx A, Gary HE Jr, Marston BJ, et al. Parainfluenza virus infection among adults hospitalized for lower respiratory tract infection. Clin Infect Dis 1999;29: 134–40.
47. Charles PG, Whitby M, Fuller AJ, et al. The etiology of community-acquired pneumonia in Australia: why penicillin plus doxycycline or a macrolide is the most appropriate therapy. Clin Infect Dis 2008;46:1513–21.
48. Templeton KE, Scheltinga SA, van den Eeden WC, et al. Improved diagnosis of the etiology of community-acquired pneumonia with real-time polymerase chain reaction. Clin Infect Dis 2005;41:345–51.
49. Pene F, Merlat A, Vabret A, et al. Coronavirus 229E-related pneumonia in immunocompromised patients. Clin Infect Dis 2003;37:929–32.
50. van der Hoek L, Pyrc K, Jebbink MF, et al. Identification of a new human coronavirus. Nat Med 2004;10:368–73.
51. Woo PC, Lau SK, Chu CM, et al. Characterization and complete genome sequence of a novel coronavirus HKU1 from patients with pneumonia. J Virol 2005;79:884–95.
52. Gaunt ER, Hardie A, Claas EC, et al. Epidemiology and clinical presentations of the four human coronaviruses 229E, HKU1, NL63, and OC43 detected over 3 years using a novel multiplex real-time PCR method. J Clin Microbiol 2010; 48:2940–7.
53. Kuypers J, Martin ET, Heugel J, et al. Clinical disease in children associated with newly described coronavirus subtypes. Pediatrics 2007;119:e70–6.
54. van der Hoek L, Ihorst G, Sure K, et al. Burden of disease due to human coronavirus NL63 infections and periodicity of infection. J Clin Virol 2010;48:104–8.
55. Dare RK, Fry AM, Chittaganpitch M, et al. Human coronavirus infections in rural Thailand: a comprehensive study using real-time reverse-transcription polymerase chain reaction assays. J Infect Dis 2007;196:1321–8.
56. Garbino J, Crespo S, Aubert JD, et al. A prospective hospital-based study of the clinical impact of non-severe acute respiratory syndrome (non-SARS)-related human coronavirus infection. Clin Infect Dis 2006;43:1009–15.
57. Mackay IM. Human rhinoviruses: the cold wars resume. J Clin Virol 2008;42: 297–320.

58. Arden KE, Mackay IM. Newly identified human rhinoviruses: molecular methods heat up the cold viruses. Rev Med Virol 2010;20:156–76.
59. Papadopoulos NG, Sanderson G, Hunter J, et al. Rhinoviruses replicate effectively at lower airway temperatures. J Med Virol 1999;58:100–4.
60. Papadopoulos NG, Bates PJ, Bardin PG, et al. Rhinoviruses infect the lower airways. J Infect Dis 2000;181:1875–84.
61. Kennedy JL, Turner RB, Braciale T, et al. Pathogenesis of rhinovirus infection. Curr Opin Virol 2012;2:287–93.
62. Falsey AR, Walsh EE, Hayden FG. Rhinovirus and coronavirus infection-associated hospitalizations among older adults. J Infect Dis 2002;185:1338–41.
63. Cheuk DK, Tang IW, Chan KH, et al. Rhinovirus infection in hospitalized children in Hong Kong: a prospective study. Pediatr Infect Dis J 2007;26:995–1000.
64. Miller EK, Lu X, Erdman DD, et al. Rhinovirus-associated hospitalizations in young children. J Infect Dis 2007;195:773–81.
65. Louie JK, Roy-Burman A, Guardia-Labar L, et al. Rhinovirus associated with severe lower respiratory tract infections in children. Pediatr Infect Dis J 2009;28:337–9.
66. Cevey-Macherel M, Galetto-Lacour A, Gervaix A, et al. Etiology of community-acquired pneumonia in hospitalized children based on WHO clinical guidelines. Eur J Pediatr 2009;168:1429–36.
67. Jain S, Ampofo K, Arnold SR, et al. Etiology of community-acquired pneumonia among hospitalized children in the United States: preliminary data from the CDC Etiology of Pneumonia in the Community (EPIC) study. Presented at the Infectious Diseases Society of America 49th Annual Meeting. Boston, October 20–23, 2011. Abstract 168.
68. Juven T, Mertsola J, Waris M, et al. Etiology of community-acquired pneumonia in 254 hospitalized children. Pediatr Infect Dis J 2000;19:293–8.
69. Michelow IC, Olsen K, Lozano J, et al. Epidemiology and clinical characteristics of community-acquired pneumonia in hospitalized children. Pediatrics 2004; 113:701–7.
70. Tsolia MN, Psarras S, Bossios A, et al. Etiology of community-acquired pneumonia in hospitalized school-age children: evidence for high prevalence of viral infections. Clin Infect Dis 2004;39:681–6.
71. Allander T. Human bocavirus. J Clin Virol 2008;41:29–33.
72. Brieu N, Guyon G, Rodiere M, et al. Human bocavirus infection in children with respiratory tract disease. Pediatr Infect Dis J 2008;27:969–73.
73. Fry AM, Lu X, Chittaganpitch M, et al. Human bocavirus: a novel parvovirus epidemiologically associated with pneumonia requiring hospitalization in Thailand. J Infect Dis 2007;195:1038–45.
74. Christensen A, Nordbo SA, Krokstad S, et al. Human bocavirus in children: mono-detection, high viral load and viraemia are associated with respiratory tract infection. J Clin Virol 2010;49:158–62.
75. Harvala H, Wolthers KC, Simmonds P. Parechoviruses in children: understanding a new infection. Curr Opin Infect Dis 2010;23:224–30.
76. Abed Y, Boivin G. Human parechovirus types 1, 2 and 3 infections in Canada. Emerg Infect Dis 2006;12:969–75.
77. McCracken GH. Diagnosis and management of pneumonia in children. Pediatr Infect Dis J 2000;19:924–8.
78. Garcia-Garcia ML, Calvo C, Pozo F, et al. Spectrum of respiratory viruses in children with community-acquired pneumonia. Pediatr Infect Dis J 2012;31:808–13.
79. Pilishvili T, Lexau C, Farley MM, et al. Sustained reductions in invasive pneumococcal disease in the era of conjugate vaccine. J Infect Dis 2010;201:32–41.

80. Ampofo K, Pavia AT, Stockmann CR, et al. Evolution of the epidemiology of pneumococcal disease among Utah children through the vaccine era. Pediatr Infect Dis J 2011;30:1100–3.
81. Falsey AR, Walsh EE. Viral pneumonia in older adults. Clin Infect Dis 2006;42: 518–24.
82. Rice TW, Rubinson L, Uyeki TM, et al. Critical illness from 2009 pandemic influenza A virus and bacterial coinfection in the United States. Crit Care Med 2012; 40:1487–98.
83. Ampofo K, Bender J, Sheng X, et al. Seasonal invasive pneumococcal disease in children: role of preceding respiratory viral infection. Pediatrics 2008;122: 229–37.
84. Talbot TR, Poehling KA, Hartert TV, et al. Seasonality of invasive pneumococcal disease: temporal relation to documented influenza and respiratory syncytial viral circulation. Am J Med 2005;118:285–91.
85. Johansson N, Kalin M, Hedlund J. Clinical impact of combined viral and bacterial infection in patients with community-acquired pneumonia. Scand J Infect Dis 2011;43:609–15.
86. Ruuskanen O, Lahti E, Jennings LC, et al. Viral pneumonia. Lancet 2011;377: 1264–75.
87. Virkki R, Juven T, Rikalainen H, et al. Differentiation of bacterial and viral pneumonia in children. Thorax 2002;57:438–41.
88. File TM Jr. New diagnostic tests for pneumonia: what is their role in clinical practice? Clin Chest Med 2011;32:417–30.
89. Nascimento-Carvalho CM, Cardoso MR, Barral A, et al. Procalcitonin is useful in identifying bacteraemia among children with pneumonia. Scand J Infect Dis 2010;42:644–9.
90. Toikka P, Irjala K, Juven T, et al. Serum procalcitonin, C-reactive protein and interleukin-6 for distinguishing bacterial and viral pneumonia in children. Pediatr Infect Dis J 2000;19:598–602.
91. Gilbert DN. Use of plasma procalcitonin levels as an adjunct to clinical microbiology. J Clin Microbiol 2010;48:2325–9.
92. Gilbert DN. Procalcitonin as a biomarker in respiratory tract infection. Clin Infect Dis 2011;52(Suppl 4):S346–50.
93. Schuetz P, Briel M, Christ-Crain M, et al. Procalcitonin to guide initiation and duration of antibiotic treatment in acute respiratory infections: an individual patient data meta-analysis. Clin Infect Dis 2012;55:651–62.
94. Franquet T. Imaging of pulmonary viral pneumonia. Radiology 2011;260:18–39.
95. Guo W, Wang J, Sheng M, et al. Radiological findings in 210 paediatric patients with viral pneumonia: a retrospective case study. Br J Radiol 2012;85(1018):1385–9.
96. Fiore AE, Fry A, Shay D, et al. Antiviral agents for the treatment and chemoprophylaxis of influenza: recommendations of the Advisory Committee on Immunization Practices (ACIP). MMWR Recomm Rep 2011;60:1–24.
97. Hayden FG, Pavia AT. Antiviral management of seasonal and pandemic influenza. J Infect Dis 2006;194(Suppl 2):S119–26.
98. Kaiser L, Wat C, Mills T. Impact of oseltamivir treatment on influenza-related lower respiratory tract complications and hospitalizations. Arch Intern Med 2003;163: 1667.
99. Lee N, Chan PK, Hui DS, et al. Viral loads and duration of viral shedding in adult patients hospitalized with influenza. J Infect Dis 2009;200:492–500.
100. McGeer A, Green KA, Plevneshi A, et al. Antiviral therapy and outcomes of influenza requiring hospitalization in Ontario, Canada. Clin Infect Dis 2007;45:1568–75.

101. Lee N, Choi KW, Chan PK, et al. Outcomes of adults hospitalised with severe influenza. Thorax 2010;65:510–5.
102. Jain S, Kamimoto L, Bramley AM, et al. Hospitalized patients with 2009 H1N1 influenza in the United States, April-June 2009. N Engl J Med 2009;361: 1935–44.
103. Bautista E, Chotpitayasunondh T, Gao Z, et al. Clinical aspects of pandemic 2009 influenza A (H1N1) virus infection. N Engl J Med 2010;362:1708–19.
104. Siston AM, Rasmussen SA, Honein MA, et al. Pandemic 2009 influenza A(H1N1) virus illness among pregnant women in the United States. JAMA 2010;303: 1517–25.
105. Yu H, Feng Z, Uyeki TM, et al. Risk factors for severe illness with 2009 pandemic influenza A (H1N1) virus infection in China. Clin Infect Dis 2011;52:457–65.
106. Yang SG, Cao B, Liang LR, et al. Antiviral therapy and outcomes of patients with pneumonia caused by influenza A pandemic (H1N1) virus. PLoS One 2012;7: e29652.
107. Louie JK, Yang S, Acosta M, et al. Treatment With neuraminidase inhibitors for critically ill patients with Influenza A (H1N1) pdm09. Clin Infect Dis 2012; 55(9):1198–204.
108. Eriksson CO, Graham DA, Uyeki TM, et al. Risk factors for mechanical ventilation in U.S. children hospitalized with seasonal influenza and 2009 pandemic influenza A. Pediatr Crit Care Med 2012;13(6):625–31.
109. Kumar A, Zarychanski R, Pinto R, et al. Critically ill patients with 2009 influenza A (H1N1) infection in Canada. JAMA 2009;302:1872–9.
110. Hsu J, Santesso N, Mustafa R, et al. Antivirals for treatment of influenza: a systematic review and meta-analysis of observational studies. Ann Intern Med 2012;156(7):512–24.
111. Randolph AG, Vaughn F, Sullivan R, et al. Critically ill children during the 2009-2010 influenza pandemic in the United States. Pediatrics 2011;128:e1450–8.
112. Harper SA, Bradley JS, Englund JA, et al. Seasonal influenza in adults and children. Diagnosis, treatment, chemoprophylaxis, and institutional outbreak management: clinical practice guidelines of the Infectious Diseases Society of America. Clin Infect Dis 2009;48:1003–32.
113. Ginocchio CC, Zhang F, Manji R, et al. Evaluation of multiple test methods for the detection of the novel 2009 influenza A (H1N1) during the New York City outbreak. J Clin Virol 2009;45:191–5.
114. Uyeki TM, Prasad R, Vukotich C, et al. Low sensitivity of rapid diagnostic test for influenza. Clin Infect Dis 2009;48:e89–92.
115. Dharan NJ, Gubareva LV, Meyer JJ, et al. Infections with oseltamivir-resistant influenza A (H1N1) virus in the United States. JAMA 2009;301:1034–41.
116. Moscona A. Global transmission of oseltamivir-resistant influenza. N Engl J Med 2009;360:953–6.
117. Fry AM, Gubareva LV. Understanding influenza virus resistance to antiviral agents: early warning signs for wider community circulation. J Infect Dis 2012; 206:145–7.
118. Hayden FG, de Jong MD. Emerging influenza antiviral resistance threats. J Infect Dis 2011;203:6–10.
119. Hurt AC, Hardie K, Wilson NJ, et al. Characteristics of a widespread community cluster of H275Y oseltamivir-resistant A (H1N1) pdm09 influenza in Australia. J Infect Dis 2012;206:148–57.
120. Krilov LR. Respiratory syncytial virus disease: update on treatment and prevention. Expert Rev Anti Infect Ther 2011;9:27–32.

121. Boeckh M, Englund J, Li Y, et al. Randomized controlled multicenter trial of aero-solized ribavirin for respiratory syncytial virus upper respiratory tract infection in hematopoietic cell transplant recipients. Clin Infect Dis 2007;44:245–9.
122. Ventre K, Randolph AG. Ribavirin for respiratory syncytial virus infection of the lower respiratory tract in infants and young children. Cochrane Database Syst Rev 2007;(1):CD000181.
123. Shachor-Meyouhas Y, Ben-Barak A, Kassis I. Treatment with oral ribavirin and IVIG of severe human metapneumovirus pneumonia (HMPV) in immune compromised child. Pediatr Blood Cancer 2011;57:350–1.
124. Refaat M, McNamara D, Teuteberg J, et al. Successful cidofovir treatment in an adult heart transplant recipient with severe adenovirus pneumonia. J Heart Lung Transplant 2008;27:699–700.
125. Doan ML, Mallory GB, Kaplan SL, et al. Treatment of adenovirus pneumonia with cidofovir in pediatric lung transplant recipients. J Heart Lung Transplant 2007; 26:883–9.
126. Darr S, Madisch I, Heim A. Antiviral activity of cidofovir and ribavirin against the new human adenovirus subtype 14a that is associated with severe pneumonia. Clin Infect Dis 2008;47:731–2.
127. Toth K, Spencer JF, Dhar D, et al. Hexadecyloxypropyl-cidofovir, CMX001, prevents adenovirus-induced mortality in a permissive, immunosuppressed animal model. Proc Natl Acad Sci U S A 2008;105:7293–7.
128. Hayden FG, Herrington DT, Coats TL, et al. Efficacy and safety of oral pleconaril for treatment of colds due to picornaviruses in adults: results of 2 double-blind, randomized, placebo-controlled trials. Clin Infect Dis 2003;36:1523–32.
129. DeVincenzo JP, El Saleeby CM, Bush AJ. Respiratory syncytial virus load predicts disease severity in previously healthy infants. J Infect Dis 2005;191: 1861–8.
130. Fodha I, Vabret A, Ghedira L, et al. Respiratory syncytial virus infections in hospitalized infants: association between viral load, virus subgroup, and disease severity. J Med Virol 2007;79:1951–8.
131. Gerna G, Piralla A, Rovida F, et al. Correlation of rhinovirus load in the respiratory tract and clinical symptoms in hospitalized immunocompetent and immunocom-promised patients. J Med Virol 2009;81:1498–507.
132. Martin ET, Kuypers J, Heugel J, et al. Clinical disease and viral load in children infected with respiratory syncytial virus or human metapneumovirus. Diagn Microbiol Infect Dis 2008;62:382–8.
133. Bradley JS, Byington CL, Shah SS, et al. The management of community-acquired pneumonia in infants and children older than 3 months of age: clinical practice guidelines by the Pediatric Infectious Diseases Society and the Infec-tious Diseases Society of America. Clin Infect Dis 2011;53:e25–76.
134. Mandell LA, Wunderink RG, Anzueto A, et al. Infectious Diseases Society of America/American Thoracic Society consensus guidelines on the management of community-acquired pneumonia in adults. Clin Infect Dis 2007;44(Suppl 2): S27–72.
135. Abed Y, Boivin G. Treatment of respiratory virus infections. Antiviral Res 2006; 70:1–16.
136. Nichols WG, Peck Campbell AJ, Boeckh M. Respiratory viruses other than influ-enza virus: impact and therapeutic advances. Clin Microbiol Rev 2008;21: 274–90.

How Important is Methicillin-Resistant *Staphylococcus aureus* as a Cause of Community-Acquired Pneumonia and What is Best Antimicrobial Therapy?

Richard G. Wunderink, MD

KEYWORDS

- Methicillin resistance • Exotoxins • Linezolid • Vancomycin
- Community-acquired MRSA • Pneumonia • Panton-Valentine leukocidin
- *Staphylococcus aureus*

KEY POINTS

- Two relative distinct types of methicillin-resistant *Staphylococcus aureus* (MRSA) pneumonia occur in patients with community-acquired pneumonia (CAP): traditional hospital-acquired strains in patients with health care–associated pneumonia risk factors, and a true community-acquired strain associated with exotoxin production.
- Despite a low frequency, community-acquired MRSA (CA-MRSA) is an important cause of CAP because of the high mortality if not suspected early, and its occurrence in young patients with long life expectancy.
- Linezolid suppresses exotoxin production in in vitro models, which may be important in CA-MRSA CAP.
- The consistent trend toward better outcomes for documented MRSA pneumonia suggests that linezolid should be considered the drug of choice for documented MRSA CAP, especially CA-MRSA.
- For suspected but undocumented MRSA, empiric vancomycin does not appear to be inferior to linezolid.

This article addresses 2 sequential questions: (1) How important is methicillin-resistant *Staphylococcus aureus* (MRSA) as a pathogen in community-acquired pneumonia (CAP)? (2) If MRSA is an important pathogen, what is the optimal antimicrobial treatment? Each of these questions is addressed separately.

Pulmonary and Critical Care Division, Northwestern University Feinberg School of Medicine, 676 North Saint Clair Street, Arkes 14-044, Chicago, IL 60611, USA
E-mail address: r-wunderink@northwestern.edu

Infect Dis Clin N Am 27 (2013) 177–188
http://dx.doi.org/10.1016/j.idc.2012.11.006
0891-5520/13/$ – see front matter © 2013 Elsevier Inc. All rights reserved.

id.theclinics.com

HOW IMPORTANT IS MRSA AS A CAUSE OF CAP?
Introduction

S aureus has always been an important cause of CAP, in many series being second only to the pneumococci. The importance of S aureus was clearly recognized during the 1918 Influenza A pandemic when a significant number of deaths were found to be caused by this pathogen. S aureus quickly developed resistance to penicillin after the introduction of this antibiotic into clinical practice in the 1940s.[1] Semisynthetic penicillins, such as methicillin, oxacillin, and nafcillin, and first-generation cephalosporins temporarily addressed the issue of antibiotic resistance. However, beginning in 1960s, case reports of methicillin resistance in hospital-acquired strains began to appear, and their frequency rapidly increased to become endemic in the 1980s.[2] Extensive use of penicillin and cephalosporin antibiotics continued to drive selection for resistance until many hospitals began reporting that 50% or more of their S aureus isolates from many sites of infection were now resistant to the marker drug, methicillin.

Once the rate of hospital S aureus isolates that were methicillin resistant exceeded 50%, case reports of MRSA pneumonia in patients who presented to the hospital with a new pneumonia began to appear. Many of these patients had previously been hospitalized or exposed to the health care system, and would currently be classified as having health care–associated pneumonia (HCAP),[3] or had specific high-risk factors such as intravenous drug abuse. These isolates typically had an antibiotic resistance pattern identical to that of hospital-acquired strains.

However, several seminal articles beginning in the early 2000s noted a highly lethal form of S aureus CAP in previously healthy, typically younger patients, some but not all of which were methicillin resistant.[4–6] Isolates in all of these highly lethal cases also carried the gene for the Panton-Valentine leukocidin (PVL) exotoxin.[5] As more cases were discovered worldwide, it became apparent that this methicillin resistance occurred against the background of strains traditionally occurring as CAP, including the USA300 and USA400 clones. A parallel marked increase in skin and soft-tissue infections with the same community-acquired MRSA (CA-MRSA) strains[7] generated tremendous concern regarding the potential increase in mortality from CAP, particularly because of an association with influenza.

A key concept in this discussion is that two relatively distinct types of MRSA pneumonia occur in patients with community-onset pneumonia. The first is due to MRSA strains traditionally causing hospital-acquired pneumonia (HAP) that now occur in patients with frequent and/or recent contact with the health care system and now classified as HCAP.[3] The second is the emergence of methicillin resistance against the background of strains long known to cause CAP and frequently capable of exotoxin production. The latter is referred to as CA-MRSA for the remainder of this article. Key distinguishing characteristics of the 2 strains are listed in **Table 1**.

Evidence that MRSA is NOT an Important Pathogen in CAP

The actual incidence of CA-MRSA CAP is fairly low. An early survey by the Centers for Disease Control and Prevention (CDC) through its Emerging Infections Network found only 51 cases from 19 states during the 2006 to 2007 influenza season.[8] Retrospective review of cases from a single United States center found only 13 cases in 18 months, fewer than 1% of patients with a discharge diagnosis of pneumonia.[9] A similar audit from a single Australian hospital identified only 16 patients older than 7.5 years.[10]

The best estimate of population-based incidence is from the prospective CDC Etiology of Pneumonia in the Community (EPIC) study, which found that only 2% to 3% of adult cases were caused by S aureus, with approximately half being MRSA.[11]

Table 1
Distinguishing characteristics of MRSA strains

	Community-Acquired (CA-MRSA)	Health Care–Associated (HCAP)
Common PFGE pattern	USA300, USA400	USA100, USA200
SCCmec type	IV, V	I, II, III
Vancomycin MIC	Usually <1 μg/mL	Often ≥1 μg/mL
Clindamycin, TMP/sulfa sensitivity	Common	Rare
PVL toxin production	Common	Rare
Other exotoxin production	Common	Rare

Abbreviations: MIC, minimum inhibitory concentration; PFGE, pulse-field gel electrophoresis; PVL, Panton-Valentine leukocidin; SCCmec, staphylococcal cassette chromosome mec gene; TMP, trimethoprim.

Because of the aggressive nature of CA-MRSA strains, gross underestimation of incidence owing to inadequate diagnoses is unlikely. A preliminary thought that the majority of these patients would be admitted to the intensive care unit (ICU)[12] was not confirmed in subsequent case series,[9,10] with approximately half of cases never admitted to the ICU, leaving open the possibility that a few cases may be missed.

Evidence that MRSA IS an Important Pathogen in CAP

The strongest evidence for the role of MRSA in CAP comes from studies of HCAP. In culture-positive cases, the incidence of MRSA in patients who meet criteria for HCAP actually exceeds that of ventilator-acquired pneumonia (VAP) (**Fig. 1**).[13,14] Many of

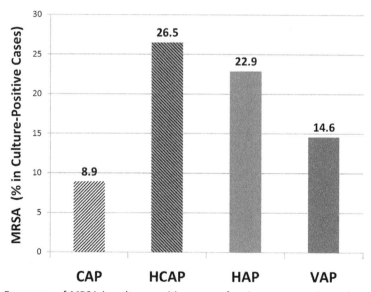

Fig. 1. Frequency of MRSA in culture-positive cases of various pneumonia syndromes. CAP, community-acquired pneumonia; HAP, hospital-acquired pneumonia (non-VAP); HCAP, health care–associated pneumonia; VAP, ventilator-associated pneumonia. (*Data from* Kollef MH, Shorr A, Tabak YP, et al. Epidemiology and outcomes of health-care-associated pneumonia: results from a large US database of culture-positive pneumonia. Chest 2005;128(6):3854–62).

these patients have been recently hospitalized and are likely to have become colonized while admitted, particularly if they have received broad-spectrum antibiotics during hospitalization. Some of the less common HCAP risk factors,[3] chronic hemodialysis, home wound care, or antibiotic infusion therapy, are more likely to select for MRSA than for other multidrug-resistant (MDR) pathogens such as *Pseudomonas* or *Acinetobacter*. However, these studies are biased owing to selection by culture positivity.[15] Prospective studies have demonstrated that the culture-positive rate for HCAP is less than 10%.[16] Even though MRSA is documented more often than typical CAP pathogens as the causative pathogen in HCAP patients, the overall rate of MRSA is 3% or less.[16,17] The main difference between *S. aureus* CAP in patients with risk factors for HCAP is that methicillin resistance is extremely high in HCAP cases, whereas 50% or more of *S. aureus* CAP without HCAP risk factors are still methicillin-sensitive *S. aureus* (MSSA). Although cases with HCAP risk factors are probably the most common cause of CAP with MRSA, true community-acquired cases appear to be increasing, whereas HCAP MRSA may be decreasing.[18]

Most cases of CAP result from aspiration of bacteria colonizing the oropharynx, including *S. aureus*.[19] The oropharynx is remarkably stable in most people, with the major disruption being associated with antibiotic therapy. However, vaccination also appears to alter the normal flora of the oropharynx and upper respiratory tract. Routine use of the highly effective conjugate pneumococcal vaccine appears to not only prevent infection but also decrease colonization. However, this may result in opportunities for other pathogens to replace the pneumococci. An increase in *S. aureus* colonization, and possibly infection, has been associated with use of the new conjugate vaccine.[20] As the vaccine expands to 13 serotypes and is released for use in adults, the incidence of *S. aureus* infections of the respiratory tract may correspondingly increase.

The incidence of CA-MRSA may also vary from year to year based on its association with influenza. The CDC EPIC study took place in the post-2009 H1N1 Influenza A pandemic, and the actual incidence of influenza was also very low in that study.[11] The ARDS Network Centers prospectively and retrospectively determined bacterial coinfections associated with critically ill patients during the 2009 H1N1 Influenza A pandemic.[21] *S. aureus* was more common than the pneumococci in these centers, with the majority being MRSA. Bacterial coinfection was associated with more shock and respiratory failure, prolonged duration of mechanical ventilation, and worse mortality. The study from the ARDS Network illustrates the possibility that the importance of MRSA CAP may be out of proportion to incidence. In the setting of influenza, CA-MRSA is associated with high mortality and affects otherwise healthy people,[22] raising greater concern and, therefore, a greater tendency to cover for this pathogen empirically.

Interpretation of Evidence

CA-MRSA as a cause of CAP has generated fear and concern out of proportion to its current status. Concern regarding CA-MRSA is based more on the case fatality rate of early case series[5,6,8,23] rather than the actual incidence, which is generally overestimated. The other factor driving disproportionate concern is that CA-MRSA CAP occurred in young patients who were immunocompetent. Despite its low frequency, CA-MRSA is an important cause of CAP, mainly because of the high mortality if not suspected early and the occurrence in younger patients with long life expectancy.

MRSA is an important concern in patients with HCAP risk factors, but once again the risk is overestimated. The main concern for coverage should be those who are critically ill, particularly those who develop respiratory failure. The greater the number of risk factors for HCAP, the greater the probability of MRSA.

Recommendations Based on Present Evidence

CA-MRSA coverage for all cases of likely bacterial CAP is unreasonable. Therefore, aggressive diagnosis combined with high clinical suspicion may be sufficient to avoid empiric MRSA coverage in the majority of patients with CAP.

Risk factors that should increase the suspicion of CA-MRSA are listed in **Table 2**. Cavitary or necrotizing CAP is very rare for other causes of CAP. The main differential diagnoses are tuberculosis in endemic countries and anaerobic pleuropneumonia. The latter can be differentiated by the foul-smelling sputum, gingivitis, and a history of loss of consciousness with risk of aspiration in the prior weeks to months. Acute aspiration does not usually result in necrotic pneumonia. A rapidly increasing pleural effusion can also be seen in β-hemolytic streptococcal pneumonia and even pneumo-coccal pneumonia. The gross hemoptysis seen in CA-MRSA CAP[23] is fairly unique among CAP pathogens, and is readily distinguished from the blood-streaked sputum occasionally seen in pneumococcal or gram-negative pneumonias. Neutropenia likely results from the PVL toxin[23] but is also rarely seen with pneumococcal, *Acinetobacter*, and other gram-negative bacterial pathogens. *S. aureus* in general appears to be significantly increased when the patient is still actively infected with influenza.[8,21] Therefore, the suspicion for CA-MRSA should increase during the peak influenza season. Conversely, CA-MRSA infections do not have a seasonal change in frequency[9,24] as CAP in general, as well as *Streptococcus pneumoniae*, appear to have. A serious pneumonia in the summer months with any of the other features should alert the clinician to possible CA-MRSA. Concurrent erythematous rash also suggests toxin-producing bacteria.[23] Prior conjugate pneumococcal vaccine, espe-cially with the expanded 13-valent vaccine, markedly decreases the likelihood of the main alternative pathogen for most of these conditions, and therefore increases the probability of CA-MRSA. Changes in the microbiome in response to this highly effective vaccination may also predispose to CA-MRSA. Simple admission to the ICU does not increase the probability of CA-MRSA sufficiently enough to warrant CA-MRSA in all cases.

Fortunately, CA-MRSA is usually easy to culture from almost any available site, and bacteremia rates are high. Even expectorated sputum can be used for diagnosis. A tracheal aspirate or bronchoalveolar lavage in an intubated patient is unlikely to not grow the pathogen, and a Gram stain is often grossly positive. Pleural fluid is another high-yield culture material. Therefore, although the indications for empiric coverage for CA-MRSA remain poorly validated, the high yield of cultures should allow safe discon-tinuation of empiric therapy in culture-negative cases.

Increasing evidence suggests that routine coverage of MDR pathogens, including MRSA, for patients with HCAP risk factors is associated with worse outcomes.[17,25] Refining HCAP to avoid routine MRSA coverage while still identifying truly high-risk patients remains controversial.[3,26] Because the main concern is critically ill, particularly intubated patients, ready access to highly diagnostic culture material can help

Table 2	
Clinical features to suggest increased risk of CA-MRSA pneumonia	
Cavitary pneumonia	Concurrent influenza
Lung necrosis in pneumonic infiltrate	Erythematous skin rash
Rapidly increasing pleural effusion	Previously healthy
Gross hemoptysis	Summer season
Neutropenia	Prior conjugate pneumococcal vaccination

significantly to avoid prolonged courses of specific MRSA treatment. Prior MRSA infections and/or documented MRSA nasal colonization may increase the probability of MRSA pneumonia for nonintubated ICU patients. Nasal MRSA colonization can be persistent and refractory to decolonization efforts, leaving the patient at risk for MRSA pneumonia.

Future Studies

The risk factors for CA-MRSA listed in **Table 2** are derived from the literature on CA-MRSA but have never been prospectively validated, particularly as a group. Given the poor ability to diagnose the cause in many cases of CAP, a randomized controlled study demonstrating improved clinical outcomes with empiric MRSA coverage in addition to standard CAP antibiotics in patients with CA-MRSA risk factors will be needed for true validation. However, the current incidence of CA-MRSA is still too low to make this feasible.

Conversely, reassessment of HCAP risk factors to select for patients at high risk for MRSA is clearly needed.[26] These risk factors are likely to be very different to those for CA-MRSA, and may be different to those for gram-negative MDR pathogens. The value of nasal screening for patients with HCAP risk factors to predict the cause of pneumonia has also not been fully explored.[27] Overuse of anti-MRSA drugs in patients with HCAP is driven by the inadequacies of culture-based diagnosis in patients who are not intubated. Alternative diagnostic tests are clearly needed.

Although the incidence of MRSA infections appears to be decreasing overall in response to better hand hygiene and other infection-control measures, the incidence of CA-MRSA infections appears to be slowly increasing.[18] Continued epidemiologic studies are therefore needed to inform empiric antibiotic recommendations.

Summary

MRSA clearly is an important pathogen in CAP. While currently causing a relatively low percentage of CAP cases, the disproportionate frequency of otherwise healthy young people with this infection drives concern and therefore empiric antibiotic therapy. **Table 2** suggests criteria to be more selective in empiric antibiotic coverage. Conversely, empiric coverage of MRSA, though very important in culture-positive HCAP, is currently excessive, and better criteria to define true risk factors can hopefully decrease the use of antibiotics directed at MRSA.

WHAT IS THE BEST ANTIMICROBIAL THERAPY FOR MRSA CAP?
Introduction

The antibiotic armamentarium to treat MRSA pneumonia is limited (**Table 3**). Quinupristin/dalfopristin (Synercid) was demonstrated to be inferior to vancomycin in patients with HAP/VAP.[28] Daptomycin has been found to be inactivated by surfactant and is therefore inappropriate for the treatment of pneumonia.[29] Clindamycin and trimethoprim/sulfamethoxazole have been used for treatment of CA-MRSA skin

Table 3
Antibiotics active against MRSA

Appropriate for Pneumonia	Unclear Pneumonia Activity	Inappropriate for Pneumonia
Linezolid	Clindamycin	Quinupristin/dalfopristin
Vancomycin	Trimethoprim/sulfamethoxazole	Daptomycin
Ceftaroline	Moxifloxacin	

infections, but substantial concern exists regarding their use as monotherapy for pneumonia. Although moxifloxacin has enhanced activity against MSSA in comparison with other fluoroquinolones, emergence of resistance when used for MRSA suggests that the fluoroquinolone class is unreliable as monotherapy. Therefore, these antibiotics should not be considered as usual treatment options for MRSA CAP. Although ceftaroline is listed as appropriate for treatment based on the study of CAP,[30] support for its use is based on activity in other MRSA infections and in vitro minimal inhibitory concentration (MIC) testing. Therefore, the controversy on treatment is whether linezolid is superior to vancomycin.

Because exotoxin production seems to play a significant role in the outcome of CA-MRSA CAP, the role of antibiotics in inducing or suppressing exotoxin production is critical in this infection. Lack of specific clinical trials on CA-MRSA limit the ability to assess this relationship, and most data are extrapolated from in vitro testing.

Evidence that Linezolid IS the Optimal Therapy for MRSA CAP

The strongest evidence for the superiority of linezolid over vancomycin for MRSA pneumonia comes from the recently published ZEPHYR trial, which was a head-to-head comparison of linezolid with adjusted-dose vancomycin.[31] Linezolid was found to be superior in clinical response rates (57.6% vs 46.6%, 95% confidence interval of the difference 0.5%–21.6%, $P<.05$) in the per-protocol population at the end of study, the a priori primary end point. Similar tends were seen in other subpopulations and in microbiologic end points. The only significant differences in toxicity were an increased rate of nephrotoxicity with vancomycin (7.3% vs 3.7% for linezolid). MRSA HCAP was included in this study.

This study confirms the results of subgroup analysis of the MRSA cases in two phase 3 clinical trials used for linezolid registration[32–35] and smaller head-to-head comparisons.[36] In addition to being a head-to-head comparison, the ZEPHYR trial also allowed adjusted-dose vancomycin, a major limitation of the prior studies.

Because neither linezolid nor vancomycin is rapidly bactericidal, ongoing exotoxin production by remaining viable CA-MRSA bacteria is possible. In vitro work has demonstrated that linezolid and clindamycin suppress PVL, hemolysins, autolysins, toxic shock syndrome toxin 1, and enterotoxin production,[37–39] consistent with their known mechanism of action of inhibiting bacterial ribosomal synthesis of proteins. In these same studies and consistent with its activity in inhibiting cell-wall synthesis, vancomycin had no effect on exotoxin production. Based on this ex vivo work, linezolid would seem to be preferable to vancomycin specifically for CA-MRSA pneumonias, although the addition of clindamycin to vancomycin may have an equivalent effect.

Evidence that Linezolid is NOT the Optimal Therapy for MRSA CAP

The greatest advantages of vancomycin over linezolid are cost and familiarity. In studies of suspected gram-positive pneumonia, the clinical response rates for vancomycin were equivalent to those of linezolid.[33,34] Previously healthy critically injured patients may be adequately treated with a high dose (up to 4.5 g/d) of vancomycin,[40] although 40% of patients still required the switch to linezolid. The ZEPHYR study did not demonstrate a mortality benefit for linezolid, despite the differences in clinical response rates.[31]

Because only 10% to 30% of patients with suspected MRSA pneumonia can be documented to actually have the pathogen,[31,35] routine use of linezolid in these patients will be extremely costly, with marginal clinical differences. In addition, increasing the use of linezolid will inevitably lead to an increasing resistance to linezolid, potentially compromising its use for vancomycin failures or infections with vancomycin-resistant bacteria such as *Enterococcus.*

One of the limitations of vancomycin is the penetration into alveolar space. Optimization of pharmacokinetics may therefore enhance vancomycin efficacy. Vancomycin may be adequate in MRSA infections caused by isolates with low MICs.[22,41] However, the MIC would likely need to be less than 1 μg/mL because most of the isolates in the ZEPHYR study had MICs of 1 μg/mL.[31] Enhanced activity by individualization of dosing to target a trough level of 15 mg/L[12] has not been clearly demonstrated to be of value, and may lead to increased nephrotoxicity.[31,42] Vancomycin activity may be enhanced by combination therapy such as the addition of rifampin[43] or by use of clindamycin for suppression of toxin production.[9]

Interpretation of Evidence

Although the superiority of linezolid over vancomycin had been questioned before the ZEPHYR trial,[31] no study of MRSA pneumonia demonstrates a clinical, microbiologic, or other relevant outcome, such as mortality or length of stay, that was superior for vancomycin in comparison with linezolid.[44] The lack of mortality benefit in the ZEPHYR trial most likely results from either the benefit of adjusted-dose vancomycin or salvage therapy with linezolid for failures in the vancomycin arm, an option that did not exist in the phase 3 trials. The consistently inferior results with vancomycin and clear nephrotoxicity raise concern that vancomycin would not even be given an indication of approval by the Food and Drug Administration for pneumonia treatment if it had not been grandfathered in as the only viable agent for MRSA infection in the past. Although no study specifically addresses the benefit of toxin suppression in CA-MRSA pneumonia, the *in vitro* work also suggests superiority of linezolid over vancomycin.

Recommendations Based on Present Evidence

The consistent trend toward better outcome for documented MRSA pneumonia suggests that linezolid should be considered the drug of choice for MRSA CAP. The cost of linezolid is likely to decrease as it goes off patent and becomes available as a generic drug. Conversely, the consistency in the quality of generic vancomycin has also raised concerns about increasing toxicity in clinical use compared with clinical trials, in which the name brand must be used as the comparator.

The major issue is suspected but undocumented MRSA. In this situation, empiric vancomycin does not appear to be inferior to linezolid. However, no study has specifically studied patients at high risk for MRSA, specifically CA-MRSA (see **Table 2**).

Once again, lack of accurate diagnostic tests for MRSA pneumonia is the major limitation for treatment recommendations. The concern about increasing linezolid resistance with indiscriminate use revolves around empiric rather than pathogen-specific therapy. Greater effort to clearly identify true MRSA pneumonias and minimize empiric antibiotic therapy is a more logical strategy to preserve linezolid sensitivity while more effectively treating true MRSA pneumonia, rather than to encourage continued empiric vancomycin use.

Future Studies

MSSA strains also produce exotoxins. The reason exotoxin production does not appear to be as significant is that MSSA is usually treated with cell-wall active antibiotics, particularly β-lactams, which are rapidly bactericidal. A cephalosporin with MRSA activity may therefore have an effect similar to that of other β-lactams in treating MSSA. The first to be approved is ceftaroline, but adequate clinical trials have not been completed to demonstrate its equivalence to linezolid for MRSA pneumonia, particularly CA-MRSA strains.[30] Such documentation would be a major advance in the management of MRSA pneumonia, and would likely minimize even more the use of vancomycin for pneumonia.

Other oxazolidinones that may have improved efficacy or decreased toxicity are also in development. Because linezolid has a defined clinical failure rate, room for improvement in this class exists as well.

The role of exotoxin production in CA-MRSA is not well defined, nor do we have complete understanding of what clinical factors enhance or initiate exotoxin production. Better characterization of not only which exotoxin is important but also whether specific measures are required to combat the release or effects of exotoxins may also define targets for further interventions.

SUMMARY

Although MRSA is an infrequent cause of CAP in general, it is a major issue for CAP in previously healthy young adults, in association with influenza, and in patients with risk factors for HCAP. Linezolid consistently demonstrates better clinical response rates than vancomycin in clinical trials of MRSA pneumonia. Linezolid also suppresses exotoxin production in *in vitro* models, which may be important in CA-MRSA CAP.

REFERENCES

1. Chambers HF. Community-associated MRSA—resistance and virulence converge. N Engl J Med 2005;352(14):1485–7.
2. Chambers HF, Deleo FR. Waves of resistance: *Staphylococcus aureus* in the antibiotic era. Nat Rev Microbiol 2009;7(9):629–41.
3. American Thoracic Society, Infectious Diseases Society of America. Guidelines for the management of adults with hospital-acquired, ventilator-associated, and healthcare-associated pneumonia. Am J Respir Crit Care Med 2005;171(4): 388–416.
4. Dufour P, Gillet Y, Bes M, et al. Community-acquired methicillin-resistant *Staphylococcus aureus* infections in France: emergence of a single clone that produces Panton-Valentine leukocidin. Clin Infect Dis 2002;35(7):819–24.
5. Gillet Y, Issartel B, Vanhems P, et al. Association between *Staphylococcus aureus* strains carrying gene for Panton-Valentine leukocidin and highly lethal necrotising pneumonia in young immunocompetent patients. Lancet 2002;359(9308):753–9.
6. Kallen AJ, Reed C, Patton M, et al. *Staphylococcus aureus* community-onset pneumonia in patients admitted to children's hospitals during autumn and winter of 2006-2007. Epidemiol Infect 2010;138(5):666–72.
7. Moran GJ, Krishnadasan A, Gorwitz RJ, et al. Methicillin-resistant *S aureus* infections among patients in the emergency department. N Engl J Med 2006;355(7): 666–74.
8. Kallen AJ, Brunkard J, Moore Z, et al. *Staphylococcus aureus* community-acquired pneumonia during the 2006 to 2007 influenza season. Ann Emerg Med 2009;53(3):358–65.
9. Lobo LJ, Reed KD, Wunderink RG. Expanded clinical presentation of community-acquired methicillin-resistant *Staphylococcus aureus* pneumonia. Chest 2010; 138(1):130–6.
10. Thomas R, Ferguson J, Coombs G, et al. Community-acquired methicillin-resistant *Staphylococcus aureus* pneumonia: a clinical audit. Respirology 2011; 16(6):926–31.

11. Jain SS, Wunderink RG, Fakhran S, et al. Etiology of community-acquired pneumonia among hospitalized adults in the United States: preliminary data from the CDC Etiology of Pneumonia in the Community (EPIC) Study. Abstract 676, Presented ID Week, San Diego, October, 2012.

12. Mandell LA, Wunderink RG, Anzueto A, et al. Infectious Diseases Society of America/American Thoracic Society consensus guidelines on the management of community-acquired pneumonia in adults. Clin Infect Dis 2007;44(Suppl 2): S27–72.

13. Kollef MH, Shorr A, Tabak YP, et al. Epidemiology and outcomes of health-care-associated pneumonia: results from a large US database of culture-positive pneumonia. Chest 2005;128(6):3854–62.

14. Micek ST, Kollef KE, Reichley RM, et al. Health care-associated pneumonia and community-acquired pneumonia: a single-center experience. Antimicrob Agents Chemother 2007;51(10):3568–73.

15. Labelle AJ, Arnold H, Reichley RM, et al. A comparison of culture-positive and culture-negative health-care-associated pneumonia. Chest 2010;137(5):1130–7.

16. Carratala J, Mykietiuk A, Fernandez-Sabe N, et al. Health care-associated pneumonia requiring hospital admission: epidemiology, antibiotic therapy, and clinical outcomes. Arch Intern Med 2007;167(13):1393–9.

17. Wilson BZ, Anzueto A, Restrepo MI, et al. Comparison of two guideline-concordant antimicrobial combinations in elderly patients hospitalized with severe community-acquired pneumonia. Crit Care Med 2012;40(8):2310–4.

18. Hadler JL, Petit S, Mandour M, et al. Trends in invasive infection with methicillin-resistant *Staphylococcus aureus*, Connecticut, USA, 2001-2010. Emerg Infect Dis 2012;18(6):917–24.

19. von Eiff C, Becker K, Machka K, et al. Nasal carriage as a source of *Staphylococcus aureus* bacteremia. Study Group. N Engl J Med 2001;344(1):11–6.

20. Bogaert D, van Belkum A, Sluijter M, et al. Colonisation by *Streptococcus pneumoniae* and *Staphylococcus aureus* in healthy children. Lancet 2004;363(9424): 1871–2.

21. Rice TW, Rubinson L, Uyeki TM, et al. Critical illness from 2009 pandemic influenza A virus and bacterial coinfection in the United States. Crit Care Med 2012;40(5):1487–98.

22. Chen SY, Liao CH, Wang JL, et al. Methicillin-resistant *Staphylococcus aureus* (MRSA) staphylococcal cassette chromosome mec genotype effects outcomes of patients with healthcare-associated MRSA bacteremia independently of vancomycin minimum inhibitory concentration. Clin Infect Dis 2012;55(10): 1329–37.

23. Gillet Y, Vanhems P, Lina G, et al. Factors predicting mortality in necrotizing community-acquired pneumonia caused by *Staphylococcus aureus* containing Panton-Valentine leukocidin. Clin Infect Dis 2007;45(3):315–21.

24. Van De Griend P, Herwaldt LA, Alvis B, et al. Community-associated methicillin-resistant *Staphylococcus aureus*, Iowa, USA. Emerg Infect Dis 2009;15(10):1582–9.

25. Kett DH, Cano E, Quartin AA, et al. Implementation of guidelines for management of possible multidrug-resistant pneumonia in intensive care: an observational, multicentre cohort study. Lancet Infect Dis 2011;11(3):181–9.

26. Ewig S, Welte T, Chastre J, et al. Rethinking the concepts of community-acquired and health-care-associated pneumonia. Lancet Infect Dis 2010;10(4):279–87.

27. Robicsek A, Suseno M, Beaumont JL, et al. Prediction of methicillin-resistant *Staphylococcus aureus* involvement in disease sites by concomitant nasal sampling. J Clin Microbiol 2008;46(2):588–92.

28. Fagon J, Patrick H, Haas DW, et al. Treatment of gram-positive nosocomial pneumonia. Prospective randomized comparison of quinupristin/dalfopristin versus vancomycin. Nosocomial Pneumonia Group. Am J Respir Crit Care Med 2000; 161(3 Pt 1):753–62.

29. Pertel PE, Bernardo P, Fogarty C, et al. Effects of prior effective therapy on the efficacy of daptomycin and ceftriaxone for the treatment of community-acquired pneumonia. Clin Infect Dis 2008;46(8):1142–51.

30. File TM Jr, Low DE, Eckburg PB, et al. FOCUS 1: a randomized, double-blinded, multicentre, Phase III trial of the efficacy and safety of ceftaroline fosamil versus ceftriaxone in community-acquired pneumonia. J Antimicrob Chemother 2011; 66(Suppl 3):iii19–32.

31. Wunderink RG, Niederman MS, Kollef MH, et al. Linezolid in methicillin-resistant *Staphylococcus aureus* nosocomial pneumonia: a randomized, controlled study. Clin Infect Dis 2012;54(5):621–9.

32. Kollef MH, Rello J, Cammarata SK, et al. Clinical cure and survival in Gram-positive ventilator-associated pneumonia: retrospective analysis of two double-blind studies comparing linezolid with vancomycin. Intensive Care Med 2004;30(3): 388–94.

33. Rubinstein E, Cammarata S, Oliphant T, et al. Linezolid (PNU-100766) versus vancomycin in the treatment of hospitalized patients with nosocomial pneumonia: a randomized, double-blind, multicenter study. Clin Infect Dis 2001;32(3):402–12.

34. Wunderink RG, Rello J, Cammarata SK, et al. Linezolid vs vancomycin: analysis of two double-blind studies of patients with methicillin-resistant *Staphylococcus aureus* nosocomial pneumonia. Chest 2003;124(5):1789–97.

35. Wunderink RG, Cammarata SK, Oliphant TH, et al. Continuation of a randomized, double-blind, multicenter study of linezolid versus vancomycin in the treatment of patients with nosocomial pneumonia. Clin Ther 2003;25(3):980–92.

36. Wunderink RG, Mendelson MH, Somero MS, et al. Early microbiological response to linezolid vs vancomycin in ventilator-associated pneumonia due to methicillin-resistant *Staphylococcus aureus*. Chest 2008;134(6):1200–7.

37. Stevens DL, Ma Y, Salmi DB, et al. Impact of antibiotics on expression of virulence-associated exotoxin genes in methicillin-sensitive and methicillin-resistant *Staphylococcus aureus*. J Infect Dis 2007;195(2):202–11.

38. Bernardo K, Pakulat N, Fleer S, et al. Subinhibitory concentrations of linezolid reduce *Staphylococcus aureus* virulence factor expression. Antimicrob Agents Chemother 2004;48(2):546–55.

39. Stevens DL, Wallace RJ, Hamilton SM, et al. Successful treatment of staphylococcal toxic shock syndrome with linezolid: a case report and in vitro evaluation of the production of toxic shock syndrome toxin type 1 in the presence of antibiotics. Clin Infect Dis 2006;42(5):729–30.

40. Hamilton LA, Christopher Wood G, Magnotti LJ, et al. Treatment of methicillin-resistant *Staphylococcus aureus* ventilator-associated pneumonia with high-dose vancomycin or linezolid. J Trauma Acute Care Surg 2012;72(6):1478–83.

41. Haque NZ, Zuniga LC, Peyrani P, et al. Relationship of vancomycin minimum inhibitory concentration to mortality in patients with methicillin-resistant *Staphylococcus aureus* hospital-acquired, ventilator-associated, or health-care-associated pneumonia. Chest 2010;138(6):1356–62.

42. Jeffres MN, Isakow W, Doherty JA, et al. A retrospective analysis of possible renal toxicity associated with vancomycin in patients with health care-associated methicillin-resistant *Staphylococcus aureus* pneumonia. Clin Ther 2007;29(6): 1107–15.

43. Jung YJ, Koh Y, Hong SB, et al. Effect of vancomycin plus rifampicin in the treatment of nosocomial methicillin-resistant *Staphylococcus aureus* pneumonia. Crit Care Med 2010;38(1):175–80.

44. Kalil AC, Murthy MH, Hermsen ED, et al. Linezolid versus vancomycin or teicoplanin for nosocomial pneumonia: a systematic review and meta-analysis. Crit Care Med 2010;38(9):1802–8.

What Is the Best Approach to the Nonresponding Patient with Community-Acquired Pneumonia?

Salvador Sialer, MD[a], Adamantia Liapikou, MD, PhD[c],
Antoni Torres, MD, PhD[a,b],*

KEYWORDS

- Community-acquired pneumonia • Treatment failure • Microbiologic diagnosis
- Biomarkers • Empiric treatment

KEY POINTS

- Treatment failure in community-acquired pneumonia is the failure to normalize the clinical features or nonresolving image in chest radiograph, despite antimicrobial therapy.
- The incidence has not been clearly established; it ranges between 6% and 15% and the mortality increases significantly, nearly 5-fold.
- There are several risk factors for treatment failure in community-acquired pneumonia (host characteristics, virulence of the pathogen, and the antimicrobial treatment administered).
- If symptoms do not improve after 72 hours of treatment, an evaluation of clinical response should be performed and changing the initial empiric antibiotic treatment must be considered.
- Measuring of serum biomarkers, procalcitonin and C-reactive protein, on the first day and on the third day have proven useful for predicting nonresponsive community-acquired pneumonia.

INTRODUCTION

The diagnosis of community acquired pneumonia (CAP) is based on the presence of clinical features (eg, cough, fever, sputum production, and pleuritic chest pain) and is supported by imaging of the lung, usually by chest radiograph. Treatment failure or nonresponse to therapy is the failure to normalize these criteria used for diagnosis.[1–3]

Given the variability in the rate of clinical response and radiographic resolution, there is no consensus on how long the physician must wait before evaluating nonresolving

[a] Pneumology Department, Clinic Institute of Thorax (ICT), Hospital Clinic of Barcelona, C/Villarroel 170, Barcelona 08036, Spain; [b] Insitut d'Investigacions Biomèdiques August Pi i Sunyer (IDIBAPS), University of Barcelona, CIBERES, C/Roselló 149-153, Barcelona 08036, Spain; [c] 3rd Pneumology Department, Sotiria Hospital, Mesogion 152, Athens 11527, Greece
* Corresponding author. Pneumology Department, Hospital Clinic, C/Villarroel 170, Barcelona 08036, Spain.
E-mail address: atorres@clinic.ub.es

Infect Dis Clin N Am 27 (2013) 189–203
http://dx.doi.org/10.1016/j.idc.2012.11.009
0891-5520/13/$ – see front matter © 2013 Elsevier Inc. All rights reserved.

pulmonary infiltrates that might be due to several causes, including inadequate antibiotic therapy, resistant or highly virulent organisms, impaired host defenses, obstructing endobronchial lesions, or noninfectious causes. The recommended time for defining therapeutic failure is 72 hours from the start of antibiotic treatment, representing the time when the patient is expected to start showing some parameters of clinical stability.

It is important to be able to identify what patients are at risk for progressive or treatment-failure pneumonia that may make them candidates for more careful monitoring. For this reason, several studies have attempted to establish risk factors, causes, and new strategies for the treatment of progressive and nonresolving pneumonia.[2,4,5]

DEFINITIONS

Treatment failure, or nonresponding CAP, is a term used to define a clinical condition whereby the response is inadequate despite antimicrobial therapy, resulting in worsening of the symptoms and slower resolution that may lead to dissemination of the infection, development of complications, and even death.[2,3,5]

There are 2 well-recognized patters of nonresponse in CAP: progressive pneumonia and persistent nonresponding pneumonia. Progressive pneumonia is characterized by a progression of the infection, resulting in clinical deterioration with acute respiratory failure requiring ventilatory support and/or septic shock, usually occurring within the first 72 hours after admission to the hospital (**Figs. 1–4**). Persistent nonresponding pneumonia is characterized by the absence or delay in achieving clinical stability. The term *early failure* is similar to progressive pneumonia, but used even before 72 hours of treatment.[2,3,5,6]

In many studies the definition of treatment failure depends on the criteria of the authors.[2,6] It is important to define when antibiotic treatment is considered to have failed because it requires some time to take effect and it also depends on the causal microorganism, the initial severity of the infection, and the conditions of the patient.

The definition of a lack of response to antibiotic treatment differs according to the site of care. The guidelines of the American Thoracic Society/Infectious Diseases Society of America suggest that treatment failure for outpatients should be considered when there is a need for hospital admission or a change in antibiotics.[7] For

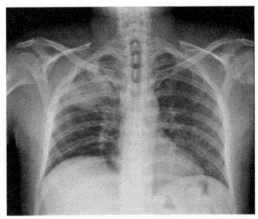

Fig. 1. Radiograph showing condensation in the right upper lobe without pleural effusion.

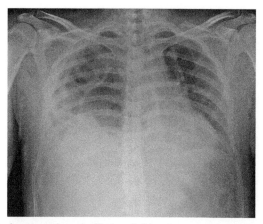

Fig. 2. Radiograph showing pleural effusion fluid.

hospitalized patients with CAP, the most frequently used period is 72 hours, in line with the median time required to achieve clinical stability, the time required to reduce bacterial concentration in the airways, or the suggested time for obtaining samples for microbiologic tests and further workup. This cutoff point (72 hours) was based in part on the study of Montravers and colleagues[8] in ventilator-associated pneumonia; the study showed that, after 72 hours of appropriate treatment, 88% of the patients had sterile cultures or insignificant bacterial growth, correlating with the clinical response.

Although the lack of clinical stability and treatment failure are closely related, they are not synonymous because they give different information on the evolution of CAP. Treatment failure leads to a delay in achieving clinical stability, whereas the delay in achieving clinical stability may be due to other causes but it is not necessarily a treatment failure.[2,3,9]

Several factors have been identified that affect clinical stability, of which the principal identified factor is the initial severity of CAP. Obviously, if the initial severity is higher (according to pneumonia severity index [PSI] risk scale or confusion, uremia, respiratory rate-low, blood pressure, age 65 years of greater score), a longer time period will be required to reach stability.[8] Other factors associated with a delay in

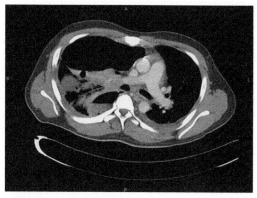

Fig. 3. CT scans showing suggested consolidation in right upper lobe, necrotizing pneumonia, and a loculated pleural empyema.

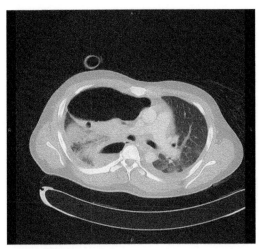

Fig. 4. CT scans showing suggested consolidation in the right upper lobe, necrotizing pneumonia, and a loculated pleural empyema.

achieving clinical stability are concomitant comorbid conditions, complications, and nonadherence to treatment guidelines.

EPIDEMIOLOGY
Incidence

The incidence of treatment failure in CAP has not been clearly established. In several multicenter studies it ranges between 6% and 24% and can potentially range up to 31% in patients with severe CAP.[10–12] A study by Aliberti and colleagues[10] of 500 patients hospitalized with CAP reported a rate of clinical failure of 13%, whereas the rate of early clinical failure was 9%. In a multicenter prospective cohort study performed in 1424 hospitalized patients, Menéndez and colleagues[13] reported treatment failure in 215 patients (15%), and early failure in 134 patients (62%), whereas Rosón and colleagues,[9] in a prospective observational study of 1383 patients, reported treatment failure in 238 patients (18%) and early failure in 6% of patients.

Prognosis

In patients with CAP, especially those with severe CAP, when a lack of treatment response occurs, the risk of complications, length of hospital stay, and death increase significantly.[1,12,13] In the study of Rosón and colleagues[9] that included 1383 immunosuppressed CAP patients, early failures had significantly higher rates of complications (58% vs 24%) and overall mortality (27% vs 4%) (P<.001 for both). In the NACE study,[14] rate of mortality in nonresponding CAP patients was significantly higher than in patients who responded to treatment (22% vs 3.5%). In a prospective multicenter study in Spain (Pneumofail), the rates were 25% and 2%, respectively. In addition, nonresponse was one of the factors associated with a worse prognosis in the multivariate analysis.[13]

Causes

It is useful to classify the etiologic cause of treatment failure in patients with CAP according to the microbiologic approach as infectious and noninfectious (**Table 1**). Infectious causes are responsible for 40% of the cases. They have been classified

Table 1	
Causes of treatment failure in communityacquired pneumonia	
Infectious	• Resistant microorganisms:
	○ *Pseudomonas aeruginosa*
	○ MRSA
	○ Beta-lactamase producing *Enterobacteriaceae*
	• Unusual microorganisms
	○ *Mycobacterium tuberculosis*
	○ *Nocardia* spp
	○ Fungi (Aspergillus spp, Histoplasma, Coccidioides)
	○ *Pneumocystis jirovecii*
	○ Hantavirus
	• Nosocomial pneumonia
	○ *Pseudomonas aeruginosa*
	○ MRSA
	○ *Acinetobacter baumanii*
	○ Anaerobes
	• Complications of pneumonia
	○ Empyema
	○ Abscess or necrotizing pneumonia
	○ Metastatic infection: endocarditis, meningitis, arthritis
Noninfectious	• Neoplasms
	• Pulmonary edema
	• Pulmonary embolism
	• Pulmonary hemorrhage
	• Cryptogenic organizing pneumonia
	• Eosinophilic pneumonia
	• Acute respiratory distress syndrome
	• Sarcoidosis
	• Vasculitis

by Arancibia and colleagues[12] as primary infections, definitive or probable persistent infections, and nosocomial infections. In this study, definite persistent infections were mostly due to microbial resistance to the administered initial empiric antimicrobial treatment and nosocomial infections were particularly frequent in patients with progressive pneumonia.

The most frequent pathogens recognized as causes of treatment failure in CAP are *Streptococcus pneumoniae*, *Legionella* species, *Staphylococcus aureus*, and *Pseudomonas aeruginosa*. In contrast, the most frequent pathogens associated with treatment failure in elderly institutionalized patients are methicillin-resistant *S aureus* (MRSA), enteric gram-negative bacilli, and *P aeruginosa*.[3,6,10]

Failures due to *S pneumoniae* highly resistant to penicillins are rare, when the treatment is according to the guidelines. Some cases of treatment failure have been described with resistance to the new fluoroquinolones, specifically, levofloxacin, and to macrolides. *P aeruginosa* represents around 5% to 8% of the cases of hospitalized CAP, whether due to persistent infection or subsequent nosocomial superinfection, with some of the *Pseudomonas* cases multiresistant.

Referring to enteric gram-negative bacilli resistance, Enterobacteriaceae β-lactam producers are increasing in the community and this could also explain treatment failure in some causes. Overall, it is important to know the risk factors for multidrug-resistant (MDR) pathogens, causing CAP to administer adequate initial antibiotic therapy.

The presence of unusual microorganisms in CAP is a cause of treatment failure because these microorganisms are not adequately covered by the recommended initial empiric therapy (Mycobacteria, *Nocardia* spp, anaerobes, fungi, *Pneumocystis jiroveci*). One example is community-acquired MRSA, which may carry a cytotoxin (Panton-Valentine leukocidin) that causes severe necrotizing pneumonia with resistance to β-lactam antibiotics.[3,15–17]

Other infectious causes of nonresponse to treatment are complications of CAP, such as empyema (see **Figs. 1–4**), endocarditis, arthritis, pericarditis, meningitis, or peritonitis, and necrotizing pneumonia (abscess).[3,6,18] Specifically, empyema is the most frequent of these complications and has to be specifically searched for in patients with CAP that initially present with pleural effusion.

Noninfectious causes can mimic CAP—especially radiologically—and behave as treatment failure. Noninfectious causes include pulmonary hemorrhage, pulmonary edema, diseases of inflammatory origin such as cryptogenic organizing pneumonia, thromboembolic diseases, eosinophilic pneumonia, and hypersensitivity pneumonitis. Also, pulmonary neoplasia, especially alveolar cell lung cancer or carcinomatous lymphangitis, is included in the differential diagnosis.[18,19]

It should also be taken into account that in up to 30% of cases, there does not seem to be any specific cause for lack of response, despite appropriate antibiotic treatment.[20,21] These cases are more frequently observed in progressive or early failure CAP.

RISK FACTORS FOR TREATMENT FAILURE

Several factors have been associated with treatment failure and may be classified as follows: factors related to initial severity of infection, host factors, factors associated with the causal microorganism, and treatment-related factors.

Initial severity is an independent risk factor for early and late treatment failure. When the authors use a risk scale, such as the Pneumonia Severity Index, it must be remembered that a higher PSI score may be more dependent on the comorbid condition and on patient age than the severity itself.[6,13]

Some previous studies[4,5,12] have shown the factors related to initial severity of infection. It has been often shown that in hospitalized patients with CAP, severe sepsis is the primary cause of clinical failure in relation to CAP. Rosón and colleagues[9] recognized uncontrolled sepsis as a cause of early clinical failure in 11% of CAP patients. In additional, in the study by Aliberti and colleagues,[10] severe sepsis was the primary cause of clinical failure related to CAP, with an incidence of up to 27%. It is known that CAP with systemic shock has a worse response to antibiotic treatment.

The complex response of the host against infection requires correct identification of the microorganism, the development of an appropriate inflammatory response, including the production of cytokines, and the ending of the inflammatory phase. Inflammatory response should be sufficient to overcome the proliferation and dissemination of the microorganism and should also remain confined to avoid dissemination into the systemic circulation, which could induce hemodynamic disorders and/or multiorgan failure.[3,6,9,10]

Despite advances in the understanding of the systemic and local inflammatory response in severe infections, it is not yet known what factors cause an excessive inflammatory response with deleterious effects. This response has been associated with the host, the bacterial load, and the virulence of the microorganisms.

Further investigation must be performed of the genetic factors related to host response against infection. Several specific mutations correspond on different inflammation phases and, because cytokine production is genetically determined, this should be the focus of this research for the future. It is confirmed that the rate of reso-lution of pneumonia depends to a large extent on host factors. Preexisting illnesses or comorbidities are present in between 50% and 80% of patients with CAP and are independent predictors of mortality. Also, many comorbidities are associated with a higher rate of infections with S aureus, enteric gram-negative bacteria, or Legionella species.[2,3,13]

A review of several studies[1,10,13] found that advanced age, serious underlying disease, congestive heart failure, hepatic disease, hypotension, hypothermia, alcohol abuse, thrombocytopenia, leukopenia or immunosuppressive therapy, multilobar involvement, pleural effusion, acidemia, and abnormal gas exchange were indepen-dent predictors of clinical failure related to CAP on admission to the hospital.

Of the factors associated with the causal microorganism of CAP, infection due to Legionella pneumonia or gram-negative microorganisms has been reported to increase the probability of treatment failure between 2-fold and 4-fold.[3,7,9,10] Legionella CAP can initially behave like a progressive pneumonia, with high mortality, and takes longer to resolve. Moreover, when the cause of CAP is mixed, resolution is delayed. Pleural effu-sion, specifically empyema caused by S pneumoniae, is associated with early and late treatment failure. Recently, the presence of community-acquired MRSA has been recognized in severe CAP, which may lead to cavitary lesions and sepsis.[3,8,20]

Among the treatment-related factors described in those patients once early signs or symptoms of severe sepsis are identified, such as problems with oxygenation, hypo-tension, or hypothermia, it is important to seek other treatment strategies. Discordant therapy and treatment that does not adhere to guidelines have been associated with treatment failure and higher mortality.[15,21]

A study by Menéndez and colleagues[22] has shown that, when the initial antibiotic treatment was selected by a pneumologist or by the clinical resident, treatment failure was lower than when selected by a nonspecialist in pneumology. Data from a prospec-tive study by Menéndez and colleagues[13] in 1424 patients hospitalized with CAP suggest that initial treatment with fluoroquinolones and influenza vaccination may confer protection against treatment failure. In this study, the failure of empiric treat-ment increased the mortality of CAP 11-fold after adjustment for risk class.

Usually pneumonia caused by MDR pathogens has been limited to the hospital stage. However, with the wide spread of health care outside the hospital, MDR path-ogens have become more frequent. Aliberti and colleagues[23] reported hospitalization in the preceding 90 days and residency in a nursing home as risk factors for acquiring MDR pathogens. In addition to these 2 factors, Shorr and colleagues[24] also found long-term hemodialysis and intensive care unit admission as risk factors for acquiring MDR pathogens. Specifically, P aeruginosa can be found in advanced and very severe chronic obstructive disease (COPD), and in patients with severe long-term bronchiectasis (**Table 2**).[7]

RECOMMENDATIONS FOR THE APPROACH TO THE NONRESPONDING PATIENT

The diagnostic approach to a patient with treatment failure requires the assessment and evaluation of several aspects, including host factors that may explain delayed resolution, clinical severity, and evolution of infiltrates in radiographs.[18,19]

If symptoms do not improve within the first 3 days of treatment, an evaluation of clin-ical response should be performed. A careful review of the clinical history and the initial microbiologic results is essential to confirm the diagnosis of CAP (**Table 3**).

The presence of some microorganisms and host factors may explain the slower resolution of infectious parameters—for example, elderly patients with comorbid

Table 2
Risk factors for multidrug-resistant (MDR) pathogens

Risk factors for all MDR	Aliberti et al,[23] 2012
	Hospitalization in the preceding 90 days
	Residency in a nursing home
	Shorr et al,[24] 2008
	Recent hospitalization
	Nursing home resident
	Long-term hemodialysis
	ICU admission
Risk factors for *Pseudomonas aeruginosa*	Mandell et al,[7] 2007
	Severe long-term bronchiectasis
	Severe COPD with frequent exacerbations leading to steroid and/or antibiotic treatment

Multidrug-resistant (MDR) pathogens (eg, methicillin-resistant *Staphylococcus aureus* [MRSA] and *Enterobacteriaceae* β-lactam producers).

conditions or immunosuppression may have a slower resolution of symptoms.[8,13] In cases like these, if there is no clinical deterioration, a conservative approach with clinical monitoring and serial radiographs may be sufficient.

Microbiology

In cases where the microbiologic cause has not been identified, when there are no host-related factors for delayed resolution, and/or on the appearance of clinical deterioration, a complete reevaluation is required to search for other alternative noninfectious diagnoses and expand the differential diagnosis. Further radiologic studies,

Table 3
Diagnostic approach in nonresponding patients

Examination	Tests
Imaging	New chest radiograph
	Thorax CT scan
Sputum	Gram stain and Giemsa stain; conventional bacteria culture; direct immunofluorescence for *Legionella*
	Ziehl–Nielsen stain for *M tuberculosis* stains for fungi and opportunists
Blood	Two sets for culture
Urine	*Legionella pneumophila* antigen
Pleural fluid	Cultures for anaerobes; bacterial cultures
Bronchoscopy	
Protected bronchial brush (PBS)	Gram stain and intracellular bacteria culture; bacteria culture; Ziehl, fungi, and Giemsa stain; direct immunofluorescence for *Legionella* and *Pneumocystis jirovesi* histologic biopsy
Bronchoalveolar lavage (BAL)	Gram-stain and bacteria culture[a]; Ziehl and modified Ziehl stain for *M tuberculosis and Nocardia spp*; cultures for mycobacteria, *Legionella*, fungi, and virus;
	Cytologic studies: Total cell count: Polymorphonuclear leukocytes, Lymphocytes—lymphocyte subpopulation, hemosiderin, eosinophils, malignant cells

[a] Quantitative criteria for the interpretation of PSB and BAL specimens are described in the text.

noninvasive samples, and endoscopic methods should be performed to evaluate the airways and to obtain samples for microbiologic tests and other studies. These studies may rule out the persistence of infection, the appearance of resistance during treatment, or the appearance of a new nosocomial infection.[1,3,8]

Microbiologic studies should include stains and cultures for the usual bacteria, fungi, virus, and opportunistic germs, including conventional and modified Ziehl-Neilson stain for *Nocardia*, and direct immunofluorescence and culture for the investigation of *Legionella*.[10,20] To differentiate between colonization and infection, the results of bacterial cultures are expressed as colony forming units per milliliter. However, the colony count of conventional bacteria should be interpreted together with other tests because previous antibiotic treatment may reduce the counts below the established cutoff point of 10^3 CFU/mL for protected brush specimens (PBS) and 10^4 CFU/mL for bronchoalveolar lavage (BAL) fluid.[25]

Radiology

The persistence of radiographic images is crucial in determining whether a patient has treatment failure in CAP. The period during which a more active diagnostic process should be performed has not been defined. The approach should be less invasive if there is a reduction of the infiltrates in the radiographs, and an improvement in symptoms. If the infiltrate does not diminish, or if symptoms persist or increase, a computed tomographic (CT) scan and bronchoscopy should be performed as part of the evaluation.[3,18,19] Radiographic resolution is significantly slower for those patients with high a comorbidity index, bacteremia, multilobar involvement, and enteric gram-negative bacillary pneumonias.[3,18,19]

Radiographic resolution is also slower in elderly people. The high prevalence of underlying COPD and smoking history in this age group has been implicated in slow radiographic resolution, 2 to 4 times as often as in younger patients. In a study by El Solh and colleagues,[26] the rate of radiographic clearance in nonimmunocompromised older patients with CAP was estimated at 35% within 3 weeks, 60% within 6 weeks, and 84% within 12 weeks. They recommended a waiting period of between 12 and 14 weeks for slowly resolving pneumonia to be considered nonresolving.

Chest radiographs may show complications of CAP as pleural effusion, lung abscess, and/or new infiltrates. Pleural effusion is frequently associated with treatment failure and thoracocentesis is required to rule out empyema (see **Figs. 1–4**).

The CT scan is useful for investigating complications such as empyema, pulmonary abscess, or other alternative diagnoses and also may suggest some specific microorganisms. For example, nodules surrounded by a halo of ground-grass attenuation with involvement near the pleura are suggestive of pulmonary *Aspergillus* and/or *Mucor* infection. Similar nodular images have been described in infections caused by *Candida* or cytomegalovirus, Wegener granulomatosis, Kaposi sarcoma, and hemorrhagic metastases. *P jiroveci* pneumonia often shows ground-glass opacity or images of interstitial pneumonia. Images of nodules or multiple masses with or without cavitation can be caused by *Nocardia* spp, *Mycobacterium tuberculosis*, or Q fever. Diffuse or mixed interstitial infiltrates may be due to virus or *M pneumoniae*. In a study by Tomiyama and colleagues[27] on the usefulness of high-resolution CT scans in acute pulmonary parenchymatous disease, the investigators were able to classify correctly the cause as infectious or noninfectious in 90% of the patients.

Fiberoptic Bronchoscopy

Bronchoscopy has to form part of the diagnostic evaluation of patients with nonresponding pneumonia if the clinical situation of the patients allows it.[28,29]

Bronchoscopy allows direct observation of the airways and makes it possible to obtain samples directly within the infected lobe. PBS and BAL reportedly have a diagnostic yield of 41% in treatment failure. A complete processing of BAL for microbiologic and nonmicrobiologic studies also provides useful diagnostic information. The study of cell counts in BAL fluid allows the orientation of a differential diagnosis of noninfectious causes. Thus, the presence of greater than 20% of eosinophils leads to causes such as pulmonary eosinophilia, fungal infection, drug-induced pneumonitis, or others. Pulmonary hemorrhage is suggested by the presence of blood or greater than 20% of hemosiderin-loaded macrophages, and hypersensitivity pneumonitis, sarcoidosis, or pulmonary fibrosis by a raised lymphocyte count.[10,20,30]

Although the diagnostic yield of invasive microbiologic samples is good, their impact on prognosis is not clear. If airway abnormalities are found, a bronchial biopsy may be performed. The role and indication of transbronchial biopsy are not clear; it should be performed if airway examination rules out other findings, and if there is no evidence of infection, as other diagnoses may be made. It has been reported in up to 57% of diagnoses with transbronchial biopsy in patients with treatment failure, although this procedure was performed in only 25% of cases. Transbronchial biopsy was particularly useful for determining noninfectious causes, including neoplasia, cryptogenic organizing pneumonia, and histiocytosis X.[3,12,20]

Biomarkers

The use of markers as an expression of inflammation is complementary to clinical parameters, alerting the clinician if they remain high—even if clinical stability is reached—and reducing the level of alert if they are reduced. The study of serum biomarkers, such as procalcitonin (PCT) and C-reactive protein (CRP), at baseline and their monitoring on day 3 or 4 of antibiotic therapy has proven useful for predicting nonresponsive CAP.[31]

PCT was a better predictor of early failure and CRP behaved in a similar way in early or late failure.[32]

Several prospective cohort studies showing that higher initial levels of CRP (>210 mg/dL; Odds Ratio, 2.6) constitute a risk factor, whereas low levels (CRP <100 mg/L; Odds Ratio, 0.21) are protective for complicated CAP.[33] Biomarker monitoring shows that the reduction of CRP after between 3 and 4 days of treatment by less than between 50% and 60% of the initial value is associated with an increased risk of having received inappropriate empiric antibiotic treatment, with an odds ratio of 6.98.[34] The behavior of several cytokines (interleukin [IL] -1, IL-6, IL-8, and IL-10), and well as CRP and PCT, was studied by Menéndez and colleagues,[32] who found that a CRP ≥219 mg/L on day 1 had an independent predictive value for identifying treatment failure.

Ruiz-González and colleagues[17] reported that changes in levels of CRP after 72 hours are useful for discriminating between true treatment failure and slow response to treatment. When levels of CRP increased between day 1 and day 4, a prediction model conducted by adding tachypnea (respiratory rate >24 breaths/min) identified patients with true treatment failure with a sensitivity of 90.9%, specificity of 58.9%, positive predictive value of 46.5%, and negative predictive value of 94.3%.

The results of another study of Menéndez and colleagues[34] have shown that both clinical criteria of stability and reduction of biomarker levels (CRP, PCT, IL-6, IL-10) after 72 hours of treatment have a high negative predictive value for ruling out subsequent severe complications.

In summary, the initial measurement of biomarkers (PCT and CRP) may help to detect some patients that might present progressive and nonresponding pneumonia.

In addition, a second measure by day 3 to 4 is also helpful to monitor the evolution of patients with CAP.

THERAPEUTIC ATTITUDE

Nonresponding patients with CAP usually require important management decisions: transfer of the patient to a higher level of care, further diagnostic testing, and/or changes in initial antibiotic treatment (**Fig. 5**).

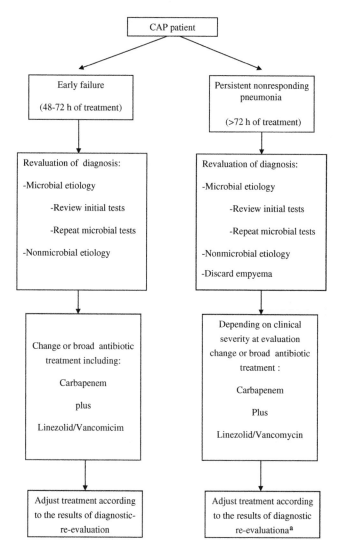

Consider treatment with steroids when COP (cryptogenic organizing pneumonia) is suspected and at least one complete course of antibiotics has been administered and infectious causes of nonresponding have been completely discarded.

Fig. 5. Approach to therapy to the nonresponding CAP patient.

If the patient develops early treatment failure, severe clinical deterioration, and/or a worsening of the radiologic infiltrates, broad antibiotic therapy may be administered even before 72 hours.[5,6]

In nonresponding CAP, the new antibiotic regimen should broaden the spectrum to cover not only the usual bacteria but also resistant S pneumoniae, P aeruginosa, S aureus (including MRSA), and anaerobic bacteria. Treatment should include anti-pseudomonal β-lactams (cefepime, imipenem, meropenem, piperacillin/tazobactam) and intravenous fluoroquinolones or aminoglycosides.

In patients with severe COPD, prolonged treatment with steroids, or those under-going immunosuppressive treatment, the coverage of Aspergillus spp should be taken into account.[2,5]

The main challenge in patients with antimicrobial treatment failures is to detect microbial resistance to the initially administered antimicrobial treatment. Despite the increase in resistance of S pneumoniae, several studies show that the increase is not influencing mortality. Current levels of β-lactam resistance do not generally result in CAP treatment failures when appropriate agents (ie, amoxicillin, ceftriaxone, or cefotaxime) and doses are used, even in the presence of bacteremia.[7]

The new broad antibiotic regimen must consist of 2 or 3 drugs and cover P aerugi-nosa, S aureus (MRSA), and Enterobacteriaceae β-lactam producers. Risk factors shown in **Table 2** may help clinicians to make the decision to cover these microorgan-isms totally or partially. the authors' personal point of view is to cover empirically all MDR and de-escalate antibiotics when the new cultures will be available. The combi-nation of an antipseudomonal carbapenem plus linezolid or vancomycin is a good option. Special attention should be given to nonresponding patients with severe COPD treated with oral steroids in whom Aspergillus spp has to be considered. Voriconazol is the best option in this case.

The beneficial effect of corticosteroid in treatment failure has not been conclusively demonstrated up to now. However, it has to be considered individually in some patients that might have noninfectious causes of chest infiltrates (eg, cryptogenic organizing pneumonia).[35,36]

NEED OR RECOMMENDATION FOR FUTURE STUDIES TO ADDRESS THE QUESTION OF BEST APPROACH TO HE NONRESPONDING PATIENT

Future studies should be focused in the following topics:

1. To determine better the risk factor for MDR (P aeruginosa, MRSA, Enterobacteria-ceae β-lactam producers) microorganisms
2. To develop and study molecular rapid techniques to detect MDR
3. To develop and validate new biomarkers able to detect CAP patients early at risk of failure to intensify treatment and monitoring
4. To investigate in animal models and humans with CAP coadjuvant (including mac-rolides as immunomodulatory agents) treatments effective in decreasing treatment failure in severe CAP and in patients at risk of failure.

CASE STUDY

A 33-year-old man without comorbid illnesses went to the emergency room (ER) with fever for 2 days. No other respiratory symptoms were present.

On arrival to the ER, the examination showed the following: respiratory rate 22/min, blood pressure 130/85 mm Hg, temperature 39°C, pulse 110/min, oxygen saturation 94%.

Laboratory findings: CRP 11.11 mg/dL, blood urea nitrogen 20 mg/dL, sodium 135 mEq/L, potassium 4.3 mEq/L, glucose 119 mg/dL, white blood cell count 21.20 × 10^9/L, hematocrit 41%.

A chest radiograph (see **Fig. 1**) showed a condensation in the right upper lobe without pleural effusion.

A diagnosis of community-acquired pneumonia was made, PSI class I. The patient was discharged with levofloxacin.

Three days later, he returned to the ER with fever, pleuritic pain, and dyspnea.

On arrival, the patient had a respiratory rate 28/min, pulse 130/min, blood pressure 100/75 mm Hg, temperature 38.5°C, oxygen saturation 88%.

Laboratory findings were as follows: CRP 33.85 mg/dL, blood urea nitrogen 40 mg/dL, sodium 133 mEq/dL, potassium 4.5 mEq/L, glucose 126 mg/dL, white blood cell count 22.8 × 109/L, hematocrit 38%.

A new chest radiograph (see **Fig. 2**) showed pleural effusion fluid level. A CT scan (see **Figs. 3** and **4**) was performed showing images suggestive of consolidation in the right upper lobe, necrotizing pneumonia, and a loculated pleural empyema.

Thoracentesis was performed confirming pleural empyema.

With the diagnosis of progressive pneumonia, patient was admitted to the intensive care unit.

In the pleural fluid culture, colonies of *Streptococcus constellatus* were isolated.

REFERENCES

1. Menéndez R, Torres A, Reyes S, et al. Initial management of pneumonia and sepsis: factors associated with improved outcome. Eur Respir J 2012;39:156–62.
2. Ewig S, Woodhead M, Torres A. Towards a sensible comprehension of severe community-acquired pneumonia. Intensive Care Med 2011;37:214–23.
3. Menendez R, Torres A. Treatment failure in community-acquired pneumonia. Chest 2007;132:1348–55.
4. Halm EA, Fine MJ, Marrie TJ, et al. Time to clinical stability in patients hospitalized with CAP. JAMA 1998;279:1452–7.
5. Low DE, Mazulli T, Marrie T. Progressive and nonresolving pneumonia. Curr Opin Pulm Med 2005;11:247–52.
6. Kheir F, Hamdi T, Khayr W, et al. Nonresolving pneumonia. Am J Ther 2011;18: 77–9.
7. Mandell LA, Wunderink RG, Anzueto A, et al. Infectious Diseases Society of America/American Thoracic Society consensus guidelines on the management of community-acquired pneumonia in adults. Clin Infect Dis 2007;44:S27–72.
8. Montravers P, Fagon JY, Chastre J, et al. Follow-up protected specimen brushes to assess treatment in nosocomial pneumonia. Am Rev Respir Dis 1993;147(1): 38–44.
9. Rosón B, Carratala J, Fernández-Sabé N, et al. Causes and factors associated with early failure in hospitalized patients with community-acquired pneumonia. Arch Intern Med 2004;164:502–8.
10. Aliberti S, Amir A, Peyrani P, et al. Incidence, etiology, timing, and risk factors for clinical failure in hospitalized patients with community-acquired pneumonia. Chest 2008;134:955–62.
11. Aliberti S, Blasi F. Clinical stability versus clinical failure in patients with community-acquired pneumonia. Semin Respir Crit Care Med 2012;33(3):284–91.
12. Arancibia F, Ewig S, Martinez JA, et al. Antimicrobial treatment failures in patients with community-acquired pneumonia. Am J Respir Crit Care Med 2000;162:154–60.

13. Menéndez R, Torres A, Zalacaín R, et al. Risk factors of treatment failure in community acquired pneumonia: implications for disease outcome. Thorax 2004;59:960–5.
14. Celis MR, Torres A, Zalacaín R, et al. Working group for the study, diagnosis and treatment of CAP in Spain (NACE). Diagnostic methods and treatment of community-acquired pneumonia in Spain: NACE study. Med Clin (Barc) 2002; 119(9):321–6.
15. McCabe C, Kirchner C, Zhang H, et al. Guideline-concordant therapy and reduced mortality and length of stay in adults with community-acquired pneumonia. Arch Intern Med 2009;169(16):1525–31.
16. Ye X, Sikirica V, Schein JR, et al. Treatment failure rates and health care utilization and costs among patients with community-acquired pneumonia treated with levofloxacin or macrolides in an outpatient setting: a retrospective claims database analysis. Clin Ther 2008;30:358–71.
17. Ruiz-González A, Falguera M, Porcel JM, et al. C-reactive protein for discriminating treatment failure from slow responding pneumonia. Eur J Intern Med 2010;21:548–52.
18. Franquet T. Imaging of pneumonia: trends and algorithms. Eur Respir J 2001;18: 196–208.
19. Washington L, Palacio D. Imaging of bacterial pulmonary infection in the immunocompetent patient. Semin Roentgenol 2007;42:122–45.
20. Pereira Gomes JC, Pedreira WL, Araujo E, et al. Impact of BAL in the management of pneumonia with treatment failure positivity of BAL culture under antibiotic therapy. Chest 2000;118:1739–46.
21. Sanyal S, Smith PR, Saha AC, et al. Initial microbiologic studies did not affect outcome in adults hospitalized with community-acquired pneumonia. Am J Respir Crit Care Med 1999;160:346–8.
22. Menéndez R, Torres A, Zalacaíín R, et al. Guidelines for the treatment of community-acquired pneumonia. Predictors of adherence and outcome. Am J Respir Crit Care Med 2005;172:757–62.
23. Aliberti S, Di Pasquale M, Zanaboni AM, et al. Stratifying risk factors for multidrug-resistant pathogens in hospitalized patients coming from the community with pneumonia. Clin Infect Dis 2012;54(4):470–8.
24. Shorr AF, Zilberberg MD, Micek ST, et al. Prediction of infection due to antibiotic-resistant bacteria by select risk factors for health care-associated pneumonia. Arch Intern Med 2008;168(20):2205–10.
25. Wu CL, Yang DI, Wang NY, et al. Quantitative culture of endotracheal aspirates in the diagnosis of ventilator-associated pneumonia in patients with treatment failure. Chest 2002;122(2):662–8.
26. El Solh AA, Aquilina AT, Gunen H, et al. Radiographic resolution of community-acquired bacterial pneumonia in the elderly. J Am Geriatr Soc 2004;52:224–9.
27. Tomiyama N, Muller NL, Johkoh T, et al. Acute parenchymal lung disease in immunocompetent patients: diagnostic accuracy of high-resolution CT. AJR Am J Roentgenol 2000;174(6):1745–50.
28. Feinsilver SH, Fein AM, Niederman MS, et al. Utility of fiberoptic bronchoscopy in nonresolving pneumonia. Chest 1990;98:1322–6.
29. El-Solh A, Aquilina A, Dhillon R, et al. Impact of invasive strategy on management of antimicrobial treatment failure in institutionalized older people with severe pneumonia. Am J Respir Crit Care Med 2002;166:1038–43.
30. Moret I, Lorenzo MJ, Sarria B, et al. Increased lung neutrophil apoptosis and inflammation resolution in nonresponding pneumonia. Eur Respir J 2011;38:1158–64.

31. Bruns AH, Oosterheert JJ, Hak E, et al. Usefulness of consecutive C-reactive protein measurements in follow-up of severe community-acquired pneumonia. Eur Respir J 2008;32:726–32.

32. Menéndez R, Cavalcanti M, Reyes S, et al. Markers of treatment failure in hospitalized community acquired pneumonia. Thorax 2008;63(5):447–52.

33. Chalmers JD, Singanayagam A, Hill AT. C-reactive protein is an independent predictor of severity in community-acquired pneumonia. Am J Med 2008; 121(3):219–25.

34. Menéndez R, Martinez R, Reyes S, et al. Stability in community-acquired pneumonia: one step forward with markers? Thorax 2009;64(11):987–92.

35. Meijvis SC, Hardeman H, Remmelts HH, et al. Dexamethasone and length of hospital stay in patients with community-acquired pneumonia: a randomized, double-blind, placebo-controlled trial. Lancet 2011;137:2023–30.

36. Confalonieri M, Urbino R, Potena A, et al. Hydrocortisone infusion for severe community-acquired pneumonia: a preliminary randomized study. Am J Respir Crit Care Med 2005;171:242–8.

What is the Association of Cardiovascular Events with Clinical Failure in Patients with Community-Acquired Pneumonia?

Paula Peyrani, MD*, Julio Ramirez, MD

KEYWORDS

- Community-acquired pneumonia • Cardiovascular events • Clinical failure
- Mortality

KEY POINTS

- An increased risk of cardiovascular events (CVEs) in hospitalized patients with community-acquired pneumonia (CAP) was recently reported.
- CVEs may be the primary determinant of clinical failure in hospitalized patients with CAP.
- Therapeutics beyond antibiotics (eg, heparin or aspirin) may be indicated during and after hospitalization.

INTRODUCTION

Cardiovascular disease, including coronary artery disease, cerebrovascular disease, and peripheral vascular disease, is the leading cause of morbidity and mortality in the United States.[1] In patients with cardiovascular disease, the main cardiovascular events (CVEs) leading to morbidity and mortality are acute myocardial infarction (AMI), sudden cardiac death, unstable angina, arrhythmias, congestive heart failure (CHF), pulmonary embolisms, claudication, transient ischemic attacks, and stroke.

Atherosclerosis, the primary factor leading to cardiovascular disease, is considered a chronic inflammatory disease.[2] Several investigators recently reported an increased risk of CVEs in hospitalized patients with community-acquired pneumonia (CAP).[3,4] High levels of proinflammatory cytokines produced during an episode of CAP are speculated to trigger CVEs from endothelial dysfunction, atheroma instability, and rupture of the atheromatous plaque.

CAP is one of the primary causes of death caused by infectious disease in the United States.[5] Most deaths occur in hospitalized patients who progress to clinical

Division of Infectious Diseases, University of Louisville, 501 East Broadway, Suite 120, Louisville, KY 40202, USA
* Corresponding author. Division of Infectious Diseases, University of Louisville, 501 East Broadway, Suite 120, Louisville, KY 40202.
E-mail address: p0peyr01@louisville.edu

Infect Dis Clin N Am 27 (2013) 205–210
http://dx.doi.org/10.1016/j.idc.2012.11.010
0891-5520/13/$ – see front matter © 2013 Elsevier Inc. All rights reserved.

id.theclinics.com

failure after hospitalization. Development of a CVE in a hospitalized patient with CAP may produce a significant decline in the clinical status, and a severe CVE may be the primary determinant of clinical failure in a patient with CAP.

This article reviews the current data on CVEs in patients with CAP and explores the association between CVEs and clinical failure in these patients.

DEFINITIONS OF CLINICAL FAILURE AND CVEs

Different criteria have been used by different investigators to define the presence of clinical failure in hospitalized patients with CAP.[6] Using a pathophysiologic approach, clinical failure can be characterized as being related to either CAP or the management of CAP (**Fig. 1**).[7] Clinical failure related to CAP is explained by the pathophysiology of the pulmonary infection with its associated local and systemic inflammatory response. Clinical failure related to CAP may develop from the progression of the local pulmonary infection (see **Fig. 1**: A.1); development of a metastatic foci of infection, such as meningitis or endocarditis (see **Fig. 1**: A.2); development of severe sepsis and/or organ failure, such as septic shock or acute respiratory distress syndrome (see **Fig. 1**: A.3); or development of a medical complication related to the systemic inflammatory response, such as a myocardial infarction, stroke, or any other cardiovascular event (see **Fig. 1**: A.4). Clinical failure related to the management of CAP, such as the development of *Clostridium difficile* colitis from antibiotics, is not associated with the pathogenesis of CAP.

According to the timing, clinical failure can be characterized as occurring during hospitalization, within 30 days of hospitalization, or during long-term follow-up. At each of these periods, clinical failure may or may not be related to the development of a CVE (**Fig. 2**).

Studies in the field of CAP evaluating the presence of CVEs have used different definitions of a CVE. Because most of these studies have been retrospectives observational studies, the definition of a CVE was based primarily on the presence of the

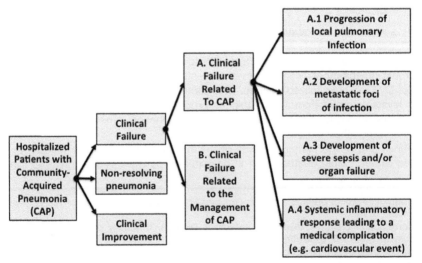

Fig. 1. Pathophysiologic classification of clinical failure in patients with CAP. (*Data from* Aliberti S, Amir A, Peyrani P, et al. Incidence, etiology, timing, and risk factors for clinical failure in hospitalized patients with community-acquired pneumonia. Chest 2008;134:955–62.)

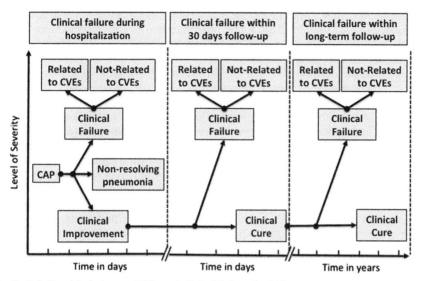

Fig. 2. Relationship between CVEs and clinical failure in CAP.

clinical diagnosis in the medical record documented by the treating physician. Clinical studies have used the following definitions for CVE[4,8–12]:

- Arrhythmias: (1) atrial flutter, atrial fibrillation, ventricular tachycardia; (2) atrial fibrillation; (3) new-onset or worsening supraventricular arrhythmias and ventricular bigeminy/tachycardia; or (4) atrial fibrillation, atrial flutter, supraventricular tachycardia, multifocal atrial tachycardia, ventricular tachycardia, or ventricular fibrillation.
- Heart failure: new or worsened CHF defined by Framingham criteria.
- AMI: (1) a typical increase and gradual decrease in biochemical markers of myocardial necrosis and ischemic symptoms, development of pathologic Q waves on electrocardiogram, electrocardiogram changes indicative of ischemia, or coronary artery intervention; (2) pathologic findings of AMI; or (3) ST elevation myocardial infarction (STEMI).
- Stroke: (1) new-onset neurologic deficit lasting more than 24 hours, with a confirmatory CT or MRI.
- Acute coronary syndrome (ACS): (1) presence of evolving diagnostic changes in electrocardiogram or diagnostic cardiac biomarkers; (2) electronic findings consistent with ischemia plus cardiac symptoms or signs; or (3) acute non-STEMI (compatible electrocardiogram changes along with positive troponin I and a clinical diagnosis of non-STEMI or unstable angina).

CVEs AND CLINICAL FAILURE WITHIN 30 DAYS' FOLLOW-UP

Most studies evaluating the association between CVEs and CAP have evaluated patients during hospitalization. Some of these studies evaluated the incidence of CVEs during hospitalization for CAP, whereas others also included the association between CVEs and clinical outcomes. Of these, only one study reported data on clinical failure.[7]

In a retrospective cohort study of 170 consecutive patients hospitalized for pneumococcal pneumonia, almost 20% developed CVEs, which included AMI, serious arrhythmias, and CHF.[8] Another retrospective cohort study of 206 patients evaluating the incidence of ACS within 15 days after hospitalization for CAP reported that 11% of the patients with pneumonia had ACS, with an 8-fold increased risk for developing CVEs compared with control patients.[10]

The association between AMI and clinical failure was evaluated in an observational study of 500 consecutive patients hospitalized with CAP. Development of AMI was diagnosed in 29 patients (5.8%). Patients who developed AMI had a longer time to clinical stability and length of stay. Clinical failure was identified in 52% of patients with AMI versus 11% in patients without AMI (P<.001). Increased mortality during hospitalization and at 30 days was also seen in patients with AMI (28% vs 7% and 31% vs 10%, respectively).[9] In another study from the same group using the same cohort of patients, the authors evaluated clinical failure as related or unrelated to CAP. Among 67 patients who developed clinical failure, 81% were related to CAP. Although AMI was the second cause of clinical failure after sepsis, all CVEs combined were the number one cause of clinical failure related to CAP.[7] More recently, data from a multicenter prospective cohort of patients with CAP showed increased mortality in patients with CAP with CVEs compared with those without CVE (15.3% vs 2.8%; odds ratio, 3.5; 95% CI, 2.3–5.2).[13] Finally, a study evaluating risk factors for acute cardiac events in hospitalized patients with CAP reported that CVEs were independently associated with 30-day mortality, with an odds ratio of 2.18 (95% CI, 1.38–3.42).[4]

CVEs AND CLINICAL FAILURE AT LONG-TERM FOLLOW-UP

Although several articles reported increased long-term mortality in hospitalized patients with CAP,[14,15] CVEs were only recently implicated as one of the possible explanations for this increased mortality.[11,16–18] In a study designed to understanding mechanisms and predictors of increased long-term mortality, the authors evaluated the association between serum markers of inflammation and mortality within the first year after an episode of pneumonia.[16] This study reported CVE as the first cause of death over 1 year, with increased interleukin (IL)-6 concentrations at the time of discharge from the hospital. The authors proposed that a persistent inflammatory response even after discharge increases the risk of CVEs and therefore mortality. In a Canadian study, patients were followed for a maximum of 5.4 years after hospitalization because of CAP.[17] All-cause mortality was reported to be 12% at 30 days, 28% within 1 year, and 53% by the end of the study. Readmissions were also evaluated, with 2% occurring within 30 days and 9% within 1 year. CVEs were the second cause after other respiratory diseases for non–pneumonia-related rehospitalizations. Another study evaluated the frequency of cardiovascular and cerebrovascular events in 4408 hospitalized patients with CAP and its association with poor outcomes at 90 days. The authors reported an increased mortality at 90 days in patients who developed CVEs and cerebrovascular events compared with those who did not.[11] Another recent study assessing the relationship between hemostasis markers and long-term mortality found that cancer was the principal cause of death over 1 year and CVEs as the second.[18]

SUMMARY

Increased incidence of CVEs associated with increased clinical failure and mortality rates has been documented in hospitalized patients with CAP.

Investigators have hypothesized that the increased risk of CVEs in this population is partly from atherosclerotic plaque instability related to the systemic inflammation from the pneumonia. This close relationship between CAP and CVEs is further evidenced by the seasonality of both processes and the reduction of CVEs seen after vaccination for influenza.[19]

Another hypothesis that can explain this association is the cardiovascular stress produce by the hypoxemia associated with pneumonia and the tachycardia associated with systemic infection. The hypercoagulability state associated with sepsis may also play a role in the development of ischemia with the subsequent development of CVEs.

More evidence is being published regarding the association between CVEs and mortality in hospitalized patients with CAP, both short- and long-term. Future research may be necessary to identify patients at risk of CVEs during or after an episode of CAP. Other interventions beyond antibiotics (eg, heparin or aspirin) may be indicated in these patients during and after hospitalization.

REFERENCES

1. World Health Organization. Cardiovascular diseases (CVDs). Available at: http://www.who.int/mediacentre/factsheets/fs317/en/index.html. Accessed October 9, 2012.
2. Ross R. Atherosclerosis is an inflammatory disease. Am Heart J 1999;138(5 Pt 2): S419–20.
3. Singanayagam A, Singanayagam A, Elder DH, et al. Is community-acquired pneumonia an independent risk factor for cardiovascular disease? Eur Respir J 2012;39(1):187–96.
4. Viasus D, Garcia-Vidal C, Manresa F, et al. Risk stratification and prognosis of acute cardiac events in hospitalized adults with community-acquired pneumonia. J Infect 2012. http://dx.doi.org/10.1016/j.jinf.2012.09.003. [Epub ahead of print].
5. Heron H. Deaths: leading causes for 2008. Natl Vital Stat Rep 2012;60(6):1–94.
6. Aliberti S, Blasi F. Clinical stability versus clinical failure in patients with community-acquired pneumonia. Semin Respir Crit Care Med 2012;33(3):284–91.
7. Aliberti S, Amir A, Peyrani P, et al. Incidence, etiology, timing, and risk factors for clinical failure in hospitalized patients with community-acquired pneumonia. Chest 2008;134(5):955–62.
8. Musher DM, Rueda AM, Kaka AS, et al. The association between pneumococcal pneumonia and acute cardiac events. Clin Infect Dis 2007;45(2):158–65.
9. Ramirez J, Aliberti S, Mirsaeidi M, et al. Acute myocardial infarction in hospitalized patients with community-acquired pneumonia. Clin Infect Dis 2008;47(2):182–7.
10. Corrales-Medina VF, Serpa J, Rueda AM, et al. Acute bacterial pneumonia is associated with the occurrence of acute coronary syndromes. Medicine (Baltimore) 2009;88(3):154–9.
11. Mandal P, Chalmers JD, Choudhury G, et al. Vascular complications are associated with poor outcome in community-acquired pneumonia. QJM 2011;104(6):489–95.
12. Corrales-Medina VF, Musher DM, Wells GA, et al. Cardiac complications in patients with community-acquired pneumonia: incidence, timing, risk factors, and association with short-term mortality. Circulation 2012;125(6):773–81.
13. Corrales-Medina VF, Suh KN, Rose G, et al. Cardiac complications in patients with community-acquired pneumonia: a systematic review and meta-analysis of observational studies. PLoS Med 2011;8(6):e1001048.
14. Mortensen EM. Potential causes of increased long-term mortality after pneumonia. Eur Respir J 2011;37(6):1306–7.
15. Bordon J, Wiemken T, Peyrani P, et al. Decrease in long-term survival for hospitalized patients with community-acquired pneumonia. Chest 2010;138(2):279–83.

16. Yende S, D'Angelo G, Kellum JA, et al. Inflammatory markers at hospital discharge predict subsequent mortality after pneumonia and sepsis. Am J Respir Crit Care Med 2008;177(11):1242–7.

17. Johnstone J, Eurich DT, Majumdar SR, et al. Long-term morbidity and mortality after hospitalization with community-acquired pneumonia: a population-based cohort study. Medicine (Baltimore) 2008;87(6):329–34.

18. Yende S, Milbrandt EB, Kellum JA, et al. Understanding the potential role of statins in pneumonia and sepsis. Crit Care Med 2011;39(8):1871–8.

19. Corrales-Medina VF, Madjid M, Musher DM. Role of acute infection in triggering acute coronary syndromes. Lancet Infect Dis 2010;10(2):83–92.

What is the Role of Antimicrobial Stewardship in Improving Outcomes of Patients with CAP?

Veronique Nussenblatt, MD, MHS[a], Edina Avdic, PharmD, MBA[b],
Sara Cosgrove, MD, MS[a],*

KEYWORDS

- Antimicrobial stewardship • Community-acquired pneumonia • CAP • Outcomes

KEY POINTS

- Adherence to antibiotic treatment guidelines is inconsistent and the erroneous diagnosis of community-acquired pneumonia (CAP) and misuse of antibiotics is prevalent.
- Short-course therapy for CAP has been shown to be as clinically effective as longer-course therapy and is associated with fewer adverse events.
- Switching from parenteral to oral antibiotics is safe at 48–72 hours even in patients with severe CAP who meet criteria for clinical stability.
- Antimicrobial stewardship programs should consider interventions to reduce duration of therapy, enhance conversion to oral therapy, and use procalcitonin to guide the need for antibiotics at the start of and during therapy. Such interventions have led to reduced antibiotic exposure without evidence of causing patient harm.

INTRODUCTION

Community-acquired pneumonia (CAP) is one of the most common infectious diagnoses encountered in clinical practice and is one of the leading causes of death in the United States, where it affects up to 4 million people a year.[1,2] It has been estimated that annual direct medical costs of health care for patients with CAP is up to $8.5 billion.[3] Given the magnitude of antibiotic use associated with treatment of CAP, ensuring that CAP is diagnosed correctly and patients receive appropriate

Disclosures: In the last two years, Dr Cosgrove has been a consultant for Merck, Novartis, Cerexa, and Ribx. She has received grants from Cubist and AdvanDx. Drs Nussenblatt and Avdic have no disclosures.
[a] Division of Infectious Diseases, Department of Medicine, The Johns Hopkins University School of Medicine, Osler 425, 600 North Wolfe Street, Baltimore, MD 21287, USA; [b] Department of Pharmacy, The Johns Hopkins Hospital, Osler 425, 600 North Wolfe Street, Baltimore, MD 21287, USA
* Corresponding author. Johns Hopkins Medical Institutions, Osler 425, 600 North Wolfe Street, Baltimore, MD 21287.
E-mail address: scosgro1@jhmi.edu

Infect Dis Clin N Am 27 (2013) 211–228
http://dx.doi.org/10.1016/j.idc.2012.11.008
0891-5520/13/$ – see front matter © 2013 Elsevier Inc. All rights reserved.

id.theclinics.com

empiric and definitive therapy for the optimal course to achieve clinical cure and reduce risk of adverse events is critical. This review summarizes interventions that may be promoted by antimicrobial stewardship programs to reduce exposure to unnecessary antibiotics, minimize adverse events, and improve outcomes for patients with CAP (**Tables 1** and **2**).

Early recognition of CAP and the administration of appropriate empiric antibiotics are essential for optimizing patient outcomes. The Infectious Diseases Society of America and American Thoracic Society guidelines provide recommendations for the empiric antibiotic treatment of patients with CAP[1] and several studies have demonstrated that adherence to antibiotic guidelines improves survival in patients with CAP.[4,5] Despite these findings, adherence to antibiotic treatment guidelines is inconsistent and the erroneous diagnosis of CAP and misuse of antibiotics is prevalent in both inpatients and outpatients.[6–11] In 2004, the requirement to administer antibiotics to patients suspected of having CAP within 4 hours of arrival to an emergency department was adopted as a reportable "core measure" by the Centers for Medicare and Medicaid Services (CMS) to enforce compliance with guidelines for the treatment of patients with CAP. Concerns by the scientific community that this core measure was based on limited scientific evidence prompted several studies demonstrating that the implementation of the measure led to the frequent misdiagnosis of CAP and the overuse of antibiotics before the establishment of the diagnosis of CAP[9,12,13] or to avoid repercussions of noncompliance with CMS CAP guidelines.[14] This core measure was subsequently changed to require that antibiotics be administered within 6 hours of presentation but were ultimately removed as of January 2012 as a core measure by CMS. Increased length of stay for hospitalized patients, risk of adverse events, and the emergence of antimicrobial resistance are negative outcomes that have been associated with unnecessary antibiotic use.[15,16] Shortening antibiotic regimens to treat CAP, "antibiotic switching" from intravenous (IV) to oral (PO) regimens, and using a procalcitonin-guided approach for the antimicrobial management of patients with suspected CAP are examples of interventions that could be incorporated into stewardship algorithms to improve patient outcomes.

Is Short-Course Antibiotic Therapy as Effective and Safe as Long-Course Antibiotic Therapy for CAP?

Several studies have shown that shorter courses of antibiotics are as effective and safe as extended courses of antibiotics and can reduce costs associated with the treatment for CAP.[17–32] Most of these studies have been randomized clinical trials performed in the inpatient setting and largely focus on antibiotic regimens containing macrolides, whereas some earlier studies examined beta-lactams and more recent studies examined quinolone-containing regimens. Most studies were performed before the most recent guideline recommendations to provide empiric therapy for CAP with a fluoroquinolone or beta-lactam-macrolide combination to provide coverage for atypical pathogens.[1]

Two meta-analyses have specifically addressed the effectiveness and safety of short-course versus long-course antibacterial therapy for CAP.[31,32] Li and colleagues[32] published a meta-analysis that included 15 randomized controlled trials comparing antibiotic courses of 7 days or fewer to extended courses of more than 7 days for mild to moderate CAP. There was no significant difference in the risk of clinical failure, mortality, or adverse events between the groups receiving short-course and extended-course therapy. Another meta-analysis by Dimopoulos and colleagues[31] looked at 7 randomized clinical trials, including 2 that included children, and also found that there was no significant difference in mortality and cure rates or adverse events for patients receiving short-course therapy, defined as 7 or fewer days, versus long courses, defined as more than 7 days, of antibiotics.

Short-course therapy with beta-lactams

Two studies performed in the 1970s and early 1980s provided initial data that use of short-course therapy for CAP is as effective as long-course therapy. Sutton and colleagues[17] showed that a single dose of long-acting or mixed long-acting and crystalline penicillin administered via intramuscular (IM) route or a day of oral penicillin in combination with probenecid was as effective as a 5-day course of standard penicillin administered IM or orally in achieving clinical cure rates for CAP of 87% to 95% among inpatients in Zimbabwe. A study performed in inpatients in Papua New Guinea by Ree and Davis[18] with 4 arms compared crystalline penicillin until 24 hours after defervescence followed by either procaine penicillin or placebo until discharge versus chloramphenicol until defervescence followed by either chloramphenicol or placebo until discharge found that in patients with moderate and severe CAP, short-course therapy (mean 2.1–2.8 days) had similar cure rates to long-term therapy (mean 5.3–6.2 days). Length of stay was similar between patients receiving short-course and long-course therapy; however, patients given shorter therapy (placebo) were kept in the hospital for several days after termination of therapy to assess the effect of treatment.

More recent studies have also demonstrated the efficacy of shorter therapy for CAP. Siegel and colleagues[19] found no significant difference in clinical cure rates for hospitalized patients receiving cefuroxime 750 mg IV q8 h for 2 days followed by cefuroxime 500 mg PO q12 h for 5 days versus 8 days. El Moussaoui and colleagues[20] randomized hospitalized patients who had received IV amoxicillin for 3 days and had clinical response to receive either 5 additional amoxicillin 750 mg PO TID or placebo; both arms had the same cure rates (89%).

Short-course therapy was not associated with increased mortality in studies that assessed this outcome, and overall, mortality rates were low (<1%). Two of 4 deaths occurred in the short-course penicillin group in the Ree and Davis study; however, this group had a greater number of patients with severe CAP compared with the other treatment groups.[18] None of the studies reported a significant difference in length of stay between patients receiving shorter versus longer treatment courses. In one study,[18] patients receiving shorter-course therapy were kept in the hospital for observation as part of the study. Three studies reported costs associated with shorter treatment.[17,19,20] Siegel and colleagues[19] estimated that treating patients with the 7-day course of antibiotics instead of a 10-day course could amount to $27,242,000 in savings a year in antibiotic costs alone. A cost analysis of the El Moussaoui and colleagues' study, however, found that the reduction in cost associated with a 1-day shorter admission for patients who received 3 days of antibiotics was offset by a slightly higher number of patient-initiated primary health care provider visits, resulting in a nonsubstantial decrease in cost and average resource use by these patients.[20] Only 1 study reported the effect of short-course therapy on adverse events.[20] Adverse events were nearly halved in the 3-day therapy group compared with the 8-day therapy group; however, this was not a significant difference (21% vs 11%, $P = .1$).

In summary, existing studies that have evaluated the effect of short-course beta-lactam treatment for CAP suggest that 3 to 5 days of therapy with beta-lactam agents is safe and has comparable cure and mortality rates compared with longer courses of therapy in most patients. It is reasonable to expect that the same duration of beta-lactam therapy would yield similar results among many current patients with CAP, particularly when a macrolide is added empirically at the start of therapy as recommended by guidelines in the United States.[1] It is important to note that 2 of the studies

Table 1
Studies evaluating short-course therapy for community-acquired pneumonia, by antibiotic

Antibiotic Group	Reference	Severity	Type of Study/ Location	Drug Regimen	Mortality	Length of Stay	Cost	Clinical Cure	Adverse Events
						Outcome			
Penicillins, cephalosporins	Sutton et al,[17] 1970	Not reported	Randomized clinical trial/In-patient	Crystalline PCN 1 million units IM q6 h × 5 d	1 death from staphylococcal empyema in hetacillin group	1 wk (average for all groups)		19/20 (95%)	Not reported
				Crystalline PCN 1 million units IM then 500,000 units IM q6 h × 4 d			$1.95	27/28 (96%)	
				Hetacillin 500 mg PO then 250 mg PO q6 h × 5 d				18/20 (90%)	
				Clemizole PCN G 1 million units IM × 1			$0.75	20/23 (87%)	
				Clemizole PCN G 1 million units IM + crystalline PCN 1 million units × 1			$0.80	18/19 (95%)	
				Bicillin 2 mL IM × 1			$0.40	18/19 (95%)	
				Ampicillin 2 g + probenacid 1 g q12 h × 24 h			$4.10	19/21 (90%)	
	Ree and Davis,[18] 1983	Moderate-severe	Not specified/ Inpatient	Crystalline PCN 4 mega units daily until 24 h after defervescence then, Procaine PCN 1.2 mega units IM daily until discharge	1 death	6.7	Not reported	Not reported	Not reported
				or Placebo	2 deaths	6.8			

Study	Severity	Study design/Setting	Regimen	Mortality/clinical failures	Length of stay	Cost	Clinical cure rate	Relapse rate
			Chloramphenicol 1.5 g PO daily until 24 h after defervescence then, 1.5 g PO daily until discharge or Placebo	1 death	5.6 6.5	No difference between groups		
Siegel et al,[19] 1999	Moderately severe	Open randomized double blind study/In-patient	Cefuroxime 750 mg IV q8 h × 2 d then, Cefuroxime 500 mg PO q12 h × 8 d or Cefuroxime 500 mg PO q12 h × 5 d	Not reported		$27 million in savings if limited to 7-d course of antibiotics	20/22 (90.9%) 21/24 (87.5%)	Not reported
El Moussaoui et al,[20] 2006	Mild to moderate-severe	Randomized double-blind placebo-controlled trial/In-patient	Amoxicillin IV × 3 d, then (if symptomatically better) 750 mg PO TID × 5 d Placebo × 5 d	1 death 1 death	8.9 7.9	Not reported	ITT: 56/63 (89%) PP: 56/60 (93%) ITT: 50/56 (89%) PP: 50/54 (93%)	21% 11%
Macrolides								
Schonwald et al,[21] 1990	Not reported	Open, randomized, multicenter study/Inpatient and outpatient	Azithromycin 250 mg PO bid on day 1, 250 mg PO daily on days 2–5 Erythromycin 500 mg PO QID × 10 d	Not reported but no clinical failures in either group	Not reported	Not reported	32/39 (82%) 27/32 (84%)	1.85% 13.6%
Kinasewitz and Wood,[22] 1991	Not reported	Randomized double-blind multicenter study/Not reported	Azithromycin 500 mg PO × 1 then 250 mg daily × 4 d Cefaclor 500 mg PO TID × 10 d	No deaths in either group	Not reported	Not reported	15/32 (46.9%) 16/39 (41.0%)	18.9% 12.1%

(continued on next page)

Table 1
(continued)

Antibiotic Group	Reference	Severity	Type of Study/Location	Drug Regimen	Mortality	Length of Stay	Cost	Clinical Cure	Adverse Events
						Outcome			
	Schonwald et al,[23] 1994	Not reported	Open, randomized multicenter study/Inpatient	Azithromycin 500 mg PO daily × 3 d; Roxithromycin 150 mg PO BID × 10 d	Not reported	Not reported	Not reported	88/89 (98.9%); 50/53 (94.3%)	16.9%; 15.1%
	Rizzato et al,[24] 1995	Low to moderately severe	Open randomized study/Inpatient	Azithromycin 500 mg PO daily × 3 d; Clarithromycin 250 mg PO BID × 8 d	Not reported	Not reported	Not reported	20/20 (100%); 17/19 (89.5%)	Not reported
	O'Doherty and Muller,[25] 1998	Mild to moderate	Randomized nonblinded/Outpatient	Azithromycin 500 mg PO daily × 3 d; Clarithromycin 250 mg PO BID × 10 d	Not reported	Not reported	Not reported	83/88 (94%); 84/88 (95%)	14%; 13%
	Rahav et al,[26] 2004	Not reported	Open, randomized open-label multicenter study/Outpatient	Azithromycin 500 mg PO daily × 3 d; Physician discretion	Not reported	Not reported	$7237.60 saved/100 treated patients	61/62 (98.4%); 40/46 (87%)	4.8%; Not reported
	Tellier et al,[27] 2004	Mild to moderate	Randomized, double-blind, active-controlled multicenter study/Inpatient and Outpatient	Telithromycin 800 mg PO daily × 5 d or 7 d; Clarithromycin 500 mg BID × 10 d	1 death; 2 deaths; 2 deaths	Not reported	Not reported	142/159 (89.3%); 143/161 (88.8%); 134/146 (91.8%)	24.4%; 21.0%; 21.9%
	D'Ignazio et al,[28] 2005	Mild to moderate	Randomized, double-blind, noninferiority multicenter study/Outpatient	Single-dose azithromycin microspheres 2.0 g; Levofloxacin 500 mg PO × 7 d	1 death; 2 deaths	Not reported	Not reported	156/174 (89.7%); 177/189 (93.7%)	19.9%; 12.3%

Fluoroquinolones	Dunbar et al,[29] 2003	Mild-severe	Randomized double-blind active treatment controlled noninferiority study/Inpatient	Levofloxacin 750 mg × 5 d Levofloxacin 500 mg × 10 d	Not reported	Not reported	Not reported	183/198 (92.4%) 175/192 (91.1%)	Similar in both groups, percentages not reported
	File et al,[30] 2007	Mild to moderate	Double-blind randomized active controlled parallel group multicenter study/ Outpatient	Gemifloxacin 320 mg PO daily × 5 d Gemifloxacin 320 mg PO daily × 7 d	Not reported	Not reported	Not reported	ITT: 237/256 (92.6%) PP: 230/242 (95.0%) ITT: 221/254 (87.0%) PP: 209/227 (92.1%)	Discontinuation rates/rash: 1.2%/0.4% 2%/2.8%
N/A	Li et al,[32] 2007	Mild to moderate	Meta-analysis/ Inpatient and outpatient	≤7 d regimen >7 d regimen	RR 0.81 (95% CI 0.46–1.43)	Not reported	Not reported	Risk of clinical failure RR 0.89 (95% CI 0.78–1.02)	RR 0.86 (95% CI 0.71–1.04)
	Dimopoulos et al,[31] 2008	Mild to moderate	Meta-analysis/ Inpatient and outpatient	≤7-d regimen >9 d	OR 0.57 (95% CI 0.23–1.43)	Not reported	Not reported	OR 0.89 (95% CI 0.74–1.07)	OR 0.9 (95% CI 0.72–1.13)

Abbreviations: BID, twice a day; CI, confidence interval; IM, intramuscular; IV, intravenous; ITT, intention to treat; OR, odds ratio; PCN, penicillin; PO, by mouth; PP, per protocol; q, every; QID, 4 times daily; TID, 3 times a day.

Table 2
Studies evaluating antimicrobial interventions targeting switch therapy or short course treatment of community-acquired pneumonia

Paper	Study Design	Intervention	Mortality	Outcomes	Complications	Length of Stay
Fine et al,[61] 2003	Cluster randomized clinical trial	1. Detailed sheet placed in chart advising conversion from IV to PO antibiotics 2. Nursing help to switch from IV to PO antibiotics and with discharge planning	No difference (5% vs 7%)	No difference in time to discontinuation of IV antibiotics (HR 1.23; 95% CI 1.00–1.52; $P = .06$)	No difference in re-hospitalization and in-hospital complications between groups	No difference between groups (median 5 d in each arm)
Schouten et al,[60] 2007	Cluster-randomized control trial	1. Key lecture 2. Distribution of consensus "critical-care pathways" 3. Hospital-specific tailored interventions	No difference between groups (7.2% vs 8.7%)	Improvement in % antibiotic therapy stopped after 3 d of defervescence (+13.3% vs −7.7%)	Less likely to be admitted to a respiratory unit (83% vs 91.3%) No differences in ICU admission rates	No difference between groups (median 8 vs 10 d)
Carratala et al,[59] 2012	Randomized trial	3-step critical pathway 1. Early mobilization 2. Switch to oral antibiotic therapy once clinically stable 3. Use of predefined criteria for deciding on hospital discharge.	No difference between groups (1.0, 95% CI −1.4 to 3.4; $P = .45$)	Shorter length of IV therapy (−2.0, 95% CI −2.0 to −1.0; $P<.001$)	Adverse events −11.4% points (95% CI, −17.2% to −5.6%; $P<.001$) No difference in readmissions	−2.1 d (95% CI −2.7 to −1.7; $P<.001$)
Avdic et al,[62] 2012	Prospective, observational	1. Educational lecture 2. Direct oral feedback regarding suggested changes in antibiotic management	Not reported	Decreased duration of antibiotic therapy (median 7 d vs 10 d, $P<.001$)	No difference in Clostridium difficile infection rates or 30-d readmission rates	No difference (median 4 vs 5 d)

Abbreviations: CI, confidence interval; HR, hazard ratio; ICU, intensive care unit; IV, intravenous; PO, by mouth.

required demonstration of clinical improvement before randomization to short-course versus long-course therapy; such an assessment also seems prudent in clinical practice when opting for shorter-course therapy. Two of the studies were performed several years ago in resource-limited settings[17,18] where comorbidities and hospital practices may differ from current practice in other settings; thus, the generalizability of their findings may be limited. Finally, certain patient populations were not reported on in the studies described, including patients with HIV and low CD4 counts and those with other forms of immunosuppression; thus, a specific recommendation regarding short-course therapy in these groups cannot be made.

Short-course therapy with macrolides

Several studies have evaluated the use of short-course azithromycin therapy (ranging from 3 to 5 days) among inpatients and have consistently shown that short-course therapy is as effective as extended courses of other macrolides[21,23,24] and cephalosporins.[22,24,26–28] A trend toward slightly higher cure rates in patients treated with shorter course therapy was noted in some studies.[22,24,26] Few of these studies specifically report mortality rates, possibly because of the low severity of CAP in their patients; although severity is not always specified, the studies that do provide this information included patients with low to moderate severity. Differences in length of stay and costs are not reported in any of the studies, except for the study by Rahav and colleagues,[26] which estimates that more than $7,000 could be saved per 100 treated patients by using short-course therapy.

Although the data are limited, the studies available in outpatients demonstrate that a 3-day to 5-day course of azithromycin for CAP should suffice to achieve comparable cure rates to an extended course. A study by O'Doherty and Muller[25] found that a 3-day course of azithromycin 500 mg daily is as effective as clarithromycin 250 mg PO twice daily for 10 days in outpatients with CAP. In 2004, a multicenter randomized open label study by Rahav and colleagues[26] reported clinical cure rates of 98.4% in outpatients with CAP treated with azithromycin 500 mg PO for 3 days compared with 87% in patients treated at the discretion of their physicians (a variety of agents from different antibiotic classes).

In summary, although short-course treatment for CAP with macrolides appears to be safe in patients with mild to moderate infection with similar cure rates to extended therapy, 5 of 8 studies were open, nonblinded randomized studies, which introduces the potential for bias when assessing patient outcomes. However, use of macrolide monotherapy for CAP among outpatients or to complete a course of therapy in hospitalized patients may become less desirable if macrolide-resistant *Streptococcus pneumoniae* or *Haemophilus influenzae* isolates are prevalent in the community, as has been reported in some areas.[33,34] Additionally, it is important to note that azithromycin reaches high lung tissue and cellular concentrations and persists at therapeutic concentrations in the lungs for up to 10 days after cessation of therapy[35]; therefore, 3 days of azithromycin may be not comparable to 3 days of beta-lactam or clarithromycin therapy. The safety of using short-course macrolide therapy in severe CAP is not known. Although there do not appear to be significant differences in adverse events between long-course and short-course therapy with macrolides, no conclusions can be made about the effect of short-course therapy on length of stay and cost given the limited data available.

Short-course therapy with fluoroquinolones

Only 2 studies have assessed short-course fluoroquinolone therapy for CAP.[29,30] Dunbar and colleagues[29] found that levofloxacin 750 mg PO for 5 days was as effective in treating CAP as 500 mg PO for 10 days in inpatients with mild to severe CAP. Cure rates were similar in the short-course and long-course arms (92.8% vs 91.1%). More recently, successful treatment with a 5-day course of gemifloxacin occurred as frequently as with a 7-day course in outpatients (92.6% vs 87.0%).[30] In that study, short-course antibiotic therapy was associated with lower antibiotic discontinuation rates (1.2% vs 2.0%) as well as rash (0.4% vs 2.8%). Neither study addressed differences in mortality or costs between the 2 treatment groups.

Is Early Transition to Oral Therapy Safe and Effective During CAP Therapy?

The early discontinuation of IV antibiotics and switch to oral antibiotics has been demonstrated to be safe in patients who meet specific criteria demonstrating clinical stability in several observational studies.[36–41] This approach, termed "switch therapy," is generally considered appropriate when a patient's respiratory symptoms have improved, they are no longer febrile or hypoxic, mental status has returned to baseline, and the patient is thought to have adequate oral intake and gastrointestinal tract absorption.[1] Several of the earlier studies demonstrating the safety of switch therapy also included the resolution of leukocytosis as a criterion for clinical stability. This approach also appears to be safe for patients with Streptococcus pneumoniae bacteremia. In a study by Ramirez and Bordon,[42] there were no clinical failures in 18 of 36 patients admitted with CAP complicated by Streptococcus pneumoniae bacteremia who met clinical criteria for stability and were switched to oral therapy.

Several randomized trials have reported decreased length of hospital stay and costs, as well decreased antibiotic-adverse events without compromising safety in patients switched to oral therapy at 48 to 72 hours.[43–47] Castro-Guardiola and colleagues[44] randomized 85 hospitalized patients with nonsevere pneumonia to receive oral antibiotics from admission or parenteral antibiotics until they had been afebrile for 72 hours before switching to oral treatment to complete a 7-day course of antibiotics. A total of 103 hospitalized patients with severe CAP (defined as having vital sign instability, altered mental status, and multilobar infection) were randomized to a 10-day course of parenteral antibiotics or parenteral antibiotics followed by early switch to oral antibiotics at 48 hours to complete a 10-day course. There were no significant differences in mortality, resolution of morbidity, or treatment failures between treatment groups for both the patients with severe and nonsevere CAP. There were fewer adverse events associated with the oral treatment among the patients with nonsevere CAP and the patients with severe CAP who were switched to oral antibiotics early, mostly because of lower rates of infusion-related phlebitis. Both of these groups also had cost savings, but this was significant only for the patients with severe pneumonia. Although the length of stay was equivalent for patients with nonsevere CAP, patients with severe CAP who received a full course of parenteral therapy had a significantly longer hospital stay (4 days) compared with those given early-switch therapy.[44]

Oosterheert and colleagues[45] randomized 302 nonintubated patients with severe CAP to receive parenteral treatment for 3 days followed by oral antibiotics when clinically stable or 7 days of parenteral antibiotics. Eighty-one percent of the patients enrolled in their study met the criteria for clinical stability at 3 days and there were no differences in clinical cure rates; however, length of hospital stay was significantly reduced. A cost-benefit analysis of a randomized study comparing a 7-day course of IV cefamandole to parenteral therapy for 2 days followed by oral therapy with cefaclor for 5 days found that hospital length of stay for patients switched to oral therapy was 2 days shorter than for the IV group only and total cost of care was reduced by 40%. In this study as well, no difference was found in cure rates or survival between the

2 groups.[46] A meta-analysis evaluating early switch to oral treatment in 1219 hospitalized patients with moderate to severe CAP enrolled in randomized clinical trials found that there was no difference in mortality, treatment success, or recurrence of CAP in patients switched to oral therapy versus those given parenteral therapy alone.[48] Duration of hospitalization was shorter for patients switched to oral therapy, and these patients had fewer antibiotic-associated adverse events. Another meta-analysis by Rhew and colleagues[49] found considerable variation in the application of early switch therapy and discharge criteria among studies evaluating switch therapy; however, the mean length of hospital stay was reduced by 3 days in patients who had early switch of oral antibiotics and early discharge when studies in which the recommended length of stay was longer than the control length of stay were excluded from the analysis.

Patient satisfaction does not appear to be affected by the early switch to oral antibiotics, as evidenced by 93% to 95% of patients treated with early switch therapy reporting that they did not feel that they were sent home too soon.[38,41]

In summary, several randomized trials including patients with both severe and non-severe CAP have shown that early switch to oral therapy is safe and associated with fewer adverse events. Most studies are more recent than those evaluating short-course therapy, potentially making their findings more generalizable to current patients with CAP; however, as clinical practice moves toward use of shorter courses of therapy overall for CAP, the benefits of decreased hospital stay and costs seen in these studies may be lost. In addition, the cost differential for parenteral and oral antibiotics used for CAP, particularly the fluoroquinolones, has diminished over the past few years, as these agents have become available generically. Nevertheless, an assessment of patients who could be on oral therapy may be a relevant activity for an antimicrobial stewardship program, as it may hasten time to discharge or limit exposure to side effects associated with parenteral therapy in patients who require continued hospitalization for other reasons.

Is Measurement of Procalcitonin Levels an Effective Way to Reduce Antibiotic Exposure in Patients with Suspected or Confirmed CAP?

The use of biomarkers in the management of infections has become prevalent, predominantly outside of the United States. Levels of procalcitonin (PCT), a calcitonin precursor, are elevated in bacterial infections.[50] Several studies have investigated its use in the management of patients with lower respiratory tract infection (LRTI) or CAP and have found it to be effective in decreasing antibiotic use for CAP compared with standard practice.[51–53] In a Swiss randomized clinical trial by Christ-Crain and colleagues,[51] patients with suspected CAP were randomized to receive antibiotics according to usual practice or antibiotic management based on serum PCT concentration measured at days 1, 4, 6, and 8 (<0.1 µg/L, strongly discouraged; <0.25 µg/L, discouraged; >0.25 µg/L, encouraged; >0.5 µg/L, strongly encouraged). Patients who received PCT-guided therapy had decreased total antibiotic exposure (Relative risk [RR] 0.52; 95% confidence interval [CI] 0.48–0.55), reduced antibiotic prescription (85% vs 99%, $P<.001$) and decreased antibiotic treatment duration (median 5 vs 12 days, $P<.001$) compared with patients treated according to standard practice. The overall clinical cure rate was 83% and was similar in both groups.

A randomized control study by Schuetz and colleagues[52] investigated the administration of antibiotics to patients with LRTIs (68% diagnosed with CAP) in 6 emergency departments based on a PCT algorithm compared with the use of standard treatment guidelines. Patients with CAP in the PCT-guided group had significantly reduced antibiotic prescription rates (90.7% vs 99.1%), antibiotic exposure (median 7.2 days vs 10.7 days), and rates of adverse events (23.5% vs 33.1%) compared with patients randomized to the usual antibiotic management approach. There were no significant differences in length of stay, mortality, or complications.

In a study of outpatients with suspected CAP by Long and colleagues,[54] subjects were randomized to receive either PCT-guided therapy or antibiotics according to current treatment guidelines. The duration of antibiotic therapy was significantly reduced for the patients receiving the PCT-guided therapy compared with patients treated according to current guidelines (median 5 days vs 7 days; $P<.001$). At 4 weeks, all patients had survived and there were no differences in clinical outcomes.

Most recently, Albrich and colleagues[53] published an observational, multinational, and multicenter study investigating the influence of PCT on the initiation and duration of antibiotics, adherence to the published PCT algorithm, and patient outcomes in patients with LRTI in Switzerland, France, and the United States. The investigators reported that the predicted mean duration of antibiotic therapy in LRTI was shorter if the PCT algorithm was followed compared with if it was not (5.9 vs 7.4 days, $P<.001$); however, they did not differentiate between patients with CAP and other LRTIs. Neither withholding antibiotics at initial presentation nor cessation of antibiotics according to the PCT protocol were associated with increased risk of in-hospital complications or mortality; patients in the former group also experienced a significant decrease in adverse events.

In summary, the experience with PCT-guided therapy in the United States is limited; however, European-based studies have demonstrated that PCT reduces antibiotic exposure in patients with CAP by decreasing the number of initial prescriptions, as well the duration of therapy, without affecting mortality and cure rates. It is important to note that the median days of therapy in the control arms of several studies evaluating the utility of PCT are quite long (10–12 days); thus, although there are significant decreases in duration of therapy in the PCT arms, the duration of antibiotic exposure remains relatively long. Indeed, the duration of therapy in the PCT arms is similar to the durations of short-course therapy that are described as being clinically effective in the studies reported previously. It may be that PCT is most helpful in distinguishing whether patients have CAP or an alternative etiology for symptoms at the time of presentation and allow for the decision to not start antibiotic therapy, thereby decreasing antibiotic exposure. In addition, it is unclear whether the use of PCT-guided therapy can be implemented in an institution as a tool to reduce antibiotic use without concomitant development of algorithms by and assistance from antimicrobial stewardship personnel. Finally, PCT-guided therapy has not been compared with other antibiotic stewardship interventions, such as postprescription review of antibiotics for patients with CAP. The benefit of PCT-guided therapy, both clinical and financial, must be assessed compared with other stewardship interventions that have been shown to be effective in decreasing antibiotic exposure before recommending that it replace them.

Are Antimicrobial Stewardship Interventions Useful to Shorten Duration of Antibiotics and Promote Switch Therapy for CAP?

Several before-and-after studies have shown that increasing awareness of CAP treatment guidelines for empiric therapy and implementing clinical pathways reinforcing these guidelines improve patient outcomes, including mortality.[55–58] Fewer studies evaluating antimicrobial stewardship efforts directed at switch therapy and reducing the duration of CAP therapy have been performed. Carratala and colleagues[59] placed a printed checklist for a 3-step critical pathway for the management of patients with CAP including the early mobilization of patients, switching to oral antibiotic therapy once clinically stable and the use of predefined criteria for deciding on hospital discharge. Patients randomized to receive the intervention received significantly fewer days of IV antibiotics (−2.0 days; 95% CI −2.0 to −1.0; P<.001), significantly reduced length of stay (−2.1 days; 95% CI −2.7 to −1.7; P<.001), and fewer adverse events, especially phlebitis. There were no significant differences in readmission or mortality rates between groups.

A cluster randomized trial performed in the Netherlands demonstrated that hospitals with educational lectures and consensus "critical-care pathways" significantly increased the rate of adherence to national guidelines for the empiric treatment of CAP compared with control hospitals. However, rates for early switch therapy, reported for patients with LRTIs, including patients with CAP and chronic obstructive pulmonary disease exacerbation combined, were higher in the control hospitals. This finding was attributed to the implementation of a switch therapy protocol in one of the control hospitals by nonstudy physicians.[60] In the same study, there was a nonsignificant 5.7% increase in the change from broad-spectrum empiric therapy to pathogen-directed therapy for patients with LRTI in the hospitals randomized to the intervention. Among patients with CAP, however, there was an improvement in the percentage of antibiotic therapies discontinued after 3 days of defervescence (+13.3% vs −7.7%). This study suggests that education and algorithms alone without active stewardship may not be an effective strategy for reducing days of parenteral therapy or streamlining therapy in hospitalized patients with CAP. In a cluster-randomized study by Fine and colleagues[61] using a multifaceted strategy, including placing a sheet in the patient's chart recommending the switch from PO to IV antibiotics and having a nurse contact the physician to discuss switching to PO antibiotics and discharge planning, there was a nonsignificant decrease in days of IV antibiotics (1 day) and length of stay and no difference in mortality or antibiotic-associated complications between groups.

One study evaluated the impact of stewardship interventions specifically targeting short course antibiotic treatment for CAP. Avdic and colleagues[62] implemented an antimicrobial intervention consisting of education and prospective feedback on antibiotic choice and duration. The mean duration of antibiotic therapy decreased significantly from 10 days to 7 days, resulting in 148 fewer days of antibiotics over a 6-month period. Duration of hospitalization (median 4 days vs 5 days) and rates of readmission (14.5% vs 7.7%) were not significantly different in the baseline and intervention periods.

RECOMMENDATION BASED ON PRESENT EVIDENCE

Sufficient evidence is available to support the promotion of short-course antibiotic therapy and switch therapy for patients with CAP as part of antimicrobial stewardship programs. These approaches have been demonstrated to be safe even in patients with severe CAP and, together, can improve patient outcomes, including adverse events, length of hospital stay, and overall hospital costs, although some of these advantages of early switch therapy may be lost as antibiotic courses are shortened. Mortality and cure rates do not appear to be improved by these approaches; however, the finding that mortality and cure rates are equivalent to those seen in patients treated with a longer course of parenteral antibiotics reinforces the safety of using these approaches in intervention programs.

Few randomized studies evaluating stewardship interventions to promote short-course therapy and de-escalation of treatment for CAP are available and the results of these studies are variable. Only 1 study[59] found that length of stay and antibiotic-associated adverse events were reduced by their stewardship intervention. This was the only study that was not cluster randomized and the discrepancy in findings may reflect differences in the receptiveness of the randomized hospitals to the interventions. Even fewer data are available regarding stewardship interventions focused on reducing the duration of antibiotics for CAP. As evidenced in the study by Avdic and colleagues,[62] direct oral feedback is an effective component of stewardship programs; however, there are few other data available on patient outcomes resulting from stewardship interventions focused on duration of therapy for CAP. In addition, whether or not rate of infection with antibiotic-resistant organisms is affected by these practices remains to be seen.

A large proportion of patients with CAP are treated as outpatients and there is a dearth of information on the effect of antibiotic therapy duration on outcomes in that population of patients. An additional advantage to short-course therapy is increased compliance with antibiotic regimens,[63] especially in outpatients in whom antibiotic stewardship may more challenging. There is also a lack of information regarding mechanically ventilated patients and immune-compromised patients, 2 patient populations that are generally excluded from studies to increase internal generalizability.

Evidence shows that patients continue to be treated with full courses of parenteral therapy despite meeting criteria for clinical stability and early switch to oral antibiotics and there is considerable variation in clinical practice preferences.[36,37,64,65] A study in the Netherlands found that the most common causes of failure to switch to oral antibiotics in eligible patients were physician opinion or preference, forgetting to switch to oral antibiotics, severity of illness on admission, and patient comorbidities,[66,67] suggesting that stewardship interventions focused on education about the safety of switch therapy even in cases of severe CAP could have significant impact. Use of PCT to guide the decisions to start and continue antimicrobial therapy is a potential resource for antimicrobial stewardship programs, although further studies are needed to understand whether it provides benefit beyond the traditional stewardship approach of providing review of therapy at 48 to 72 hours. In addition, successful implementation of PCT use in an institution to reduce antimicrobial exposures in patients with suspected or confirmed CAP in the absence of carefully designed protocols and/or concomitant stewardship team assistance with interpretation has not been described.

NEED FOR FUTURE STUDIES

Implementation of treatment guidelines through active antimicrobial stewardship has raised awareness by clinicians of the importance of timely and appropriate treatment of CAP and has successfully improved outcomes in these patients. Implementation of the individual interventions described in this review could further improve outcomes; however, the best method of implementing these approaches as part of stewardship interventions and data on whether or not these interventions will improve patient outcomes are lacking. Further robust studies are needed across different patient populations and settings to address that question.

SUMMARY

- Adherence to antibiotic treatment guidelines is inconsistent and the erroneous diagnosis of CAP and misuse of antibiotics is prevalent.
- Short-course therapy for CAP has been shown to be as clinically effective as longer-course therapy and is associated with fewer adverse events.
- Switching from parenteral to oral antibiotics is safe at 48 to 72 hours even in patients with severe CAP who meet criteria for clinical stability.

- Antimicrobial stewardship programs should consider interventions to reduce duration of therapy, enhance conversion to oral therapy, and use procalcitonin to guide the need for antibiotics at the start of and during therapy. Such interventions have led to reduced antibiotic exposure without evidence of causing patient harm.

REFERENCES

1. Mandell LA, Wunderink RG, Anzueto A, et al. Infectious Diseases Society of America/ American Thoracic Society consensus guidelines on the management of community-acquired pneumonia in adults. Clin Infect Dis 2007;44(Suppl 2):S27–72.
2. Buie VC, Owings MF, DeFrances CJ, et al. National hospital discharge survey: 2006 summary. National Center for Health Statistics. Vital Health Stat 2010;13:168.
3. Bonafede MM, Suaya JA, Wilson KL, et al. Incidence and cost of CAP in a large working-age population. Am J Manag Care 2012;18:380–7.
4. McCabe C, Kirchner C, Zhang H, et al. Guideline-concordant therapy and reduced mortality and length of stay in adults with community-acquired pneumonia: playing by the rules. Arch Intern Med 2009;169:1525–31.
5. Arnold FW, LaJoie AS, Brock GN, et al. Improving outcomes in elderly patients with community-acquired pneumonia by adhering to national guidelines: community-acquired pneumonia organization international cohort study results. Arch Intern Med 2009;169:1515–24.
6. Fakih MG, Hilu RC, Savoy-Moore RT, et al. Do resident physicians use antibiotics appropriately in treating upper respiratory infections? A survey of 11 programs. Clin Infect Dis 2003;37:853–6.
7. Fok MC, Kanji Z, Mainra R, et al. Characterizing and developing strategies for the treatment of community-acquired pneumonia at a community hospital. Can Respir J 2002;9:247–52.
8. Schouten JA, Hulscher ME, Kullberg BJ, et al. Understanding variation in quality of antibiotic use for community-acquired pneumonia: effect of patient, professional and hospital factors. J Antimicrob Chemother 2005;56:575–82.
9. Kanwar M, Brar N, Khatib R, et al. Misdiagnosis of community-acquired pneumonia and inappropriate utilization of antibiotics: side effects of the 4-h antibiotic administration rule. Chest 2007;131:1865–9.
10. Kuyvenhoven MM, van Balen FA, Verheij TJ. Outpatient antibiotic prescriptions from 1992 to 2001 in the Netherlands. J Antimicrob Chemother 2003;52:675–8.
11. Roumie CL, Halasa NB, Grijalva CG, et al. Trends in antibiotic prescribing for adults in the United States—1995 to 2002. J Gen Intern Med 2005;20:697–702.
12. File TM Jr, Gross PA. Performance measurement in community-acquired pneumonia: consequences intended and unintended. Clin Infect Dis 2007;44:942–4.
13. Welker JA, Huston M, McCue JD. Antibiotic timing and errors in diagnosing pneumonia. Arch Intern Med 2008;168:351–6.
14. Nicks BA, Manthey DE, Fitch MT. The Centers for Medicare and Medicaid services (CMS) community-acquired pneumonia core measures lead to unnecessary antibiotic administration by emergency physicians. Acad Emerg Med 2009; 16:184–7.
15. Polk RE, Fishman N. Antimicrobial stewardship. 7th edition. In: Mandell GL, Bennett JC, Dolin R, editors. Mandell, Douglas and Bennett's principles and practice of infectious disease. Orlando, Florida: Churchill Livingstone; 2010. No 1.
16. Weber DJ. Collateral damage and what the future might hold. The need to balance prudent antibiotic utilization and stewardship with effective patient management. Int J Infect Dis 2006;10:S17–24.

17. Sutton DR, Wicks AC, Davidson L. One-day treatment for lobar pneumonia. Thorax 1970;25:241–4.
18. Ree GH, Davis M. Treatment of lobar pneumonia in Papua New Guinea: short course chemotherapy with penicillin or chloramphenicol. J Infect 1983;6:29–32.
19. Siegel RE, Alicea M, Lee A, et al. Comparison of 7 versus 10 days of antibiotic therapy for hospitalized patients with uncomplicated community-acquired pneumonia: a prospective, randomized, double-blind study. Am J Ther 1999;6:217–22.
20. el Moussaoui R, de Borgie CA, van den Broek P, et al. Effectiveness of discontinuing antibiotic treatment after three days versus eight days in mild to moderate-severe community acquired pneumonia: randomised, double blind study. BMJ 2006;332:1355.
21. Schonwald S, Gunjaca M, Kolacny-Babic L, et al. Comparison of azithromycin and erythromycin in the treatment of atypical pneumonias. J Antimicrob Chemother 1990;25(Suppl A):123–6.
22. Kinasewitz G, Wood RG. Azithromycin versus cefaclor in the treatment of acute bacterial pneumonia. Eur J Clin Microbiol Infect Dis 1991;10:872–7.
23. Schonwald S, Barsic B, Klinar I, et al. Three-day azithromycin compared with ten-day roxithromycin treatment of atypical pneumonia. Scand J Infect Dis 1994;26:706–10.
24. Rizzato G, Montemurro L, Fraioli P, et al. Efficacy of a three day course of azithromycin in moderately severe community-acquired pneumonia. Eur Respir J 1995;8:398–402.
25. O'Doherty B, Muller O. Randomized, multicentre study of the efficacy and tolerance of azithromycin versus clarithromycin in the treatment of adults with mild to moderate community-acquired pneumonia. Azithromycin Study Group. Eur J Clin Microbiol Infect Dis 1998;17:828–33.
26. Rahav G, Fidel J, Gibor Y, et al. Azithromycin versus comparative therapy for the treatment of community acquired pneumonia. Int J Antimicrob Agents 2004;24:181–4.
27. Tellier G, Niederman MS, Nusrat R, et al. Clinical and bacteriological efficacy and safety of 5 and 7 day regimens of telithromycin once daily compared with a 10 day regimen of clarithromycin twice daily in patients with mild to moderate community-acquired pneumonia. J Antimicrob Chemother 2004;54:515–23.
28. D'Ignazio J, Camere MA, Lewis DE, et al. Novel, single-dose microsphere formulation of azithromycin versus 7-day levofloxacin therapy for treatment of mild to moderate community-acquired pneumonia in adults. Antimicrob Agents Chemother 2005;49:4035–41.
29. Dunbar LM, Wunderink RG, Habib MP, et al. High-dose, short-course levofloxacin for community-acquired pneumonia: a new treatment paradigm. Clin Infect Dis 2003;37:752–60.
30. File TM Jr, Mandell LA, Tillotson G, et al. Gemifloxacin once daily for 5 days versus 7 days for the treatment of community-acquired pneumonia: a randomized, multicentre, double-blind study. J Antimicrob Chemother 2007;60:112–20.
31. Dimopoulos G, Matthaiou DK, Karageorgopoulos DE, et al. Short- versus long-course antibacterial therapy for community-acquired pneumonia: a meta-analysis. Drugs 2008;68:1841–54.
32. Li JZ, Winston LG, Moore DH, et al. Efficacy of short-course antibiotic regimens for community-acquired pneumonia: a meta-analysis. Am J Med 2007;120:783–90.
33. Jenkins SG, Brown SD, Farrell DJ. Trends in antibacterial resistance among Streptococcus pneumoniae isolated in the USA: update from PROTEKT US Years 1-4. Ann Clin Microbiol Antimicrob 2008;7:1.

34. Ehrhardt AF, Russo R. Clinical resistance encountered in the respiratory surveillance program (RESP) study: a review of the implications for the treatment of community-acquired respiratory tract infections. Am J Med 2001;111:30S–5S.
35. Lode H, Borner K, Koeppe P, et al. Azithromycin—review of key chemical, pharmacokinetic and microbiological features. J Antimicrob Chemother 1996;37(Suppl C): 1–8.
36. Ramirez JA, Cooper AC, Wiemken T, et al. Switch therapy in hospitalized patients with community-acquired pneumonia: tigecycline vs. levofloxacin. BMC Infect Dis 2012;12:159.
37. Mertz D, Koller M, Haller P, et al. Outcomes of early switching from intravenous to oral antibiotics on medical wards. J Antimicrob Chemother 2009;64:188–99.
38. Ramirez JA, Vargas S, Ritter GW, et al. Early switch from intravenous to oral antibiotics and early hospital discharge: a prospective observational study of 200 consecutive patients with community-acquired pneumonia. Arch Intern Med 1999;159:2449–54.
39. Ramirez JA. Switch therapy in community-acquired pneumonia. Diagn Microbiol Infect Dis 1995;22:219–23.
40. Ramirez JA, Srinath L, Ahkee S, et al. Early switch from intravenous to oral cephalosporins in the treatment of hospitalized patients with community-acquired pneumonia. Arch Intern Med 1995;155:1273–6.
41. Lee RW, Lindstrom ST. Early switch to oral antibiotics and early discharge guidelines in the management of community-acquired pneumonia. Respirology 2007; 12:111–6.
42. Ramirez JA, Bordon J. Early switch from intravenous to oral antibiotics in hospitalized patients with bacteremic community-acquired Streptococcus pneumoniae pneumonia. Arch Intern Med 2001;161:848–50.
43. Yaqub A, Khan Z. Comparison of early intravenous to oral switch amoxicillin/clavulanate with parenteral ceftriaxone in treatment of hospitalized patients with community acquired pneumonia. Pak J Med Sci 2005;21:259–66.
44. Castro-Guardiola A, Viejo-Rodriguez AL, Soler-Simon S, et al. Efficacy and safety of oral and early-switch therapy for community-acquired pneumonia: a randomized controlled trial. Am J Med 2001;111:367–74.
45. Oosterheert JJ, Bonten MJ, Schneider MM, et al. Effectiveness of early switch from intravenous to oral antibiotics in severe community acquired pneumonia: multicentre randomised trial. BMJ 2006;333:1193.
46. Omidvari K, de Boisblanc BP, Karam G, et al. Early transition to oral antibiotic therapy for community-acquired pneumonia: duration of therapy, clinical outcomes, and cost analysis. Respir Med 1998;92:1032–9.
47. Norrby SR, Petermann W, Willcox PA, et al. A comparative study of levofloxacin and ceftriaxone in the treatment of hospitalized patients with pneumonia. Scand J Infect Dis 1998;30:397–404.
48. Athanassa Z, Makris G, Dimopoulos G, et al. Early switch to oral treatment in patients with moderate to severe community-acquired pneumonia: a meta-analysis. Drugs 2008;68:2469–81.
49. Rhew DC, Tu GS, Ofman J, et al. Early switch and early discharge strategies in patients with community-acquired pneumonia: a meta-analysis. Arch Intern Med 2001;161:722–7.
50. Muller B, Becker KL, Schachinger H, et al. Calcitonin precursors are reliable markers of sepsis in a medical intensive care unit. Crit Care Med 2000;28:977–83.
51. Christ-Crain M, Stolz D, Bingisser R, et al. Procalcitonin guidance of antibiotic therapy in community-acquired pneumonia: a randomized trial. Am J Respir Crit Care Med 2006;174:84–93.

52. Schuetz P, Christ-Crain M, Thomann R, et al. Effect of procalcitonin-based guidelines vs standard guidelines on antibiotic use in lower respiratory tract infections: the ProHOSP randomized controlled trial. JAMA 2009;302:1059–66.

53. Albrich WC, Dusemund F, Bucher B, et al. Effectiveness and safety of procalcitonin-guided antibiotic therapy in lower respiratory tract infections in "Real Life": an International, Multicenter Poststudy Survey (ProREAL). Arch Intern Med 2012;172:715–22.

54. Long W, Deng X, Zhang Y, et al. Procalcitonin guidance for reduction of antibiotic use in low-risk outpatients with community-acquired pneumonia. Respirology 2011;16:819–24.

55. Capelastegui A, Espana PP, Quintana JM, et al. Improvement of process-of-care and outcomes after implementing a guideline for the management of community-acquired pneumonia: a controlled before-and-after design study. Clin Infect Dis 2004;39:955–63.

56. Hauck LD, Adler LM, Mulla ZD. Clinical pathway care improves outcomes among patients hospitalized for community-acquired pneumonia. Ann Epidemiol 2004; 14:669–75.

57. Marrie TJ. Experience with levofloxacin in a critical pathway for the treatment of community-acquired pneumonia. Chemotherapy 2004;50(Suppl 1):11–5.

58. Blasi F, Lori I, Bulfoni A, et al. Can CAP guideline adherence improve patient outcome in internal medicine departments? Eur Respir J 2008;32:902–10.

59. Carratala J, Garcia-Vidal C, Ortega L, et al. Effect of a 3-step critical pathway to reduce duration of intravenous antibiotic therapy and length of stay in community-acquired pneumonia: a randomized controlled trial. Arch Intern Med 2012;172: 922–8.

60. Schouten JA, Hulscher ME, Trap-Liefers J, et al. Tailored interventions to improve antibiotic use for lower respiratory tract infections in hospitals: a cluster-randomized, controlled trial. Clin Infect Dis 2007;44:931–41.

61. Fine MJ, Stone RA, Lave JR, et al. Implementation of an evidence-based guideline to reduce duration of intravenous antibiotic therapy and length of stay for patients hospitalized with community-acquired pneumonia: a randomized controlled trial. Am J Med 2003;115:343–51.

62. Avdic E, Cushinotto LA, Hughes AH, et al. Impact of an antimicrobial stewardship intervention on shortening the duration of therapy for community-acquired pneumonia. Clin Infect Dis 2012;54:1581–7.

63. Cockburn J, Gibberd RW, Reid AL, et al. Determinants of non-compliance with short term antibiotic regimens. Br Med J (Clin Res Ed) 1987;295:814–8.

64. Halm EA, Switzer GE, Mittman BS, et al. What factors influence physicians' decisions to switch from intravenous to oral antibiotics for community-acquired pneumonia? J Gen Intern Med 2001;16:599–605.

65. Peyrani P, Christensen D, LaJoie AS, et al. Antibiotic therapy of hospitalized patients with community-acquired pneumonia: an international perspective from the CAPO Cohort Study. J Ky Med Assoc 2006;104:513–7.

66. Engel MF, Postma DF, Hulscher ME, et al. Barriers to an early switch from intravenous to oral antibiotic therapy in hospitalised patients with community-acquired pneumonia. Eur Respir J 2012. [Epub ahead of print].

67. Schouten JA, Hulscher ME, Natsch S, et al. Barriers to optimal antibiotic use for community-acquired pneumonia at hospitals: a qualitative study. Qual Saf Health Care 2007;16:143–9.

How Effective is Vaccination in Preventing Pneumococcal Disease?

Daniel M. Musher, MD

KEYWORDS

- *Streptococcus pneumoniae* • Pneumococcus • Vaccine • Pneumonia
- Community-acquired pneumonia

KEY POINTS

- Although some controversy persists, the 23-valent pneumococcal polysaccharide vaccine (PPV23) provides 50% to 80% protection in adults against pneumococcal infection, and vaccination with PPV23 is recommended for immunocompromised adults as well as all adults >65 years of age.
- Infants and toddlers do not make antibody after vaccination with PPV23, and this vaccine is not recommended for them.
- Vaccination with protein-conjugated pneumococcal polysaccharides (PCV) stimulates good antibody responses in infants and toddlers. Vaccination with PCVs also stimulates mucosal antibody and suppresses colonization.
- Beginning in 2000, widespread use of a vaccine containing 7 common PCVs (PCV7) greatly decreased disease caused by these vaccine serotypes, not only in those infants and children who were vaccinated but also in older children and in adults.
- Widespread vaccination with PCV13, which contains 13 PCVs is expected to greatly reduce disease caused by these serotypes in all sectors of the population at large.
- Based on evidence for modestly better antibody levels and possible better persistence of antibody in adults after PCV, as well as on the suggestion that PCV primes for enhanced response to PPV, the Centers for Disease Control and Prevention (CDC) have recently recommended that all immunocompromised adults aged 19 to 64 years receive PCV13 followed 8 weeks later by PPV23.
- Some experts predict that the use of PCV13 in adults will rapidly become irrelevant as the prevalence of these serotypes diminishes.

Infectious Disease Section, Michael E. DeBakey Veterans Affairs Medical Center, 2002 Holcombe Blvd, Houston, TX 77030, USA
E-mail address: Daniel.musher@va.gov

Infect Dis Clin N Am 27 (2013) 229–241
http://dx.doi.org/10.1016/j.idc.2012.11.011
0891-5520/13/$ – see front matter © 2013 Elsevier Inc. All rights reserved.

id.theclinics.com

AVAILABLE PNEUMOCOCCAL VACCINES

In the United States, the following 2 pneumococcal vaccines are currently approved for use:

1. PPV23, marketed as Pneumovax or Pnu-Immune, consists of capsular material from 23 pneumococcal types that have historically caused about 75% to 85% of pneumococcal disease in children or adults.
2. Protein-conjugate pneumococcal vaccine (PCV, initially marketed as Prevnar or Prevnar7 [PCV7], now replaced by Prevnar13 [PCV13]). PCV13 contains capsular polysaccharides from the 13 most common types that cause disease in children, covalently linked to a nontoxic protein that is nearly identical to diphtheria toxin. Many of the types covered by PCV13 are also common causes of adult infections.

PPV23 has been used in adults for decades and is not recommended for infants or toddlers. PCV7 was recommended of use in infants and toddlers in 2000; since 2011, PCV13 has been recommended in its place. PCV13 has also recently been recommended for limited use in adults. All these recommendations are discussed below.

INTRODUCTION

As has been shown in other articles within this issue, *Streptococcus pneumoniae* remains an important cause of community-acquired pneumonia (CAP), even though the proportion of CAP caused by pneumococcus has steadily decreased in the past 50 years. This section discusses the use of pneumococcal vaccination as a means of preventing pneumococcal pneumonia or, more broadly, as a means of preventing CAP. Clearly, the efficacy of pneumococcal vaccine in any given population will vary with the proportion of CAP cases that are attributable to *S. pneumoniae*.

BRIEF HISTORY OF PNEUMOCOCCAL VACCINATION

The understanding of humoral immunity arose from experiments performed by the Klemperers in the 1890s. This uncle and nephew team, members of the distinguished German-Jewish family that included conductor Otto Klemperer and pathologist Paul Klemperer, followed principles that had been elucidated by Pasteur. The team boiled pneumococci, injected them repeatedly into rabbits, and then challenged the rabbits with live organisms; these immunized animals were resistant to infection. The investigators transferred serum (the "humoral factor") from immunized rabbits to unimmunized ones, thereby conferring protection and showing that resistance could be transferred with serum from immune animals ("humoral immunity"). When immunized rabbits were challenged with certain other pneumococci, they were not protected, but they could be immunized with repeated injection of killed organisms from the new strain. This finding led to the concept of type-specific immunity; the first strain was called type (or serotype) I and the second was called type II. At first, all others were called type III. In the ensuing 100 years, some 91 distinct types of *S. pneumoniae* have been identified.

In 1911, Lister and Wright began studies in which they injected killed pneumococci into South African miners, a group of men in whom the rate of pneumococcal disease was as high as 50 to 60 cases per 1,000 miners per year.[1,2] These attempts seemed to be quite successful in reducing morbidity and mortality of pneumococcal pneumonia, although later authorities criticized their lack of scientific rigor and interpretation of results.[3] By the 1930s, investigators at the Rockefeller Institute found that the capsular material was the immunizing substance, and, soon thereafter, Felton succeeded in extracting sufficient amounts of capsular polysaccharide to use as a vaccine. In 1937, Smillie and colleagues[4] used Felton's preparation of capsular polysaccharide from S. pneumoniae type I as a vaccine to abort outbreaks of pneumococcal pneumonia in an institutional setting. Studies during the Second World War showed that vaccination with capsular polysaccharide from 4 prevalent serotypes could prevent outbreaks of pneumococcal infection in military recruits.[5]

Pneumonia had always been a major cause of death in persons of all ages, and many studies had shown that more than 90% of all recognized cases were caused by S. pneumoniae.[2] In the early 1960s, nearly all CAP was thought to be due to pneumococcus. Textbook chapters on pneumonia focused on pneumococcus, referring the reader to sections on other microorganisms to learn about other causes of pulmonary infection. For a variety of reasons, including but not limited to the aging of the population, the increasing prevalence of comorbid conditions and medications that reduce immunity predisposing to other kinds of pneumonia, and the use of pneumococcal vaccine, this is no longer the case. Recent studies suggest that about 30% to 50% of CAP leading to hospitalization is caused by pneumococcus, with *Staphylococcus aureus, Haemophilus influenzae*, respiratory viruses, and gram-negative bacteria causing most of the rest (see related articles within this issue for additional information).

PNEUMOCOCCAL POLYSACCHARIDE VACCINE (PPV)

The discovery of penicillin greatly reduced the frequency and serious complications of pneumococcal pneumonia in otherwise healthy adults, thereby reducing interest in pneumococcal vaccine. Only in the 1960s when it became clear that despite available antibiotic therapy pneumococcal disease remained a common and life-threatening problem[6] was there a renewed interest in pneumococcal polysaccharide vaccine (PPV). Austrian[7] worked to develop a vaccine consisting of capsular polysaccharides from the 14 serotypes (PPV14) that most commonly caused pneumonia; this vaccine

Group Studied	Percentage Reduction
Pneumococcal disease due to a vaccine type	
Invasive disease	82%
Bacteremic pneumonia	87%
Nonbacteremic pneumonia	73%
All pneumococcal disease	
Invasive disease	74%
Pneumonia	76%
Nonbacteremic pneumonia	53%
All-cause pneumonia	
All results	29%
Low-income countries	46%
High-income countries	26% (not significant)
All-cause mortality	
All results	13% (not significant)
Low-income countries	21%
High-income countries	0% (not significant)

Table 1
Incidence per 1000 person-years

Condition observed	Vaccine $n = 502$	Placebo $n = 504$	Percentage Reduction
Pneumococcal pneumonia	12	32	63.8% ($P = .002$)
Nonpneumococcal pneumonia	43	59	29.4% ($P = .08$)
All-cause pneumonia	55	91	44.8% ($P < .001$)
All-cause death	89	80	NS ($P = .46$)

Abbreviation: NS, nonsignificant.

was later expanded to include capsule from 23 types that, until the late 1990s, caused more than 85% of disease. PPV23 is currently marketed in the United States as PNEUMOVAX 23 (Merck) or Pnu-Immune 23 (Lederle).

Many studies have examined the efficacy of PPV, and a range of results has been observed, depending on the end point being investigated. In general, the more specific the end point, the better is the efficacy. A 2008 Cochrane review by Moberley and colleagues[8] analyzed the protective effects of PPV in published randomized control trials as follows (reductions in disease were significant unless otherwise noted):

These data show that PPV clearly reduces the rate of pneumococcal infection, whether invasive (positive blood cultures or isolation of the organism from a normally sterile site) or noninvasive, due to vaccine strains. Substantial protection, albeit to a somewhat lesser degree, is still apparent if infecting strains have not been typed. In fact, these results are precisely what might be expected if PPV23 contains capsular material from types that cause about 80% of all pneumococcal disease. Because all-cause pneumonia comprises an umbrella diagnosis with many potential causes, it is not surprising that a protective effect is not so clearly discernible. It is also reasonable to expect that the overall socioeconomic conditions and a higher rate of vaccination in high-income countries have reduced the frequency of pneumococcal disease, thereby blunting the efficacy of PPV23, when compared with developing countries. A subsequent review by Huss and colleagues[9] found that the PPV was not protective, but this review was seriously flawed, as has been shown elsewhere.[10]

More recent studies have essentially confirmed these results. In a prospective study involving 8 Japanese nursing homes, subjects were randomized to receive PPV23 or placebo[11]; the incidences of pneumonia and death were then studied, with the results given in **Table 1**.

A cohort study of community-living adults in the Kaiser Permanente system[12] showed similar results, but it should be noted that a case-control study of persons hospitalized in Edmonton, Alberta, Canada[13] found no significant protection. The investigators of this last-named study reported separately that even though PPV did not prevent hospitalization for CAP, it reduced complications and mortality from that disease,[14] a result also reported by Fisman and colleagues.[15]

Many case-control studies of PPV have also been reported, showing protection rates of 50% to 60% (range 40%–90%).[16–22] Some results have suggested that PPV23 protects against invasive pneumococcal infection (defined as pneumococcal disease with isolation of the infecting organisms from a normally sterile body site), but not against nonbacteremic pneumococcal pneumonia.[20,21] However, this concept is not biologically plausible and results are opposed by those cited above.

In an important case-control study, Shapiro and colleagues[18] showed that the benefit of PPV23 decreases with age and with time after vaccination. The investigators found that PPV23 was about 90% protective in adults aged 50 to 60 years, with protection persisting for 5 years. With aging, and presumably in the face of comorbid and/or immune-compromising conditions, the initial rate of protection is much lower and falls off far more rapidly, so that in persons older than 90 years, the rate of protection was about 20% in the first year after vaccination and was not detectable after that.

POLYSACCHARIDE VACCINE IN IMMUNOCOMPROMISED PERSONS

Unfortunately, patients who, because of an immunocompromising condition, are most in need of protection against pneumococcal infection are the least likely to benefit from PPV. Hodgkin disease, multiple myeloma, and lymphoma block the ability of the immune system to respond appropriately to new antigenic stimuli, especially to polysaccharides, and patients with these diseases respond to few or no capsular polysaccharides contained in PPV23. Drugs that are immunosuppressive also suppress responses to PPV23, and patients who have received a solid-organ or a bone marrow transplant do not respond well,[23] hence the recommendation that transplant candidates be vaccinated before transplantation. Even persons with advanced heart failure and those who have increasing age and frailty respond only poorly to PPV23, with no response to a varying number of antigens and a low antibody level to the rest.[24] Patients who recover from pneumococcal pneumonia also respond very poorly to PPV23.[25] Even when persons with all these conditions make antibody in response to PPV, the antibody may not be as effective in opsonizing bacteria and, therefore, in protecting the vaccinated subject.[24,26] Patients with untreated human immunodeficiency virus (HIV) infection and low CD4 counts also respond poorly or not at all to PPV23[27]; once effective antiviral treatment has been given, responses are partially restored, but are still not normal.[28]

RECOMMENDATIONS FOR USE OF POLYSACCHARIDE VACCINE

The CDC's Immunization Practices Advisory Committee[29] recommends PPV23 for all persons older than 2 years who are at substantially increased risk of developing pneumococcal infection and/or of having a serious complication of such an infection. Perhaps most important are those with anatomic or functional asplenia. Others include persons (1) older than 65 years; (2) with cerebrospinal fluid (CSF) leak, diabetes mellitus, alcoholism, cirrhosis, chronic renal insufficiency, chronic pulmonary disease, or advanced cardiovascular disease; (3) who have an immunocompromising condition associated with increased risk of pneumococcal disease, such as multiple myeloma, lymphoma, Hodgkin disease, HIV infection, organ transplantation, or chronic use of glucocorticoids; or (4) who live in environments in which outbreaks are particularly likely to occur, such as nursing homes. Recommendations for pneumococcal vaccination for adults are summarized in **Table 2**.

REVACCINATION WITH POLYSACCHARIDE VACCINE

After healthy adults older than 50 years of age are vaccinated, antibody levels peak at 1–2 months, thereafter declining rapidly over a 1- to 2-year period, persisting at very low levels for 5 to 10 years.[30,31] It is not known what level of antibody is protective. The CDC recommends that "All persons should be vaccinated with PPV23 at the age of 65 years. Those who have received PPV23 before the age of 65 years for any indication

Table 2
Indications for administration of PPV23 and PCV13 in adults aged 19 to 64 years

Risk Group	Medical Condition	PCV13	PPV23	PPV23 Revax[a]
Presumed Immunocompetent	Asplenia (including hemoglobinopathies)	X	X	X
	CSF leaks	X	X	—
	Cochlear implant	X	X	—
	Chronic heart disease	—	X	—
	Cigarette smoking	—	X	—
	Chronic lung disease	—	X	—
	Diabetes	—	X	—
	Alcoholism	—	X	—
	Chronic liver disease	—	X	—
Immunocompromised	Congenital or acquired immunodeficiencies	X	X	X
	HIV infection	X	X	X
	Chronic renal failure	X	X	X
	Nephrotic syndrome	X	X	X
	Leukemia	X	X	X
	Lymphoma	X	X	X
	Hodgkin disease	X	X	X
	Generalized malignancy	X	X	X
	Iatrogenic immunosuppression	X	X	X
	Solid organ transplant	X	X	X
	Multiple myeloma	X	X	X

[a] Single revaccination 5 years after a prior vaccination.

should receive another dose of the vaccine at the age of 65 years or later if at least 5 years have passed since the previous dose. Those who receive PPV23 at or after the age of 65 years should receive only a single dose."[29]

Patients who have undergone splenectomy are under special risk for overwhelming pneumococcal infection, and some experts think that such patients should be revaccinated at 5- to 6-year intervals.[32] The same might be said for adults in their 70s and 80s who were vaccinated at the age of 65 years. The concern, largely theoretical, that repeated vaccination may lead to hypresponsiveness[33] does not seem to be relevant if vaccine is given at less than 5-year intervals[31,34,35]; administration at closer intervals has been shown in selected groups of patients to be successful.[36]

PROTEIN-CONJUGATE POLYSACCHARIDE VACCINE (PCV)

Children younger than 2 years do not respond well to polysaccharide antigens. However, when a polysaccharide is covalently conjugated to a carrier protein, the resulting antigen is recognized as T-cell dependent, stimulating a good antibody response in children younger than 2 years and inducing immunologic memory. In the 1990s, a study of PCV7 in 38,000 infants and toddlers in the Kaiser Permanente system yielded spectacular results, showing a 98% reduction in bacteremia and meningitis[37] and a 67% reduction in otitis media due to vaccine serotypes. Within a few years after PCV7 was marketed in 2000 as Prevnar 7, its widespread use in the United States brought about the near disappearance of serious disease caused by vaccine strains in children nationwide (**Fig. 1**).[38] A 13-valent vaccine, marketed as Prevnar 13, was approved in 2010, and is expected to cause the same kinds of decreases in incidence of infection due to these strains.

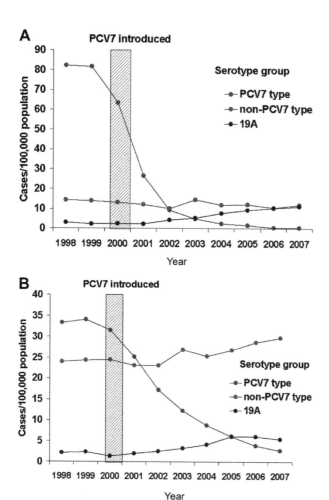

Fig. 1. Infections due to serotypes of pneumococcus included in PCV7 occurring in children younger than 5 years (A) or adults older than 65 years (B) between 1998 and 2007. (*Data from* Pilishvili T, Lexau C, Farley MM, et al. Sustained reductions in invasive pneumococcal disease in the era of conjugate vaccine. J Infect Dis 2010;201:32–41.)

OTHER EFFECTS OF CONJUGATE PNEUMOCOCCAL VACCINE
Indirect Effect

A second property of PCV that distinguishes it from PPV23 is that it stimulates mucosal immunity, protecting against pneumococcal colonization.[39] In an Alaskan village, after administration of PCV7, carriage of vaccine strains decreased remarkably, not only in vaccinated children but also in adults.[40] This effect on colonization explains the very important indirect effects of conjugate vaccine (sometimes called the "herd effect"). As shown in **Fig. 1**, widespread vaccination of infants and toddlers with PCV7 has also led to a remarkable decrease in pneumococcal infection in older persons who did not, themselves, receive the vaccine. This decrease resulted from a lower rate of colonization among infants and toddlers who had received the vaccine and a consequent lower rate of spread to the rest of the population. At present, in the

United States, the incidence of pneumonia in adults caused by pneumococcal types included in PCV7 has been reduced by more than 90%.[38] These same direct and indirect effects are anticipated for the 13 serotypes contained in PCV13, as a result of the widespread use of this vaccine since 2010,[41] a factor that must be considered in any discussion of PCV13 for adults.

Comparison of PCV with PPV in Adults

Many investigators have postulated that, by altering the nature of the antigenic stimulation, PCV might stimulate higher levels of antibody that persist longer than those after PPV. The author and his colleagues recently reviewed all comparative studies of PPV and PCV, whether in normal or immunocompromised adults, that were published through 2010.[42] All studies were based on in vitro assays of antibody levels or antibody opsonic activity. It was concluded that up to 6 months after PCV, antibody levels were similar or slightly higher than those after PPV, but no definitive or consistent advantage was demonstrated. In 2 reports of antibody persistence 1 year after vaccination, antibody levels were similar and opsonic activity was slightly greater after PCV.[43,44] Data, as yet unpublished, obtained by the manufacturer of PCV13 are based on study of 924 subjects who were randomized to receive PPV23 or PCV13. This large study seems to show slight but significant differences favoring PCV13 1 month after vaccination; whether these differences are clinically meaningful is entirely unknown.

As far as the actual efficacy of PCV is concerned, only 1 study has been carried out. PCV7 was clearly protective against pneumococcal infection when given to patients with AIDS in Malawi[45]; however, the efficacy waned dramatically after the first year. Although the investigators did not directly compare PCV7 to PPV23, they had previously reported that PPV23 failed to protect patients with AIDS in Uganda.[46] Taken together, these 2 studies by the same group of investigators influenced the Advisory Council on Immunization Practices (ACIP) of the CDC to make its recommendations, released in October 2012, that are summarized in **Table 2**.

Immunologic Priming by PCV

The third property of PCV is that, by virtue of stimulating long-lived memory cells,[47] this vaccine may prime for a better response to a second administration of vaccine than does PPV. Studies to date do not strongly support this suggestion; some have found a priming effect, whereas others have not.[42] However, it is possible that the antibody persists better after PCV, and it seems well established that PCV primes the immunologic system for better responses to subsequent challenge with PPV.

Replacement Serotypes

An undesired effect of vaccination with PCV has been an increase in infection caused by serotypes that are not included in the vaccine (called replacement serotypes). Unlike PPV, PCV stimulates mucosal immunity and therefore prevents colonization by vaccine types. In doing so, an ecological niche for colonization by nonvaccine strains is created. The result has been the emergence of new serotypes as common causes of pneumococcal disease. For example, the most common cause of pneumococcal infection in persons of all ages in the past few years has been type 19F, which rose to prominence as a replacement strain after implementation of routine vaccination with PCV7. This type is contained in PCV13, but it seems very likely that other replacement strains will emerge as PCV13 is widely used.

RECOMMENDATIONS FOR USE OF PCV13 IN ADULTS

The basic recommendation has been that adults older than 65 years receive a single dose of PPV23. If they have previously been vaccinated within 5 years and are now older than 65 years, physicians should wait 5 years before recommending revaccination. This recommendation is unchanged.

In October, 2012, the ACIP of the CDC recommended[48] the following:

1. Adults 19 years or older with immunocompromising conditions, functional or anatomic asplenia, CSF leaks, or cochlear implants and those who have not previously received PCV13 or PPSV23 receive a single dose of PCV13 followed by a dose of PPSV23 at least 8 weeks later.
2. Adults 19 years or older with immunocompromising conditions, functional or anatomic asplenia, CSF leaks, or cochlear implants and those who have previously received one or more doses of PPSV23 receive a dose of PCV13 1 or more years after the last PPSV 23 dose. For those who require additional doses of PPSV23, the first such dose should be given no sooner than 8 weeks after PCV13 and at least 5 years since the most recent dose of PPSV23. These recommendations are given in **Table 2**.

CONTROVERSIES AND UNRESOLVED PROBLEMS

There are several problems with the official recommendation. First, as noted above, it is not at all clear that PCV stimulates better antibody responses than PPV. Second, the importance of pneumococcal pneumonia has steadily diminished in recent years. Third, emphasis on PCV13 for the pediatric population will almost certainly lead to the near disappearance of these vaccine strains from the adult population, so a program based on vaccinating adults with PCV13 may be unimportant. Fourth, the cost analysis[49] that showed significant (albeit modest) benefit to the final recommendations was based on projected figures derived from a Delphi analysis, in which experts estimate a predicted efficacy for various approaches. The experts who comprised the Delphi panel had generally accepted the view of Huss and colleagues[9] that PPV23 only prevented bacteremic, but not nonbacteremic, pneumococcal pneumonia. Finally, PCV13 is recommended for the groups of patients for whom there is simply no evidence that they will respond, for example, those with multiple myeloma.

For these reasons, the author is unenthusiastic about recommendations that advocate a set of 2 vaccinations—conjugate followed by unconjugated polysaccharide vaccine. Much greater effort needs to be expended on new approaches to pneumococcal vaccination involving common conserved proteins (see next section) (**Box 1**).

Box 1
Potential problems with new ACIP recommendations

Logistical

    Compliance with 2 vaccinations 8 weeks apart

    Costs (to individual patients and to society)

Usefulness

    Data on which recommendations are based are not solid

    Continuing decline in prevalence of vaccine strains in the population

    No data that some of the most severely immunosuppressed persons will respond

NEWER VACCINES

The principal advantage of the conjugate vaccine seems to be that it primes for a better immunologic response with revaccination, but a multiple vaccine approach greatly increases the cost of vaccination while decreasing the likelihood of compliance, and one is still left with the issue of replacement strains now that PCV13 has been adopted. With all the concerns over indirect effects and replacement strains following the use of polysaccharide vaccines, it seems appropriate to direct efforts toward developing vaccines that use highly conserved pneumococcal proteins such as detoxified pneumolysin, pneumococcal histidine triad protein D, pneumococcal surface protein A, or other surface-expressed proteins as their basis. Several such vaccines are currently under study,[50–52] and any discussion of new approaches should address their use.

REFERENCES

1. Musher DM, Watson DA, Dominguez EA. Pneumococcal vaccination: work to date and future prospects. Am J Med Sci 1990;300(1):45–52.
2. Heffron R. Pneumonia with special reference to pneumococcus lobar pneumonia. New York: The Commonwealth Fund; 1939.
3. Orenstein AJ. Vaccine prophylaxis in pneumonia: a review of fourteen years' experience with inoculation of native mine workers on the Witwatersrand against pneumonia. J Med Assoc South Africa 1931;5:339–46.
4. Smillie WG, Wornock GH, White HJ. A study of a type I pneumococcus epidemic at the State Hospital at Worcester, Mass. Am J Public Health Nations Health 1938; 28:293–302.
5. MacLeod CM, Hodges RG, Heidelberger M, et al. Prevention of pneumococcal pneumonia by immunization with specific capsular polysaccharides. J Exp Med 1945;82:445–65.
6. Austrian R, Gold J. Pneumococcal bacteremia with especial reference to bacteremic pneumococcal pneumonia. Ann Intern Med 1964;60:759–76.
7. Austrian R. Some observations on the pneumococcus and on the current status of pneumococcal disease and its prevention. Rev Infect Dis 1981;3(Suppl):S1–17.
8. Moberley SA, Holden J, Tatham DP, et al. Vaccines for preventing pneumococcal infection in adults. Cochrane Database Syst Rev 2008;(1):CD000422.
9. Huss A, Scott P, Stuck AE, et al. Efficacy of pneumococcal vaccination in adults: a meta-analysis. CMAJ 2009;180(1):48–58.
10. Musher DM. Editorial commentary: should 13-valent protein-conjugate pneumococcal vaccine be used routinely in adults? Clin Infect Dis 2012;55(2):265–7.
11. Maruyama T, Taguchi O, Niederman MS, et al. Efficacy of 23-valent pneumococcal vaccine in preventing pneumonia and improving survival in nursing home residents: double blind, randomised and placebo controlled trial. BMJ 2010;340:c1004.
12. Hechter RC, Chao C, Jacobsen SJ, et al. Clinical effectiveness of pneumococcal polysaccharide vaccine in men: California Men's Health Study. Vaccine 2012; 30(38):5625–30.
13. Johnstone J, Eurich DT, Minhas JK, et al. Impact of the pneumococcal vaccine on long-term morbidity and mortality of adults at high risk for pneumonia. Clin Infect Dis 2010;51(1):15–22.
14. Johnstone J, Marrie TJ, Eurich DT, et al. Effect of pneumococcal vaccination in hospitalized adults with community-acquired pneumonia. Arch Intern Med 2007;167(18):1938–43.

15. Fisman DN, Abrutyn E, Spaude KA, et al. Prior pneumococcal vaccination is associated with reduced death, complications, and length of stay among hospitalized adults with community-acquired pneumonia. Clin Infect Dis 2006;42(8): 1093–101.
16. Bolan G, Broome CV, Facklam RR, et al. Pneumococcal vaccine efficacy in selected populations in the United States. Ann Intern Med 1986;104(1):1–6.
17. Sims RV, Steinmann WC, McConville JH, et al. The clinical effectiveness of pneumococcal vaccine in the elderly. Ann Intern Med 1988;108(5):653–7.
18. Shapiro ED, Berg AT, Austrian R, et al. The protective efficacy of polyvalent pneumococcal polysaccharide vaccine. N Engl J Med 1991;325(21):1453–60.
19. Farr BM, Johnston BL, Cobb DK, et al. Preventing pneumococcal bacteremia in patients at risk. Results of a matched case-control study. Arch Intern Med 1995; 155(21):2336–40.
20. Jackson LA, Neuzil KM, Yu O, et al. Effectiveness of pneumococcal polysaccharide vaccine in older adults. N Engl J Med 2003;348(18):1747–55.
21. Musher DM, Rueda-Jaimes AM, Graviss EA, et al. Effect of pneumococcal vaccination: a comparison of vaccination rates in patients with bacteremic and nonbacteremic pneumococcal pneumonia. Clin Infect Dis 2006;43(8):1004–8.
22. Dominguez A, Izquierdo C, Salleras L, et al. Effectiveness of the pneumococcal polysaccharide vaccine in preventing pneumonia in the elderly. Eur Respir J 2010;36(3):608–14.
23. Blumberg EA, Brozena SC, Stutman P, et al. Immunogenicity of pneumococcal vaccine in heart transplant recipients. Clin Infect Dis 2001;32(2):307–10.
24. Ridda I, Macintyre CR, Lindley R, et al. Immunological responses to pneumococcal vaccine in frail older people. Vaccine 2009;27(10):1628–36.
25. Musher DM, Rueda AM, Nahm MH, et al. Initial and subsequent response to pneumococcal polysaccharide and protein-conjugate vaccines administered sequentially to adults who have recovered from pneumococcal pneumonia. J Infect Dis 2008;198(7):1019–27.
26. Romero-Steiner S, Musher DM, Cetron MS, et al. Reduction in functional antibody activity against Streptococcus pneumoniae in vaccinated elderly individuals highly correlates with decreased IgG antibody avidity. Clin Infect Dis 1999;29(2):281–8.
27. Rodriguez-Barradas MC, Musher DM, Lahart C, et al. Antibody to capsular polysaccharides of Streptococcus pneumoniae after vaccination of human immunodeficiency virus-infected subjects with 23-valent pneumococcal vaccine. J Infect Dis 1992;165(3):553–6.
28. Rodriguez-Barradas MC, Alexandraki I, Nazir T, et al. Response of human immunodeficiency virus-infected patients receiving highly active antiretroviral therapy to vaccination with 23-valent pneumococcal polysaccharide vaccine. Clin Infect Dis 2003;37(3):438–47.
29. Centers for Disease Control and Prevention. Updated recommendations for prevention of invasive pneumococcal disease among adults using the 23-valent pneumococcal polysaccharide vaccine (PPSV23). MMWR Morb Mortal Wkly Rep 2010;59(34):1102–6.
30. Musher DM, Manoff SB, Liss C, et al. Safety and antibody response, including antibody persistence for 5 years, after primary vaccination or revaccination with pneumococcal polysaccharide vaccine in middle-aged and older adults. J Infect Dis 2010;201:515–24.
31. Musher DM, Manoff SB, McFetridge RD, et al. Pneumococcal polysaccharide vaccine, and immunogenicity and safety of 2nd and 3d doses in older adults. Hum Vaccin 2011;7:919–28.

32. Musher DM. Streptococcus pneumoniae. In: Mandell GL, Bennett JE, Dolin R, editors. Principles and practice of infectious diseases. 7th edition. Philadelphia: Churchill Livingstone; 2010. p. 2623–42.

33. O'Brien KL, Hochman M, Goldblatt D. Combined schedules of pneumococcal conjugate and polysaccharide vaccines: is hyporesponsiveness an issue? Lancet Infect Dis 2007;7(9):597–606.

34. Hammitt LL, Bulkow LR, Singleton RJ, et al. Repeat revaccination with 23-valent pneumococcal polysaccharide vaccine among adults aged 55-74 years living in Alaska: no evidence of hyporesponsiveness. Vaccine 2011;29(12):2287–95.

35. Torling J, Hedlund J, Konradsen HB, et al. Revaccination with the 23-valent pneumococcal polysaccharide vaccine in middle-aged and elderly persons previously treated for pneumonia. Vaccine 2003;22(1):96–103.

36. Rodriguez-Barradas MC, Groover JE, Lacke CE, et al. IgG antibody to pneumococcal capsular polysaccharide in human immunodeficiency virus-infected subjects: persistence of antibody in responders, revaccination in nonresponders, and relationship of immunoglobulin allotype to response. J Infect Dis 1996; 173(6):1347–53.

37. Black SB, Shinefield HR, Ling S, et al. Effectiveness of heptavalent pneumococcal conjugate vaccine in children younger than five years of age for prevention of pneumonia. Pediatr Infect Dis J 2002;21(9):810–5.

38. Pilishvili T, Lexau C, Farley MM, et al. Sustained reductions in invasive pneumococcal disease in the era of conjugate vaccine. J Infect Dis 2010;201:32–41.

39. Kayhty H, Auranen K, Nohynek H, et al. Nasopharyngeal colonization: a target for pneumococcal vaccination. Expert Rev Vaccines 2006;5(5):651–67.

40. Hammitt LL, Bruden DL, Butler JC, et al. Indirect effect of conjugate vaccine on adult carriage of Streptococcus pneumoniae: an explanation of trends in invasive pneumococcal disease. J Infect Dis 2006;193(11):1487–94.

41. Dagan R, Patterson S, Juergens C, et al. The efficacy of the 13-valent conjugate pneumococcal polysaccharide vaccine (PCV13) additional serotypes on nasopharyngeal colonization; a randomized double-blind pediatric trial. In: 8th International Symposium on Pneumococci and Pneumococcal Diseases. Iguazu Falls (Brazil), 2012. Abstract #58.

42. Musher DM, Sampath R, Rodriguez-Barradas MC. The potential role for protein-conjugate pneumococcal vaccine in adults: what is the supporting evidence? Clin Infect Dis 2011;52(5):633–40.

43. Jackson LA, Neuzil KM, Nahm MH, et al. Immunogenicity of varying dosages of 7-valent pneumococcal polysaccharide-protein conjugate vaccine in seniors previously vaccinated with 23-valent pneumococcal polysaccharide vaccine. Vaccine 2007;25(20):4029–37.

44. de Roux A, Schmole-Thoma B, Siber GR, et al. Comparison of pneumococcal conjugate polysaccharide and free polysaccharide vaccines in elderly adults: conjugate vaccine elicits improved antibacterial immune responses and immunological memory. Clin Infect Dis 2008;46(7):1015–23.

45. French N, Gordon SB, Mwalukomo T, et al. A trial of a 7-valent pneumococcal conjugate vaccine in HIV-infected adults. N Engl J Med 2010;362(9):812–22.

46. French N, Nakiyingi J, Carpenter LM, et al. 23-valent pneumococcal polysaccharide vaccine in HIV-1-infected Ugandan adults: double-blind, randomised and placebo controlled trial. Lancet 2000;355(9221):2106–11.

47. Clutterbuck EA, Lazarus R, Yu LM, et al. Pneumococcal conjugate and plain polysaccharide vaccines have divergent effects on antigen-specific B cells. J Infect Dis 2012;205:1408–16.

48. Use of 13-Valent Pneumococcal Conjugate Vaccine and 23-Valent Pneumococcal Polysaccharide Vaccine for Adults with Immunocompromising Conditions: Recommendations of the Advisory Committee on Immunization Practices (ACIP). Morb Mortal Wkly 2012;61(40):816–9.
49. Smith KJ, Wateska AR, Nowalk MP, et al. Cost-effectiveness of adult vaccination strategies using pneumococcal conjugate vaccine compared with pneumococcal polysaccharide vaccine. JAMA 2012;307:804–12.
50. Moffitt KL, Malley R. Next generation pneumococcal vaccines. Curr Opin Immunol 2011;23(3):407–13.
51. Denoel P, Philipp MT, Doyle L, et al. A protein-based pneumococcal vaccine protects rhesus macaques from pneumonia after experimental infection with *Streptococcus pneumoniae*. Vaccine 2011;29(33):5495–501.
52. Salha D, Szeto J, Myers L, et al. Neutralizing antibodies elicited by a novel detoxified pneumolysin derivative, PlyD1, provide protection against both pneumococcal infection and lung injury. Infect Immun 2012;80(6):2212–20.

Index

Note: Page numbers of article titles are in **boldface** type.

Infect Dis Clin N Am 27 (2013) 243–252
http://dx.doi.org/10.1016/S0891-5520(13)00009-3
0891-5520/13/$ – see front matter © 2013 Elsevier Inc. All rights reserved.

id.theclinics.com

Moving?

Make sure your subscription moves with you!

To notify us of your new address, find your **Clinics Account Number** (located on your mailing label above your name), and contact customer service at:

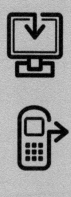

Email: journalscustomerservice-usa@elsevier.com

800-654-2452 (subscribers in the U.S. & Canada)
314-447-8871 (subscribers outside of the U.S. & Canada)

Fax number: 314-447-8029

Elsevier Health Sciences Division
Subscription Customer Service
3251 Riverport Lane
Maryland Heights, MO 63043

Printed and bound by CPI Group (UK) Ltd, Croydon, CR0 4YY

03/10/2024

01040436-0004